Minimally Invasive Surgical Operations

Minimally Invasive Surgical Operations

Edited by Warren Guerra

hayle medical

New York

Hayle Medical,
750 Third Avenue, 9th Floor,
New York, NY 10017, USA

Visit us on the World Wide Web at:
www.haylemedical.com

ISBN: 978-1-63241-766-4

The publisher's policy is to use permanent paper from mills that operate a sustainable forestry policy. Furthermore, the publisher ensures that the text paper and cover boards used have met acceptable environmental accreditation standards.

Printed in China.

Cataloging-in-Publication Data

Minimally invasive surgical operations / edited by Warren Guerra.
p. cm.
Includes bibliographical references and index.
ISBN 978-1-63241-766-4
1. Endoscopic surgery. 2. Endoscopy. 3. Surgery, Operative. 4. Microsurgery. I. Guerra, Warren.
RD33.53 .M45 2019
617.05--dc23

Table of Contents

Preface

The world is advancing at a fast pace like never before. Therefore, the need is to keep up with the latest developments. This book was an idea that came to fruition when the specialists in the area realized the need to coordinate together and document essential themes in the subject. That's when I was requested to be the editor. Editing this book has been an honour as it brings together diverse authors researching on different streams of the field. The book collates essential materials contributed by veterans in the area which can be utilized by students and researchers alike.

Minimally invasive surgical operations are the surgical procedures, which limit the size of incisions required. Consequently, they reduce the risk of infections, pain and wound healing time. Angioplasty and endovascular aneurysm repair are some examples. Such surgeries are guided by tracked surgical instruments in addition to preoperative or intraoperative images. Using cameras, ultrasonic and electromagnetic fields or a combination of these, the patient's anatomy and the surgeon's precise movements are captured and relayed in real-time. This book brings forth some of the most innovative concepts and elucidates the unexplored aspects of minimally invasive surgical operations. The various studies that are constantly contributing towards advancing technologies and evolution of this field are examined in detail. As this field is emerging at a fast pace, this book will help the readers to better understand the concepts of minimally invasive surgical operations.

Each chapter is a sole-standing publication that reflects each author´s interpretation. Thus, the book displays a multi-facetted picture of our current understanding of application, resources and aspects of the field. I would like to thank the contributors of this book and my family for their endless support.

Editor

Minimally Invasive Midvastus versus Standard Parapatellar Approach in Total Knee Arthroplasty

San-Zhong Xu, Xiang-Jin Lin*, Xiang Tong, Xuan-Wei Wang

Department of Orthopaedics, First Affiliated Hospital, College of Medicine, Zhejiang University, Hangzhou City, Zhejiang Province, China

Abstract

Objective: Minimally invasive midvastus approach (mini-midvastus) has been widely used in total knee arthroplasty (TKA). However, the clinical effects still remains controversial. This meta-analysis was based on randomized controlled trials (RCTs) aiming to quantitatively analyze the clinical efficacy of mini-midvastus versus standard parapatellar approach in TKA.

Methods: This meta-analysis was performed according to the PRISMA guidelines. A literature search for the eligible RCTs was carried out in the databases of PubMed, the Cochrane library, EMBASE and Web of Science. Two independent reviewers independently completed the study selection, data extraction, and the assessment of methodological quality. Meta-analysis was conducted by the RevMan 5.2 software.

Results: A total of 18 RCTs (937 patients with 1093 TKAs) published from 2007 to 2013 were included. The meta-analysis suggested that the mini-midvastus approach significantly improved knee range of motion (ROM) and decreased visual analog score (VAS) at postoperative 1–2 weeks ($p<0.05$), and there were no statistical differences in terms of knee society score (KSS) (6 weeks to 1 year), VAS (6 weeks to 6 months), ROM (6 weeks to 6 months), lateral retinacular release, blood loss, straight leg raise, hospital stay and postoperative complications between the mini-midvastus and standard parapatellar approach ($p>0.05$). However, the operative time was significantly longer when performing the mini-midvastus group than the parapartellar approach ($p<0.05$).

Conclusion: This meta-analysis found that compared with the standard parapatellar approach, the mini-midvastus approach had early advantages in the VAS and ROM, but had the disadvantage in the operative time.

Level of Evidence: Therapeutic study Level I.

Editor: Joel Joseph Gagnier, University of Michigan, United States of America

Funding: The authors have no support or funding to report.

Competing Interests: The authors have declared that no competing interests exist.

* E-mail: xuszzju@126.com

Introduction

Minimally invasive surgery (MIS) in total knee arthroplasty (TKA) has been a safe and effective technique for patients with end-stage arthritis [1]. It was originally defined as a small surgical incision less than 14 cm during TKA [2]. However, the current view tends to describe it as a technique which minimizes the disruption of muscle, soft tissue and blood supply during operation. The previous studies have confirmed the MIS technique was associated with less pain, earlier recovery and better quadriceps function than the conventional TKA [2–4].

In MIS TKA, subvastus, midvastus and quads-sparing approaches are the most commonly alternatives to standard parapatellar approach [5,6]. Subvastus and quads-sparing approaches preserved the knee extensor mechanism, and thus were regarded as more minimally invasive than the parapatrllar approach. However, the small surgical field and the increasing operative difficulty limit the popularity theses two approach [7,8]. As a compromise of these approaches, mini-midvastus approach was introduced as it minimized the vascular and muscular disruption of knee and provided a relatively better operative exposure [6,9]. Therefore, mini-midvastus approach has probably been the most popular approach in MIS TKA [10].

Currently, numerous well-designed studies have compared the clinical results of mini-midvastus with medial parapatellar approach. However, the conclusions among studies are still controversial. Some studies found no differences between mini-midvastus and parapatellar approaches [5,11–13], whereas others supported the mini-midvastus [14,15] or standard parapatellar approach [11,16,17]. Therefore, we designed this meta-analysis to quantitatively compare the clinical efficacy and safety of mini-midvastus and parapatellar approach in TKA.

Materials and Methods

Our meta-analysis was strictly conducted according to PRISMA(Preferred Reporting Items for Systematic Reviews and Meta-Analyses) statement – a reporting guideline for meta-analysis [18].

Inclusion criteria for this meta-analysis

To improve the level of evidence, this study only included published randomized controlled trials (RCTs), but retrospective study, quasi- or non-RCTs were not considered for inclusion. The patients participated in RCT must be adult patients who underwent the primary TKA. All the patients should be divided into two groups: one performed the mini-midvastus approach, and the other performed the standard parapatellar approach. All the parameters of patients such as patient number, age and body mass index (BMI) should be comparable in both groups. The following outcomes were extracted for meta-analysis: (1). Primary outcomes: Knee Society Score (KSS) and Visual analog score (VAS); (2). Secondary outcomes: knee range of motion (ROM), operative time, lateral retinacular release, blood loss, straight leg raise, hospital stay and postoperative complications (total complications, deep vein thrombosis and wound infection).

Search strategies for identification of studies

A systematic literature search was conducted in PubMed (1950-October, 2013), EMBASE (1974-October, 2013), Cochrane Library (issue 9, 2013) and Web of Science (SCI) (1980- October, 2013). The following search strategies were used in the search: #1. Arthroplasty, Replacement, Knee [Mesh] OR knee arthroplasty OR knee replacement; #2. parapatellar OR standard OR conventional; #3. midvastus OR mini-midvastus OR vastus splitting; #4. #1 AND #2 AND #3. Furthermore, the references lists of included studies and Google scholar were also searched. All the processes were performed by two blinded authors.

Data extraction and quality assessment

Data was extracted using a pre-designed sheet. The quality assessment of the included studies was evaluated by the Tool recommended by the Cochrane Collaboration [19]. The items, including randomization; allocation concealment; blinding of participants; blinding of outcome assessors; incomplete outcome data; selective reporting; and other bias, were assessed by "Yes", "No" or "Unclear" by two independent authors. Disagreement was resolved by discussion among authors.

Statistical analysis

The dichotomous outcomes (lateral retinacular release and postoperative complications) were analyzed with odds ratios (OR) and 95% confidence interval (95% CI). The continuous outcomes (KSS, VAS, ROM, SLR, operative time, blood loss and hospital stay) were analyzed using mean difference (MD) and 95% CI. Statistical heterogeneity were tested with the χ^2 test and I^2 statistic: $I^2>50\%$ meaning significant heterogeneity, and $I^2\leq 50\%$ meaning no significant heterogeneity [20]. When heterogeneity was not significant, a fixed effect model was used for meta-anlysis, otherwises a random-effect model was used. Subgroup analysis was conducted in the different types of complications and outcomes at different time points. Meta-analysis was done using the software of Review Manager 5.2.

Results

Literature search

Figure 1 showed the flow chart of the literature search. The initial search found 307 potentially relevant citations from PubMed, EMBASE, Cochrane Library and Web of Science. After carefully screening the title, abstract and full text, 18 RCTs were finally included [5,11–17,21–30].

The characteristics of included RCTs

Table 1 summarized the basic characteristics of included studies. All the studies were published in 7 years (2007–2013) recently. There were a total of 937 patients (female: 70.2%, male: 29.8%) with 1093 TKAs in the included 18 RCTs. All the included RCTs were small trials with patients' number ranging from 20 to 100. The mean age of the included patients ranged from 62.6 to 71.5 years, BMI 24.4 to 34.8 kg/m^2, and the follow-up duration 3 months to 3 years. Both groups were well matched in patient number, age, BMI and preoperative knee function and flexion.

Methodological quality assessment

The methodological quality of the included studies was shown in Table 2. All the studies reported that the included participates were randomly assigned to two groups, but four [11,14,21,27] did not mentioned the method of randomization. The method of blinding was performed in 12 of 18 RCTs (66.7%), but allocation concealment was in 5 studies (27.8%).

Results of meta-analysis

Table 3 showed the results of meta-analysis.

Primary outcomes

KSS. Six studies were available for meta-analysis of KSS [12–14,17,26,29]. Subgroup analyses found no differences between the min-midvastus and standard groups in postoperative 6 weeks ($p=0.24$), 3 months ($p=0.59$), 6 months ($p=0.26$) and 1 year ($p=0.33$). The heterogeneity was statistically significant in KSS at 6 week ($I^2=89\%$). (Table 3)

VAS. Five studies were included for meta-analysis of VAS [12,22–24,27]. Subgroup analyses suggested that the mini-midvastus approach significantly decreased VAS at postoperative 2 weeks ($p<0.01$), and no differences were seen between the two groups at the time points of 3 day ($p=0.42$), 6 week ($p=0.22$), 3 month ($p=0.82$), 6 month ($p=0.80$). The heterogeneity was statistically significant in VAS at 3 days ($I^2=80\%$). (Table 3)

Secondary outcomes

Meta-analysis revealed that the mini-midvastus group showed significantly better ROM at postoperative 2 weeks ($p<0.05$) but required longer operative time ($p<0.05$). There were no differences in lateral retinacular release ($p=0.12$), blood loss ($p=0.33$), straight leg raise ($p=0.13$), hospital stay ($p=0.79$) and postoperative complications (total postoperative, $p=0.88$; wound infection, $p=0.64$; deep vein thrombosis, $p=0.22$). The significant heterogeneity was found in ROM at 6 weeks ($I^2=86\%$), operative time ($I^2=93\%$) and hospital stay ($I^2=53\%$). (Table 3)

Discussion

The major finding of this study was that the midvastus approach was superior to the standard parapatellar approach in VAS and ROM in the short term (postoperative 2 weeks). There were no statistical differences between the mini-midvastus and parapatellar approach in terms of KSS (6 weeks to 1 year) VAS (6 weeks to 6 months), ROM (6 weeks to 6 months), lateral retinacular release, blood loss, straight leg raise, hospital stay and postoperative complications. In addition, the midvastus approach was found to be associated with significantly longer operative time in TKA.

An earlier meta-analysis [31] had compared the short-term results of the midvastus with the standard approach. Their results showed that the midvastus approach obtained better postoperative recovery, less lateral release and complication rates than the

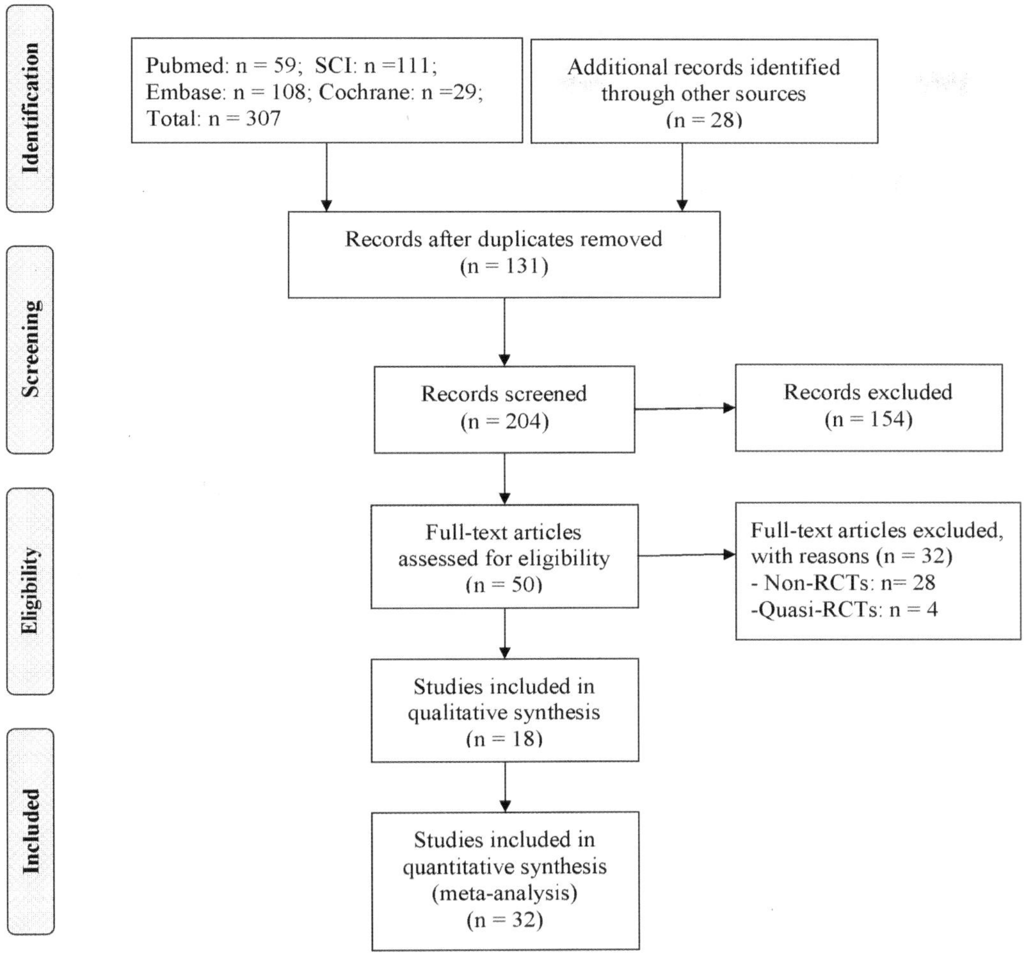

Figure 1. Flow chart of literature screening.

standard approach. However, there were several obvious limitations related to this published meta-analysis. First, that study only analyzed the short-term outcomes without the analysis of the long-term results; second, the data of meta-analysis was based on not only RCTs but also quasi-RCTs, which might lower the strength of evidence; third, the studies which did not use MIS technique in midvastus approach was also included in meta-anlysis, which might effect the specificity of the mini-midvastus; fourth, the meta-analysis should be updated as a number of well-designed RCTs were recently published [5,11–14,21,22]. Compared with the published meta-analysis, we included 7 more RCTs [5,11–14,21,22] and excluded 4 RCTs [32–35] who did not use MIS in the midvastus group. Therefore, we believe our evidence was stronger on the efficiency of the mini-midvastus approach in TKA.

Our meta-analysis was based on 18 RCTs published from 2007 to 2013. The primary outcomes, VAS and KSS, were the top concerns by the patients undergoing primary TKA. However, we only found that the VAS in the mini-midvastus group was reduced in the early period postoperatively. This results were similar with the previous study of Fu et al [27]. In this randomized controlled study with 68 bilateral TKAs, the VAS score of the midvastus group was significantly decreased in the first week after surgery. With regard to KSS, we did not observe any differences between the mini-midvastus and standard approach up to 1 year postoperatively. This corresponded well with the recent studies [5,11]. Zhang et al. [11] compared 45 midvastus TKAs with 44 parapatellar TKAs and found no significant difference in KSS during the follow-up period (7 days, 6 weeks, 3 months and 6 months). Guy et al. [5] randomized 80 patients to perform mini-midvastus approach or standard parapatellar approach, and also did not find statistical difference in KSS at intervals up to 1 year.

With regard to the secondary outcomes, the current study found significantly higher ROM in the mini-midvastus group than the standard group in the short term (2 weeks), while no differences were found in the later period (6 weeks to 6 months). In addition, we found the mini-midvastus approach significantly increased operative time. That was understandable as the MIS technique in the mini-midvastus group needed more operative procedure and surgical skills. There were no differences in lateral retinacular release, blood loss, straight leg raise, hospital stay and postoperative complications. These results were mostly in accordance well with the previous meta-analysis [31]. In that meta-analysis, the authors found that the midvastus group significantly decreased lateral release rate compared with the standard group, while our result did not find different between two groups. The possible reason was for a quasi-randomized trial [36] they included, in which, the lateral release rate was significantly higher in the midvastus (1/22) than that in the parapatellar group (13/29). When excluding this quasi-randomized trial, the difference disappeared.

Table 1. Characteristics of included studies.

Study-year	Year	Country	Group	Age	BMI	Patients	Male	Female	Total TKA	Follow-up
Chin	2007	Singapore	Mini-MV	67.4 (56–80)	28.50(22.1–40.0)	30	6	24	30	3 months
			MP	69.0 (57–80)	27.5 (18.6–34.2)	30	3	27	30	
Cho	2013	Korea	Mini-MV	65.5±5.1	29.1±3.9	33	1	32	33	1 year
			MP	67.0±5.7	28.0±4.1	33	2	31	33	
Dalury	2008	USA	Mini-MV	67 (53–86)	30 (23.6–39)	20	6	14	20	3 months
			MP						20	
Fu	2008	China	Mini-MV	67 (53–86)	30 (23.6–39)	34	7	27	34	3 months
			MP						34	
Guy	2012	UK	Mini-MV	71.2	28.2±3.0	40	38	42	40	1 year
			MP	69.1	28.9±3.8	40			40	
Heekin	2013	USA	Mini-MV	65.13±6.49	30.98±5.44	40	26	14	40	2 years
			Mini-MP						40	
Hernandez-Vaquero	2010	Spain	Mini-MV	70.8±5.9	32.1±6	26	5	21	26	6 months
			MP	70.5±6.9	30.8±3.3	36	6	30	36	
Juosponis	2009	Lithuania	Mini-MV	72±5.5	27.95±3.2	35	5	30	35	3 months
			MP	71.4±5.04	29.08±2.7	35	5	30	35	
Karachalios	2008	Greece	Mini-MV	71.1 (52–78)	32 (27–35)	50	19	31	50	3 years
			MP	70.8 (54–77)	31.5 (28–35)	50	15	35	50	
Karpman	2009	USA	Mini-MV	74±7.7	30±7.3	20	7	13	20	6 months
			MP	73±5.1	29±4.6	19	9	10	19	
Kim	2011	Korea	Mini-MV	67±6	27.1±3	23	0	23	23	1 year
			MP	68±7	28.4±5	22	0	22	22	
Kolisek	2007	USA	Mini-MV	67 (48–84)	32 (19–49)	40	29	11	40	3 months
			MP	70 (54–79)	30 (20–40)	40	24	15	40	
Lee	2011	Korea	Mini-MV	67 (54–73)	27.5 (23.1–33.8)	30	2	28	30	6 months
			MP						30	
Nestor	2010	USA	Mini-MV	66.7±9.6	29.6±5.6	27	9	18	27	6 months
			MP						27	
Pongcharoen	2013	Thailand	Mini-MV	67±4.9	27±2.4	30	5	25	30	1 year
			MP	67±6.0	26±2.3	30	7	23	30	
Varnell	2011	Italy	Mini-MV	75±7	29.5±4.59	20	6	14	20	6 months
			Mini-SV	71±6	30.96±6.16	18	11	7	20	
Walter	2007	USA	Mini-MV	71.5 (53–85)	31.8 (26.2–43.9)	25	6	19	25	3 months
			MP	66.6 (50–80)	34.8 (22.3–59.4)	19	7	12	19	
Zhang	2013	China	Mini-MV	62.6 (48–70)	24.8 (19.6–29.4)	45	14	31	45	6 months
			MP	63.7 (47–74)	24.4(19.2–28.6)	44	14	30	44	

*.Mini-MV = mini-midvastus, MP = medial parapatellar, NR = not report

Table 2. Risk of bias in included studies.

Study	Random Sequence Generation	Allocation concealment	Blinding of participants	Blinding of outcome assessment	Incomplete Outcome data	Selective reporting	Other bias
Zhang 2013	Yes (Not reported)	Unclear	Unclear	Unclear	Yes	Unclear	Unclear
Pongcharoen 2013	Yes (Computer-generated numbers)	Unclear	Unclear	Unclear	Yes	Unclear	Unclear
Heekin 2013	Yes (Randomization table)	Unclear	Yes	Unclear	Yes	Unclear	Unclear
Cho 2013	Yes (Not reported)	Unclear	Unclear	Unclear	Yes	Unclear	Unclear
Guy 2012	Yes (Randomization table)	Yes (Sealed envelope)	Unclear	Yes	Yes	Unclear	Unclear
Varnell 2011	Yes (Not reported)	Unclear	Unclear	Unclear	Yes	Unclear	Unclear
Lee 2011	Yes (Computer-generated numbers)	Yes (Sealed envelope)	Unclear	Yes	Yes	Unclear	Unclear
Kim 2011	Yes (Randomization table)	Yes (Sealed envelope)	Yes	Yes	Yes	Unclear	Unclear
Hernandez-Vaquero 2010	Yes (Randomization table)	Unclear	No	Yes	Unclear	Unclear	Unclear
Nestor 2010	Yes (Randomization table)	Unclear	Yes	Yes	Yes	Unclear	Unclear
Karpman 2009	Yes (Computer-generated numbers)	Unclear	Yes	Yes	Yes	Unclear	Unclear
Juosponis 2009	Yes (Randomization table)	Yes (Sealed envelope)	Unclear	Unclear	Yes	Unclear	Unclear
Dalury 2008	Yes (Randomization table)	Unclear	Unclear	Yes	Yes	Unclear	Unclear
Karachalios 2008	Yes (Computer-generated numbers)	Yes (Sealed envelope)	Unclear	Yes	Yes	Unclear	Unclear
Fu 2008	Yes (Not reported)	Unclear	Yes	Yes	Yes	Unclear	Unclear
Walter 2007	Yes (Randomization table)	Yes (Sealed envelope)	Unclear	Yes	Yes	Unclear	Unclear
Kolisek 2007	Yes (Randomization table)	Yes (Sealed envelope)	Unclear	Unclear	Yes	Unclear	Unclear
Chin 2007	Yes (Randomization table)	Yes (Sealed envelope)	Yes	Yes	Yes	Unclear	Unclear

Table 3. Meta-analysis of nini-midvastus versus medial parapatellar approach.

Results	TKAs		Included studies	MD or OR (95% CI); p value	Heterogeneity
	MV	MP			
KSS 6 weeks	168	168	5 [11,15,20,26,29]	5.15 (−3.36, 13.66); $p=0.24$	$I^2=89\%$
KSS 3 months	168	168	5 [11,15,20,26,29]	0.55 (−1.41, 2.50); $p=0.59$	$I^2=0\%$
KSS 6 months	73	73	2 [11,20]	−2.15 (−5.92, 1.62); $p=0.26$	$I^2=30\%$
KSS 1 year	103	103	3 [11,19,20]	0.66 (−0.68, 1.99); $p=0.33$	$I^2=26\%$
VAS 3 days	91	91	3 [22,23,27]	−0.27 (−0.91, 0.37); $p=0.42$	$I^2=80\%$
VAS 1–2 weeks	91	91	3 [22,23,27]	−0.20 (−0.29, 0.11); $p<0.01$	$I^2=0\%$
VAS 6 weeks	87	87	3 [19,22,23]	−0.12 (−0.32, 0.07); $p=0.22$	$I^2=0\%$
VAS 3 months	87	87	3 [19,22,23]	−0.02 (−0.21, 017); $p=0.82$	$I^2=0\%$
VAS 6 months	86	96	3 [19,22,24]	−0.02 (−0.20, 015); $p=0.80$	$I^2=0\%$
ROM 1–2 week	146	145	5 [22,23,25–27]	7.45 (3.26, 11.64); $p<0.05$	$I^2=26\%$
ROM 6 weeks	272	268	8 [15,20,22,23,26,27,33,34]	2.12 (−2.42, 6.66); $p=0.36$	$I^2=86\%$
ROM 3 months	151	151	5 [15,20,22,23,27]	0.72 (−1.20, 2.65); $p=0.46$	$I^2=0\%$
ROM 6 months	66	76	2 [20,24]	1.03 (−1.77, 3.83); $p=0.47$	$I^2=0\%$
Operative time	255	264	8 [14,19,22,24–27,30]	11.64(5.50, 17.78); $p<0.05$	$I^2=93\%$
Lateral retinacular release	329	318	7 [13,15,20,27,28]	0.67 (0.41, 1.11); p = 0.12	$I^2=0\%$
Blood loss	268	266	8 [5,11,13,19,22,25,29,30]	1.73 (−1.79, 5.25); $p=0.33$	$I^2=0\%$
Straight leg raise	144	137	4 [13,27,28,34]	0.43 (0.15, 1.27); $p=0.13$	$I^2=0\%$
Hospital stay	141	144	5 [20,24,25,28,30]	1.46(−9.03, 11.94); $p=0.79$	$I^2=53\%$
Total Complication	405	413	12 [5,11,13,14,19,22–25,27,29,30]	0.95 (0.53, 1.71); $p=0.88$	$I^2=0\%$
Wound infection	430	432	13 [5,11,13,14,19,22–25,27–30]	1.22(0.52, 2.90); $p=0.64$	$I^2=0\%$
Deep vein thrombosis	254	253	7 [5,11,14,23,27,29,30]	0.46 (0.13, 1.59); p = 0.22	$I^2=0\%$

This meta-analysis has some limitations. First, despite 18 RCTs were included, the data for meta-analysis was still insufficient, especially for the primary outcomes. Second, the heterogeneity among studies was significant in the KSS at 6 weeks, VAS at 3 days, ROM at 6 weeks and operative time. Although a random-effect model was applied to incorporate heterogeneity in meta-analysis, the readers still should be cautious with these results. Furthermore, some RCTs included for meta-analysis did not carry out binding method and allocation concealment, which might increase a risk of performance and selection bias.

Additionally, there are several strengths in this present meta-analysis. First, the evidence is based on the meta-analysis of RCTs, which is the highest level of evidence (Level I). Second, in order to ensure the accuracy of data, a thorough literature search was conducted for the published studies only, and unpublished studies were not included. Third, we compared the clinical outcomes in the long-term period by subgroup analysis, which was very important to evaluate the safety of a new technique. Fourth, we excluded the studies without using MIS in the midvastus approach, minimized the bias from the differences in the operative procedures, and specially focused on efficacy of the mini-midvastus versus standard approach.

Conclusions

Based on the meta-analysis of RCTs, we conclude that the mini-midvastus approach is associated with the short-term advantages in the VAS and ROM, but has significantly longer operative time compared with the standard parapatellar approach. There are no statistically differences in KSS lateral retinacular release, blood loss, straight leg raise, hospital stay and postoperative complications between groups.

Author Contributions

Conceived and designed the experiments: SZX XJL XT. Performed the experiments: SZX XJL XT XWW. Analyzed the data: SZX XJL XWW. Contributed reagents/materials/analysis tools: SZX XJL XT. Wrote the paper: SZX XJL XT XWW.

References

1. Costa CR, Johnson AJ, Harwin SF, Mont MA, Bonutti PM (2013) Critical review of minimally invasive approaches in knee arthroplasty. J Knee Surg 26: 41–50.
2. Adams J, Ryall C, Pandyan A, Metcalf C, Stokes M, et al. (2012) Proximal interphalangeal joint replacement in patients with arthritis of the hand: a meta-analysis. J Bone Joint Surg Br 94: 1305–1312.
3. Granchi D, Cenni E, Giunti A, Baldini N (2012) Metal hypersensitivity testing in patients undergoing joint replacement: a systematic review. J Bone Joint Surg Br 94: 1126–1134.
4. Yin ZG, Zhang JB, Kan SL, Wang XG (2012) Diagnostic accuracy of imaging modalities for suspected scaphoid fractures: meta-analysis combined with latent class analysis. J Bone Joint Surg Br 94: 1077–1085.

5. Guy SP, Farndon MA, Conroy JL, Bennett C, Grainger AJ, et al. (2012) A prospective randomised study of minimally invasive midvastus total knee arthroplasty compared with standard total knee arthroplasty. Knee 19: 866–871.
6. Chang CH, Yang RS, Chen KH, Liu TK, Chen WC, et al. (2010) Muscle torque in total knee arthroplasty: comparison of subvastus and midvastus approaches. Knee Surg Sports Traumatol Arthrosc 18: 934–938.
7. Wegrzyn J, Parratte S, Coleman-Wood K, Kaufman KR, Pagnano MW (2013) The John Insall award: no benefit of minimally invasive TKA on gait and strength outcomes: a randomized controlled trial. Clin Orthop Relat Res 471: 46–55.
8. Varela-Egocheaga JR, Suarez-Suarez MA, Fernandez-Villan M, Gonzalez-Sastre V, Varela-Gomez JR, et al. (2010) Minimally invasive subvastus approach: improving the results of total knee arthroplasty: a prospective, randomized trial. Clin Orthop Relat Res 468: 1200–1208.
9. Alshryda S, Sarda P, Sukeik M, Nargol A, Blenkinsopp J, et al. (2011) Tranexamic acid in total knee replacement: a systematic review and meta-analysis. J Bone Joint Surg Br 93: 1577–1585.
10. Tria AJ Jr (2007) Minimally invasive total knee arthroplasty: past, present, and future. Am J Orthop (Belle Mead NJ) 36: 6–7.
11. Zhang Z, Zhu W, Gu B, Zhu L, Chen C (2013) Mini-midvastus versus mini-medial parapatellar approach in total knee arthroplasty: a prospective, randomized study. Arch Orthop Trauma Surg 133: 389–395.
12. Pongcharoen B, Yakampor T, Charoencholvanish K (2013) Patellar tracking and anterior knee pain are similar after medial parapatellar and midvastus approaches in minimally invasive TKA. Clin Orthop Relat Res 471: 1654–1660.
13. Heekin RD, Fokin AA (2013) Mini-Midvastus Versus Mini-Medial Parapatellar Approach for Minimally Invasive Total Knee Arthroplasty: Outcomes Pendulum Is at Equilibrium. J Arthroplasty doi:10.1016/j.arth.2013.05.016.
14. Cho KY, Kim KI, Umrani S, Kim SH (2013) Better quadriceps recovery after minimally invasive total knee arthroplasty. Knee Surg Sports Traumatol Arthrosc doi:10.1007/s00167-013-2556-2.
15. Kim JG, Lee SW, Ha JK, Choi HJ, Yang SJ, et al. (2011) The effectiveness of minimally invasive total knee arthroplasty to preserve quadriceps strength: a randomized controlled trial. Knee 18: 443–447.
16. Karachalios T, Giotikas D, Roidis N, Poultsides L, Bargiotas K, et al. (2008) Total knee replacement performed with either a mini-midvastus or a standard approach: a prospective randomised clinical and radiological trial. J Bone Joint Surg Br 90: 584–591.
17. Dalury DF, Snow RG, Adams MJ (2008) Electromyographic evaluation of the midvastus approach. J Arthroplasty 23: 136–140.
18. Moher D, Liberati A, Tetzlaff J, Altman DG (2009) Preferred reporting items for systematic reviews and meta-analyses: the PRISMA statement. J Clin Epidemiol 62: 1006–1012.
19. Higgins JPT, Green S (2011) Cochrane Handbook for Systematic Reviews of Interventions Version 5.1.0. The Cochrane Collaboration. Available at: www.cochrane-handbook.org. Accessed September 2, 2013.
20. Higgins JP, Thompson SG (2002) Quantifying heterogeneity in a meta-analysis. Stat Med 21: 1539–1558.
21. Varnell MS, Bhowmik-Stoker M, McCamley J, Jacofsky MC, Campbell M, et al. (2011) Difference in stair negotiation ability based on TKA surgical approach. J Knee Surg 24: 117–123.
22. Lee DH, Choi J, Nha KW, Kim HJ, Han SB (2011) No difference in early functional outcomes for mini-midvastus and limited medial parapatellar approaches in navigation-assisted total knee arthroplasty: a prospective randomized clinical trial. Knee Surg Sports Traumatol Arthrosc 19: 66–73.
23. Nestor BJ, Toulson CE, Backus SI, Lyman SL, Foote KL, et al. (2010) Mini-midvastus vs standard medial parapatellar approach: a prospective, randomized, double-blinded study in patients undergoing bilateral total knee arthroplasty. J Arthroplasty. 25: 5–11, 11 e11.
24. Hernandez-Vaquero D, Noriega-Fernandez A, Suarez-Vazquez A (2010) Total knee arthroplasties performed with a mini-incision or a standard incision. Similar results at six months follow-up. Bmc Musculoskeletal Disorders 11: 27.
25. Karpman RR, Smith HL (2009) Comparison of the early results of minimally invasive vs standard approaches to total knee arthroplasty: a prospective, randomized study. J Arthroplasty 24: 681–688.
26. Juosponis R, Tarasevicius S, Smailys A, Kalesinskas RJ (2009) Functional and radiological outcome after total knee replacement performed with mini-midvastus or conventional arthrotomy: controlled randomised trial. Int Orthop 33: 1233–1237.
27. Fu Pei-liang, Li Xiao-hua, Wu Yu-li, Xie Qing-yun, Sun Jiu-yi, et al. (2008) Comparison of midvastus and standard medial parapatellar approaches in total knee arthroplasty. Journal of Clinical Rehabilitative Tissue Engineering 12: 1793–1796.
28. Walter F, Haynes MB, Markel DC (2007) A randomized prospective study evaluating the effect of patellar eversion on the early functional outcomes in primary total knee arthroplasty. J Arthroplasty 22: 509–514.
29. Kolisek FR, Bonutti PM, Hozack WJ, Purtill J, Sharkey PF, et al. (2007) Clinical experience using a minimally invasive surgical approach for total knee arthroplasty: early results of a prospective randomized study compared to a standard approach. J Arthroplasty 22: 8–13.
30. Chin PL, Foo LS, Yang KY, Yeo SJ, Lo NN (2007) Randomized controlled trial comparing the radiologic outcomes of conventional and minimally invasive techniques for total knee arthroplasty. J Arthroplasty 22: 800–806.
31. Alcelik I, Sukeik M, Pollock R, Misra A, Naguib A, et al. (2012) Comparing the mid-vastus and medial parapatellar approaches in total knee arthroplasty: a meta-analysis of short term outcomes. Knee 19: 229–236.
32. Ozkoc G, Hersekli MA, Akpinar S, Ozalay M, Uysal M, et al. (2005) Time dependent changes in patellar tracking with medial parapatellar and midvastus approaches. Knee Surg Sports Traumatol Arthrosc 13: 654–657.
33. Bathis H, Perlick L, Blum C, Luring C, Perlick C, et al. (2005) Midvastus approach in total knee arthroplasty: a randomized, double-blinded study on early rehabilitation. Knee Surg Sports Traumatol Arthrosc 13: 545–550.
34. Keating EM, Faris PM, Meding JB, Ritter MA (1999) Comparison of the midvastus muscle-splitting approach with the median parapatellar approach in total knee arthroplasty. J Arthroplasty 14: 29–32.
35. Dalury DF, Jiranek WA (1999) A comparison of the midvastus and paramedian approaches for total knee arthroplasty. J Arthroplasty 14: 33–37.
36. Kelly MJ, Rumi MN, Kothari M, Parentis MA, Bailey KJ, et al. (2006) Comparison of the vastus-splitting and median parapatellar approaches for primary total knee arthroplasty: a prospective, randomized study. J Bone Joint Surg Am 88: 715–720.

2

Biomechanical Effects of a Unilateral Approach to Minimally Invasive Lumbar Decompression

Zachary A. Smith[1], Georgios A. Vastardis[2,3], Gerard Carandang[2,3], Robert M. Havey[2,3], Sean Hannon[2,3], Nader Dahdaleh[1], Leonard I. Voronov[2,3], Richard G. Fessler[1], Avinash G. Patwardhan[2,3]*

1 Northwestern Feinberg School of Medicine, Department of Neurological Surgery, Northwestern University, Chicago, Illinois, United States of America, **2** Loyola University Stritch School of Medicine, Department of Orthopaedic Surgery, Maywood, Illinois, United States of America, **3** Edward Hines Jr. VA Hospital, Hines, Illinois, United States of America

Abstract

Minimally invasive (MI) lumbar decompression became a common approach to treat lumbar stenosis. This approach may potentially mitigate postoperative increases in segmental motion. The goal of this study was to evaluate modifications to segmental motion in the lumbar spine following a MI unilateral approach as compared to traditional facet-sparing and non-facet sparing decompressions. Six human lumbar cadaveric specimens were used. Each specimen was tested in flexion-extension 0 N and 400 N of follower preload), axial rotation, and lateral bending. Each testing condition was evaluated following three separate interventions at L4–L5: 1) Minimally invasive decompression, 2) Facet-sparing, bilateral decompression, and 3) Bilateral decompression with a wide facetectomy. Range of motion following each testing condition was compared to intact specimens. Both MI and traditional decompression procedures create significant increases in ROM in all modes of loading. However, when compared to the MI approach, traditional decompression produces significantly larger increase in ROM in flexion-extension ($p<0.005$) and axial rotation ($p<0.05$). It additionally creates increased ROM with lateral bending on the approach side ($p<0.05$). Lateral bending on the non-approach side is not significantly changed. Lastly, wide medial facet removal (40% to 50%) causes significant hypermobility, especially in axial rotation. While both MI and traditional lumbar decompressions may increase post-operative ROM in all conditions, a MI approach causes significantly smaller increase in ROM. With an MI approach, increased movement with lateral bending is only toward the approach side. Further, non-facet sparing decompression is further destabilizing in all loading modes.

Editor: Carlos M. Isales, Georgia Regents University, United States of America

Funding: The first author (Dr. Smith) was supported by the AANS/CNS Apfelbaum Award and the CNS Spine Fellowship Award. The last author (Dr. Patwardhan) received funding from the US Department of Veterans Affairs, Washington, DC. The funders had no role in study design, data collection and analysis, decision to publish, or preparation of the manuscript.

* E-mail: apatwar@lumc.edu

Introduction

Minimally invasive spine surgery (MISS) techniques are being increasingly utilized in practice.[1,2,3,4,5,6,7,8,9] Of these MISS techniques, the minimally invasive decompression of lumbar stenosis is both one of the most frequently utilized and "mature" techniques.[3,7] Favorable clinical outcomes have been reported with this decompression technique, even in more challenging patient populations [10,11]. The most prominent of its advantages is a decrease in iatrogenic soft-tissue injury, a difference that is often reflected in peri-operative outcome measures [10,12,13].

The potential biomechanical implications of this surgical approach are less understood. While there are several described variants, the focus of this report is that of a unilateral approach to single-level bilateral lumbar decompression. This technique utilizes sequential tubular muscle dilation and either a microscope or endoscope. There are two anatomic features of this technique that may help to maintain native biomechanics [14]. Firstly, the trajectory of decompression allows for an internal decompression. This requires only a partial *ipsilateral* facetectomy and preserves the contralateral facet. As the facet joints are critical to lumbar stability, especially in axial rotation, this may minimize post-operative instability. Secondly, the spinous processes and the midline ligaments are well preserved. When these midline structures are removed, this may negatively impact native spinal biomechanics.

The goal of this study is to evaluate the biomechanical effects of a modern technique for minimally invasive lumbar decompression. Previous studies have evaluated the role of graded facet removal [15,16]; however, to our knowledge, a minimally invasive model using complete lumbar spines has not been investigated. In this biomechanical cadaver study, we evaluated the effects of minimally invasive decompression (MI-D) on native lumbar spine mechanics.

Materials and Methods

Specimens and Experimental Setup

Six fresh-frozen human cadaveric lumbar spine specimens (L1-sacrum, age 56.5±15.7, 4 males, 2 females) were used for this

Table 1. Specimen demographics for six lumbar spine segments.

Specimen	Age (years)	Sex	Cause of Death
1	73	M	Lung Cancer
2	79	M	Lung Cancer
3	41	M	Cardiac Arrest
4	44	M	GSW to the Head
5	52	F	Colon Cancer
6	50	F	Breast Cancer

Abbreviations:
M = Male, F = Female.
GSW = Gun shot wound.

study (Table 1). Specimens were procured from the GenLife Institute tissue bank (Phoenix, AZ).

Radiographic screening was performed to exclude specimens with fractures, metastatic disease and bridging osteophytes. The specimens were thawed and stripped of the paraspinal musculature while preserving the discs, facet joints, and osteoligamentous structures. All tests were performed at room temperature.

Specimens were fixed to the apparatus at the caudal end and free to move in any plane at the proximal end. A moment was applied by applying an offset vertical load for flexion, extension, and lateral bending. Axial rotation was produced by applying two equal and opposite forces (**Fig. 1**). The specimen was cycled between specified maximum moment endpoints in flexion, extension, lateral bending, and axial rotation.

The angular motion of the L1 to L5 vertebrae relative to Sacrum was measured using an optoelectronic motion measurement system (Model Certus, Optotrak, Northern Digital, Waterloo, Ontario). In addition, bi-axial angle sensors (Model 902-45, Applied Geomechanics, Santa Cruz, CA) were mounted on each vertebra to allow real-time feedback for the optimization of the preload path. A six-component load cell (Model MC3A-6-1000, AMTI Inc., Newton, MA) was placed under the specimen to measure the applied compressive preload and moments. Fluoroscopic imaging (GE OEC 9800 Plus digital fluoroscopy machine) was used to document implant position.

The follower load technique was used to apply compressive preloads to the lumbar spine during the range of motion experiments in flexion and extension [17]. The compressive preload was applied along a path that follows the lordotic curve of the lumbar spine. By applying a compressive load along the follower load path the segmental bending moments and shear forces due to the preload application were minimized. This allowed the lumbar spine to support physiologic compressive preloads without damage or instability.

The follower load cable guides were attached to the vertebral bodies of L2–L5. The preload was applied using bilateral loading cables that were attached to the cup holding L1 vertebra. The cables passed freely through guides anchored to each vertebra and were connected to a loading hanger under the specimen. The cable guide mounts allowed anterior-posterior adjustments of the follower load path within a range of about ten millimeters. The preload path was optimized by adjusting the cable guides to minimize changes in lumbar lordosis when a compressive load of up to 400 N was applied to the specimen beginning in its neutral posture. Our previous experience demonstrated that the optimization of the follower preload path minimizes the effects of artifact moment and shear force on the range of motion of the spine in flexion-extension.

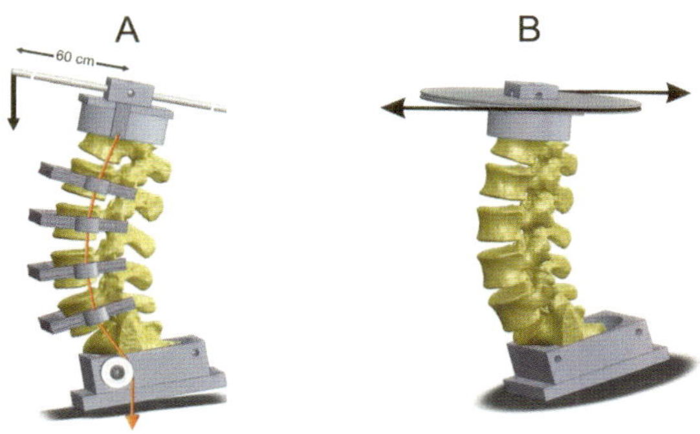

Figure 1. Schematic of the loading apparatus for range of motion tests in flexion-extension and axial rotation. Testing for ROM in lateral bending was performed using an offset-loading arm in the frontal plane.

Experimental Protocol

All specimens were tested in each of the three conditions: intact, following minimally invasive surgery, and after open laminectomy. Each condition was tested under moments of +8 Nm in flexion and −6 Nm in extension with compressive follower preloads of 0 N and 400 N. Previous biomechanical studies on human lumbar spine specimens have used moments ranging from 5 Nm to 10 Nm, depending on the specific goals of their experimental studies.[18] In our experience, maximum moments of 8 Nm in flexion and 6 Nm in extension are generally adequate to capture the vast majority of the available ROM of the cadaveric lumbar spine specimen without the risk of causing tissue damage. This is particularly important if multiple test runs on the same specimen are planned, as in the case of the present study. The load-displacement data were first collected on the intact specimen until two reproducible loops were obtained for each loading case. This was then repeated after each surgical technique. This protocol was also performed for lateral-bending (±6 Nm) and axial rotation (±5 Nm).

Surgical Techniques

Three testing conditions were compared to the intact condition. A minimally invasive L4/L5 decompression was patterned after a minimally invasive unilateral approach for bilateral internal decompression, which can be aided by either microscope or endoscope. A 18 mm×6 cm METRx portal was docked (Figure 1) from a left-approach at L4/L5. A unilateral L4 hemilaminotomy with a partial superior L5 hemilaminotomy was completed through the METRx tube, using standard operative tools, including a hand-held drill. The ligamentum flavum was completely removed and bilateral L4/L5 foramina were opened. Confirmation of a "pedicle-to-pedicle" decompression, including an evaluation of the contralateral foramina, was undertaken with a lateral fluoroscopy (Figure 1).

The second surgical condition patterned a standard midline L4/L5 decompression with an 80% removal of the L4 lamina and 20% removal of the superior portion of L5. The supraspinous and intraspinous ligaments were cut and the L4 spinous process removed. For both minimally invasive and traditional decompressions, facet removal was carefully checked. Two independent observers marked and confirmed the medial (most medial facet fiber attachments) and lateral extent of the facets. For the first two

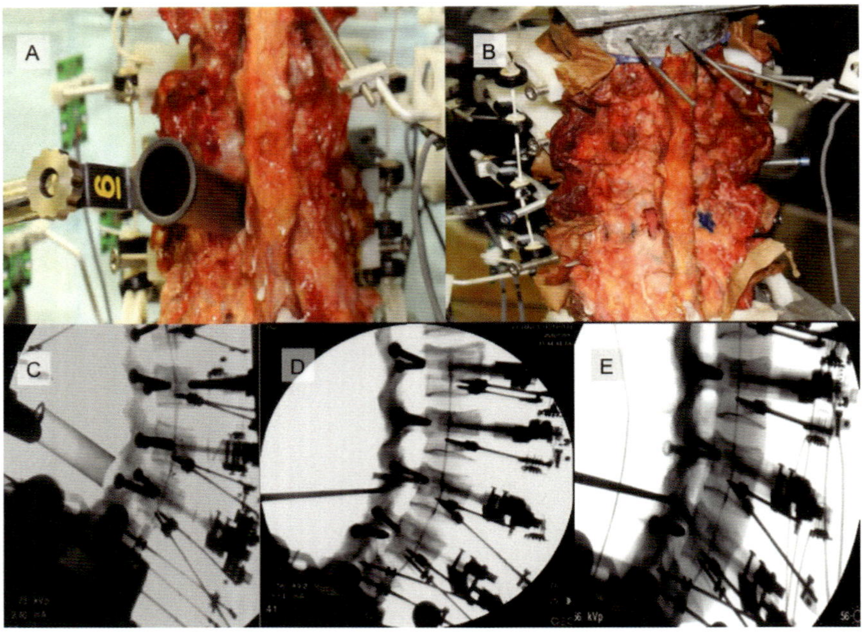

Figure 2. Images demonstrating testing of the minimally invasive surgical procedure. Unilateral docking of the METRx tube at L4/L5 is shown (A) as well as post-procedural anatomic changes following decompression (B). A radiograph demonstrating tubular docking is shown in C. Following complete removal of the ligamentum flavum and internal bony decompression, a curette was placed at the superior and inferior extent of decompression to confirm a "pedicle-to-pedicle" dural decompression.

testing conditions, 15–20% of medial facet was removed. Markings of these facet lines are shown in Figure 2.

The final testing condition was a "wide" decompression (Figure 2 and 3). The second operative condition was extended to involve a 20% greater removal of the medial facets (40% resection). The capsule of the facet was only disrupted to this line and the midline capsule was undisturbed.

Experimental Protocol

Analysis of variance (ANOVA) was used to assess the effects of various surgical steps on the range of motion in flexion-extension, left and right lateral bending, and left and right axial rotation. Where indicated by the results of the ANOVA, statistical analyses with one-tailed Bonferroni-adjusted p values were used to evaluate significant differences in ROM between each testing condition.

Results

Flexion and extension ROM values for each surgical condition are reported for testing with and without a 400 N follower preload (Table 2). In general, the effect of the follower preload was to attenuate post-operative hypermobility. Given the stabilizing forces of the muscles *in vivo*, this would be expected.

A traditional decompression produced significant differences in range of motion in flexion-extension ($p<0.01$), lateral bending ($p<0.05$) and axial rotation ($p<0.01$) (Table 2). It should be noted that a MI-decompression also produced significant ROM changes in each of these same conditions ($p<0.05$); however, the traditional decompression creates significantly more mobility as compared to MI-D at L4/L5 in flexion-extension ($p<0.01$) and axial rotation ($p<0.05$) (Table 2).

When the effect of MI-D was evaluated separately for left and right lateral bending, the ROM increase, as compared to the intact condition, was isolated to bending toward the side of the approach ($p<0.05$). Lateral bending to the opposite direction was not significant ($p>0.05$).

As mentioned in the Surgical Techniques section, less than 25% of the medial facet was removed in the initial two testing conditions. However, we found that a more extensive resection of the facet (40% resection) resulted in additional ROM increases that were significant (Table 2). This effect was most evident in axial rotation.

Discussion

While the technique of minimally invasive lumbar decompression has been well described [12], the effect of this approach on spinal biomechanics remains poorly understood. It is quite difficult to evaluate how this surgical approach, as well as other techniques, impacts the spine *in vivo*. As such, the testing of a cadaveric model that represents the anatomic changes enacted by this surgical approach may help us better understand how this surgery changes native spinal biomechanics. In this study, we have evaluated a cadaveric lumbar spine following minimally invasive decompression.

In general, the lumbar spine specimens used in this study were without evidence of significant degenerative disease and adequate bone quality. Each full lumbar spine segment was first tested intact with a follower preload, to simulate *in vivo* conditions with load-bearing musculature, and then after each surgical condition. The results of this study demonstrate that a minimally invasive approach produces a significantly smaller increase in segmental spine motion in flexion-extension and axial rotation when compared to a traditional, midline laminectomy. In right lateral bending, there was a significantly smaller increase in motion from intact after minimally invasive surgery as compared to traditional decompression. However, with lateral bending to the side of the

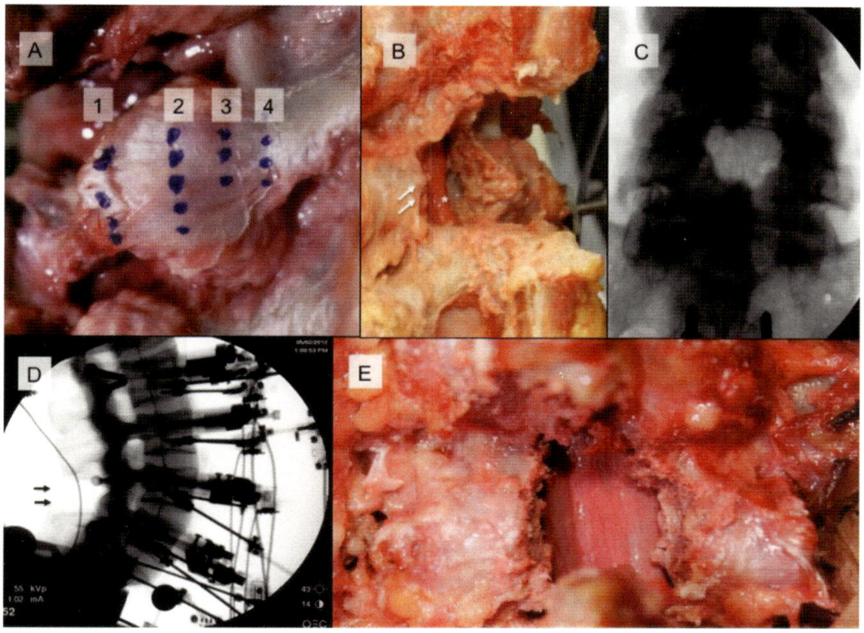

Figure 3. Capsular facet fibers were marked in each specimen by two observers. As shown in A, Line 1 and 4 correspond to the lateral and medial facet extent with line 2 the midpoint and 3 at 25% distance from midline. An oblique view in B, shows "traditional open L4/L5 decompression with extent of facet removal (double arrows) and dural decompression (*) shown). AP and lateral radiographs of this decompression are in C and D. Image E represents "wide factectomy" of 40% bilateral medial facet removal.

surgical approach (in our case, from the left), both approaches were equally destabilizing.

From our results, it also seems that even partial facet removal can have implications upon post-operative spinal mobility. With the MI approach, even removal of less than 15–25% of the facet can instigate mild hypermobility with lateral bending to the approach side. However, lateral bending to the contralateral side is not affected. This implies that the MI approach may preserve the biomechanics of the opposite facet. Further, our results further validate previous reports demonstrating that graded removal of

Table 2. L4–L5 range of motion (in degrees), corresponding to a moment of 8 Nm in flexion and 6 Nm in extension, ±6 Nm in lateral bending, and ±5 Nm in axial rotation.

Testing Condition	Intact	MI-D	TD	WTD
Total FE (no follower preload)	9.4 (1.3)	10.2* (1.4)	11.2*† (1.2)	11.2*† (1.2)
Total FE with 400 N follower preload	9.2 (1.7)	9.6* (1.9)	10.7*† (1.9)	12.3*† (1.9)
Flexion (400 N follower preload)	6.1 (1.8)	6.3 (1.7)	6.7* (1.6)	8.1*†(0.8)
Extension (400 N follower preload)	3.0 (0.8)	3.3 (0.8)	4.0*† (1.0)	4.3* (1.4)
Total Axial Rotation	3.7 (1.3)	4.0* (1.4)	4.5*† (1.5)	6.3*† (2.5)
Left Axial Rotation	1.7 (0.6)	1.9* (0.8)	2.3*† (0.9)	3.3* (1.4)
Right Axial Rotation	2.0 (0.7)	2.1 (0.7)	2.2* (0.8)	3.0† (1.1)
Total Lateral Bending	8.0 (2.8)	8.4* (2.8)	8.6* (2.7)	10.4*† (1.9)
Left Lateral Bending	4.0 (1.3)	4.3* (1.4)	4.4† (1.2)	5.4*† (1.2)
Right Lateral Bending	3.9 (1.6)	4.0 (1.5)	4.2* (1.6)	5.0 (0.7)

Abbreviations:
FE = Flexion-Extention.
MI –D= Minimally invasive decompression.
TD = Traditional decompression.
WTD = Wide traditional decompression.
(SD) = Standard deviation.
(*denotes statistically significant difference from the intact condition;
†denotes statistically significant difference from the MI-D condition).
The values in parentheses denote one standard deviation of the mean.

bilateral facets will result in predictable post-operative hypermobility, especially with axial rotation. Abumi, et al. [15] demonstrated significant instability created by unilateral complete facet removal. Our model differs, as we tested a full lumbar segment with a follower preload; however, our results show similar effects from aggressive facet removal.

In the clinical setting, increased segmental mobility may influence clinical outcomes. While decompressive laminectomy is generally a highly successful operation, clinical outcomes commonly deteriorate with longer follow-ups [18,19,20]. As reported in by Iguchi et al. [21], sustained long-term outcomes following non-instrumented decompression may be limited by post-operative spinal instability. This finding was especially prominent in patients with evidence of pre-operative instability. Further, the incidence of lumbar spondylolisthesis following laminectomy, even with facet preserving techniques, has been reported from 8% to 31% [22,23]. These clinical findings parallel reported data from *in vitro* models. Bisschop et al. recently demonstrated that following single-level laminectomy, there was a significant decrease in both segmental shear stiffness as well as shear-yield force [24,25].

Clinically significant spinal stenosis is more common to older patients. Thus, pre-operative risk factors, such as medical co-morbidities, increased body habitus, and underlying degenerative spinal changes (including segmental instability) are more common in surgical candidates for lumbar decompression. Uniquely, these patients may be the ones who benefit most from minimally invasive techniques. Rosen et al. found excellent clinical outcomes, with few complications, in a study of 57 patients over 75 years of age, treated with MI lumbar decompression [11]. This same finding has been shown in obese patients with both instrumented [26] and non-instrumented techniques.[28] Many reports have questioned the role of non-instrumented decompression in patients with pre-operative spondylolisthesis. However, in a recent report on minimally invasive lumbar decompression, only a single case (1.8%) in 54 treated patients required subsequent spinal fusion. This was in spite of 27 patients (50%) having a grade I (or greater) spondylolisthesis at baseline [10].

There are multiple modern variants of MI lumbar decompression. Minimally invasive techniques have been described using a microscope [27,28] or an endoscope [12,13]. While we evaluated a unilateral approach to bilateral decompression in this study, surgical approaches utilizing bilateral hemilaminotomies have also been described. Fundamental to each of these approaches is preservation of the midline bones and ligaments and judicious medial facetectomy. We feel that both approaches allow for an adequate decompression of the dura. However, a potential limitation of our work is that we have not studied the bilateral approach in our biomechanical model.

A notable limitation in our study is that we used only one minimally invasive technique for decompression. For instance, Lee et. al studied a bilateral laminotomy technique that preserves the midline osteo-ligamentous complex [29]. In their cadaveric simulation model, they a significant decrease in motion for this simulated surgery when compared to a traditional laminectomy. Although there are differences between the decompression in our study and that of Lee et.al, we believe that the preservation of the midline ligamentous complex is a shared component of successful minimally invasive lumbar decompressions. As can be seen in clinical practice, technical variants can be applied equally with success and less injury to the native spinal anatomy.

The methodology of our study also presents other limitations. For instance, cadaveric studies cannot account for the effect of muscular forces on each spinal segment. However, the implementation of full lumbar segments using the follower preload technique, which serves to simulate these forces, may minimize this limitation [17]. In addition, our study primarily used younger specimens. Although this is ideal for studying native spinal biomechanics, this may not model the patients who are commonly candidates for surgery.

Conclusions

1. A minimally invasive, unilateral approach to treat lumbar stenosis produces significantly less biomechanical instability than a traditional midline laminectomy, in all modes of testing.
2. MI decompression does increase ROM in most testing conditions.
3. Lateral bending and axial rotation are only affected on the side of the approach with MI decompression.
4. Wide bilateral facetectomy, even when comprising <50% of the facet, is progressively destabilizing, especially in axial rotation.

Author Contributions

Conceived and designed the experiments: ZS RH ND LV RF AP. Performed the experiments: GV SH. Analyzed the data: GC ZS RH ND LV RF AP. Wrote the paper: ZS GC RH ND LV RF AP.

References

1. Fessler R (2002) Minimally invasive spine surgery. Neurosurgery 51: Siii-iv.
2. Isaacs R, Podichetty VK, Santiago P, Sandhu FA, Spears J, et al (2005) Minimally invasive microendoscopy-assisted transforaminal lumbar interbody fusion. J Neurosurg Spine 3: 98–105.
3. Khoo L, Fessler RG (2002) Microendoscopic decompressive laminotomy for the treatment of lumbar stenosis. Neurosurgery 51: S145–S154.
4. Khoo L, Smith ZA, Asgarzadie F, Barlas Y, Armin SS, et al (2011) Minimally invasive extracavitary approach for thoracic discectomy and interbody fusion: 1-year clinical and radiographic outcomes compared with a cohort of traditional anterior trans-thoracic approaches. J Neurosurg Spine 14: 250–260.
5. Lawton C, Smith ZA, Barnawi A, Fessler RG (2011) The surgical technique of minimally invasive transforaminal lumbar interbody fusion. J Neurosurg Sci 55: 259–264.
6. Ogden A, Bresnahan L, Smith JS, Natarajan R, Fessler RG (2009) Biomechanical comparison of traditional and minimally invasive intradural exposures using finite element analysis. Clin Biomech 24: 143–147.
7. Palmer S, Turner R, Palmer R (2002) Bilateral decompression of lumbar spinal stenosis involving a unilateral approach with the microscope and tubular retractor system. J Neurosurg 97: 213–217.
8. Perez-Cruet M, Foley KT, Isaacs RE, Rice-Wyllie L, Wellington R, et al (2002) Microendoscopic lumbar discectomy: technical note. Neurosurgery 51: S129–136.
9. Billinghurst J, Akbarnia BA (2009) Extreme lateral interbody fusion - XLIF. Curr Orthop Pract 20: 238–251.
10. Palmer S, Davison L (2012) Minimally invasive surgical treatment of lumbar spinal stenosis: Two-year follow-up in 54 patients. Surg Neurol Int 3.
11. Rosen D, O'Toole JE, Eicholz KM, Hrubes M, Huo D, et al. (2007) Minimally invasive lumbar spinal decompression in the elderly: Outcomes of 50 patients aged 75 years and older. Neurosurgery 60: 503–510.
12. Khoo L, Fessler RG (2002) Microendoscopic decompressive laminotomy for the treatment of lumbar stenosis. Neurosurgery 51: S146–S154.
13. Ikuta K, Arima J, Tanaka T, Oga M, Nakano S, et al (2005) Short-term results of micro-endoscopic posterior decompression for lumbar spinal stenosis. Technical note. J Neurosurg Spine 2: 624–633.
14. Bresnahan L, Ogden AT, Natarajan RN, Fessler RG (2008) A biomechanical evaluation of graded posterior element removal for treatment of lumbar stenosis: Comparison of a minimally invasive approach with two standard laminectomy techniques. Spine 34: 17–23.
15. Abumi K, Panjabi MM, Kramer KM, Duranceau J, Oxland T, et al (1990) Biomechanical evaluation of lumbar spinal stability after graded facetectomies. Spine 15: 1142–1147.
16. Hamasaki T, Tanaka N, Kim J, Okada M, Ochi M, et al (2009) Biomechanical assessment of minimally invasive decompression for lumbar spinal canal stenosis. Spine 22: 486–491.

17. Patwardhan A, Havey RM, Meade KP, Lee B, Dunlap B (1999) A follower-load increases load-carrying capacity of the lumbar spine in compression. Spine 24: 1003–1009.
18. Jonsson B, Annertz M, Sjoberg C, Stromqvist B (1997) A prospective and consecutive study of surgically treated lumbar spinal stenosis. Part II: Five-year follow-up by an independent observer. Spine 11: 107–110.
19. Katz J, Lipson SJ, Larson MG, McInnes JM, Fossel AH, et al (1991) The outcome of decompressive laminectomy for degenerative lumbar stenosis. J Bone Joint Surg [Am] 73-A: 809–816.
20. Scholz M, Firsching R, Lanksch WR (1998) Long term follow-up in lumbar spinal stenosis. Spinal Cord: 200–204.
21. Iguchi T, Kurihara A, Nakayama J, Sato K, Kurosaka M, et al (2000) Minimum 10-year outcome of decompressive laminectomy for degenerative lumbar spinal stenosis. Spine 25: 1754–1759.
22. Fox M, Onofrio BM, Hanssen AD (1996) Clinical outcomes and radiological instability following decompressive lumbar laminectomy for degenerative spinal stenosis: a comparison of patients undergoing concomitant arthrodesis versus decompression alone. J Neurosurg 85: 793–802.
23. Fu Y, Zeng BF, Xu JG (2008) Long-term outcomes of two different decompressive techniques for lumbar spinal stenosis. Spine 33: 514–518.
24. Bisschop A, Mullender MG, Kingma I, Jiya TU, van der Veen AJ, et al. (2011) The impact of bone mineral density and disc degeneration on shear strength and stiffness of the lumbar spine following laminectomy. Eur Spine J 21: 530–536.
25. Bisschop A, van Royen BJ, Mullender MG, Paul CP, Kingma I, et al (2012) Which factors prognosticate spinal instability following lumbar laminectomy. Eur Spine J.
26. Rosen D, Ferguson SD, Ogden AT, Huo D, Fessler RG (2008) Obesity and self-reported outcome after minimally invasive lumbar spinal fusion. Neurosurgery 63: 956–960; discussion 960.
27. Weiner B, Walker M, Brower RS, McCulloch JA (1999) Microdecompression for lumbar spinal canal stenosis. Spine 24: 2268–2272.
28. McCulloch J, Young PH (1998) Essentials of Microsurgery. Philadelphia, PA: Lippincott. 453–486. p.
29. Lee M, Bransford RJ, Bellabarba C, Chapman, J, R, Cohen AM, et al (2010) The effect of bilateral laminotomy versus laminectomy on the motion and stiffness of the human lumbar spine: a biomechanical comparison. Spine 35: 1789–1793.

3

Minimally Invasive Surgical Approaches and Traditional Total Hip Arthroplasty: A Meta-Analysis of Radiological and Complications Outcomes

Baohui Yang, Haopeng Li*, Xijing He, Guoyu Wang, Siyue Xu

Department of Orthopaedic Surgery, The 2nd Affiliated Hospital of Medical College, Xi'an Jiaotong University, Xi'an, Shaanxi Province, People's Republic of China

Abstract

Background: Minimally invasive total hip arthroplasty (MITHA) remains considerably controversial. Limited visibility and prosthesis malposition increase the risk of post-surgical complications compared to those of the traditional method.

Methods: A meta-analysis was undertaken of all published databases up to May 2011. The studies were divided into four subgroups according to the surgical approach taken. The radiological outcomes and complications of minimally invasive surgery were compared to traditional total hip arthroplasty (TTHA) using risk ratio, mean difference, and standardized mean difference statistics.

Results: In five studies involving the posterolateral approach, no significant differences were found between the MITHA groups and the TTHA groups in the acetabular cup abduction angle ($p = 0.41$), acetabular anteversion ($p = 0.96$), and femoral prosthesis position ($p = 0.83$). However, the femoral offset was significantly increased (WMD = 3.00; 95% CI, 0.40–5.60; $p = 0.02$). Additionally, there were no significant differences among the complications in both the groups (dislocations, nerve injury, infection, deep vein thrombosis, proximal femoral fracture) and revision rate ($p > 0.05$). In three studies involving the posterior approach, there were no significant differences in radiological outcomes or all other complications between MITHA or TTHA groups ($p > 0.05$). Three studies involved anterolateral approach, while 2 studies used the lateral approach. However, the information from imaging and complications was not adequate for statistical analysis.

Conclusions: Posterior MITHA seems to be a safe surgical procedure, without the increased risk of post-operative complication rates and component malposition rates. The posterolateral approach THA may lead to increased femoral offset. The current data are not enough to reach a positive conclusion that lateral and anterolateral approaches will result in increased risks of adverse effects and complications at the prosthesis site.

Editor: Joel Joseph Gagnier, University of Michigan, United States of America

Funding: The authors have no support or funding to report.

Competing Interests: The authors have declared that no competing interests exist.

* E-mail: LHP-3993@163.com

Introduction

Total hip arthroplasty (THA) is considered one of the most successful operations in orthopedic surgery for over 40 years, during which improvements in the design of implants and biological materials have resulted in positive clinical outcomes. However, for the past decade, considerable interest has been devoted to the development of minimally invasive surgical techniques [1]. Minimally invasive total hip arthroplasty (MITHA) has now become popular around the world. It is defined as the use of a 10 cm or even smaller incision to complete the total hip joint replacement [2,3,4].

The advantages of minimally invasive surgeries include less soft-tissue trauma (smaller skin incision and less muscle damage), reduced blood loss and fewer blood transfusion requirements. Postoperative benefits include less pain, shorter hospital stay, quicker return to function and a better cosmetic appearance [2,4,5].

Despite the increase in adopting MITHA, its risks and benefits still generate debates among orthopedic surgeons. Many of them believe that MITHA introduces additional risks due to the limited visibility of anatomical landmarks and vital structures [6]. Higher risks for thromboembolism, infection, neurovascular injury, femoral fracture and component malposition leading to increased prosthetic wear, are the various complications that have been documented [7]. Bradley P et al [8] retrospectively reviewed 46 revision THAs performed during a 3-year period and concluded that MITHA may be a risk factor for early revision surgery and the long-term survival therefore may be lower than that for non-minimal invasive surgery. Another drawback seems to be the learning curve, which tends to be longer for surgeons with little experience of hip prosthetic surgery. Some other randomized, case-control studies also reveal inconsistent results regarding these issues [9–12]. Therefore, it remains controversial whether MITHA increases post-operative complications and prosthesis malposition.

There have been several related meta-analysis studies [13,14]. These analyses seem to have simply pooled the results together without an explicitly defined sub-group analysis of the surgical approach. Clearly, a 12 cm posterior approach would have very different risks and complications than an 8 cm direct anterior, or two incision approach. A very recent study [15] also pointed this issue. Therefore, to group all MITHA approaches together and make comparisons in a pooled analysis is unsound since differences in technique (e.g. between the mini-anterior, mini-posterior, mini-anterolateral approaches) are significant and need to be analyzed separately. The purpose of this meta-analysis was to compare the MITHA with conventional, or traditional total hip arthroplasty (TTHA) with respect to complications and post-operative results through imaging, of subgroups formed by the surgical approaches taken.

Materials and Methods

We conducted a meta-analysis using the guidelines of the Cochrane Collaboration [16], and our findings were reported according to the Quality of Reporting of Meta-analyses statement [17].

Types of studies included

Any randomized controlled trials comparing MITHA and TTHA for the treatment of hip disease.

Types of Participants

Participants of the 2 treatment groups were similar demographically, and there were no statistically significant differences with respect to the variables of age, gender, body mass index (<35.0).

Types of interventions

We focused on comparing MITHA and TTHA with a common operation approach that is, posterior, posterolateral:, anterolateral, lateral, so that there would be a consistency between the two groups.

We excluded studies in which the surgical approach was inconsistent (for example, if the minimally invasive group used the anterolateral approach, and the traditional group used the posterior approach, etc.). In addition, we also excluded studies that examined the double incision surgical approach.

Types of outcome measures

The primary outcomes were:

1. Imaging outcomes (acetabular abduction angle, acetabular anteversion, femoral prosthesis position (varus or valgus), and femoral offset.
2. Postoperative complications (dislocation, iatrogenic nerve injury, infection, deep vein thrombosis, proximal femoral fracture, and revision rate).

Search strategy

The following search terms were used: total hip arthroplasty (or THA), total hip replacement (or THR), prosthesis (or prostheses or implant), minimally invasive (or less invasive), mini-incision (or MIS or minimal incision or small incision). The literature range was defined as between February 1990 and May 2011. The databases searched included PubMed, Cochrane Central Register of Controlled Trials, Embase, and CBMdisc. A manual search was performed for relevant publications from European Federation of National Associations of Orthopaedics and Traumatology and British Hip Society.

Data collection and analysis

Both review authors (BaoHui Yang and HaoPeng LI) assessed potentially eligible trials for inclusion, any disagreement were resolved through discussion. Titles of journals, names of authors or supporting institutions were not masked at any stage.

Data extraction and management

Data were extracted independently by both authors using piloted forms. The data included the general characteristics of each study and the outcomes measured. General characteristics included study design, first author, year of publication, sample size, and interventions. Only the primary outcomes were measured.

Assessment of risk of bias in included studies

To avoid inherent problems with scale validity [17], we did not use a quality scale or a checklist. We assessed the methodological quality as described by the Cochrane Reviews Handbook 5.0.2 [17], Methodological quality assessment scheme (Table S1). The studies were classified into A: low risk of bias and each of the criteria was appropriate, B: medium risk of bias and most of the criteria were appropriate, and C: high risk of bias and most of the criteria were not appropriate.

Measures of treatment effect

For continuous data such as acetabular cup abduction angle, the mean and standard deviation were used to calculate the weighted mean difference (WMD) and 95% confidence interval (CI); for count data such as post-operative complications, the odds ratio (OR) or relative risk (RR) and 95% CI were used. Data processing was performed using Review Manager 5.0 software (the Cochrane Collaboration).

Assessment of heterogeneity. The heterogeneity test P values revealed by the forest plot were used to determine the heterogeneity of the included studies. I^2 was used to estimate the size of the heterogeneity. $I^2>50\%$ indicated considerable heterogeneity among the included studies.

Subgroup analysis and investigation of heterogeneity

We planned separate outcome analyses according to the different surgical approaches, and if there is no heterogeneity internal each groups, data were pooled using the fixed-effect model and 95% confidence intervals. Where there was clear or significant heterogeneity, we viewed the results of the random-effects model, but in such cases opted not to pool data where the outcome measures were clearly different.

Results

Description of studies

A total of 552 citations were identified from the search strategy. Twelve studies were deemed appropriate (Figure 1). Eleven were written in English, one was in Chinese, and a total of 1077 cases were reported in the included studies. The basic characteristics of the 12 included studies are summarized in Table S2. The diseases included: osteoarthritis, rheumatoid arthritis, traumatic arthritis, congenital dislocation of the hip, femoral head necrosis, femoral neck fracture and other types. Consistent baselines were observed for all patients.

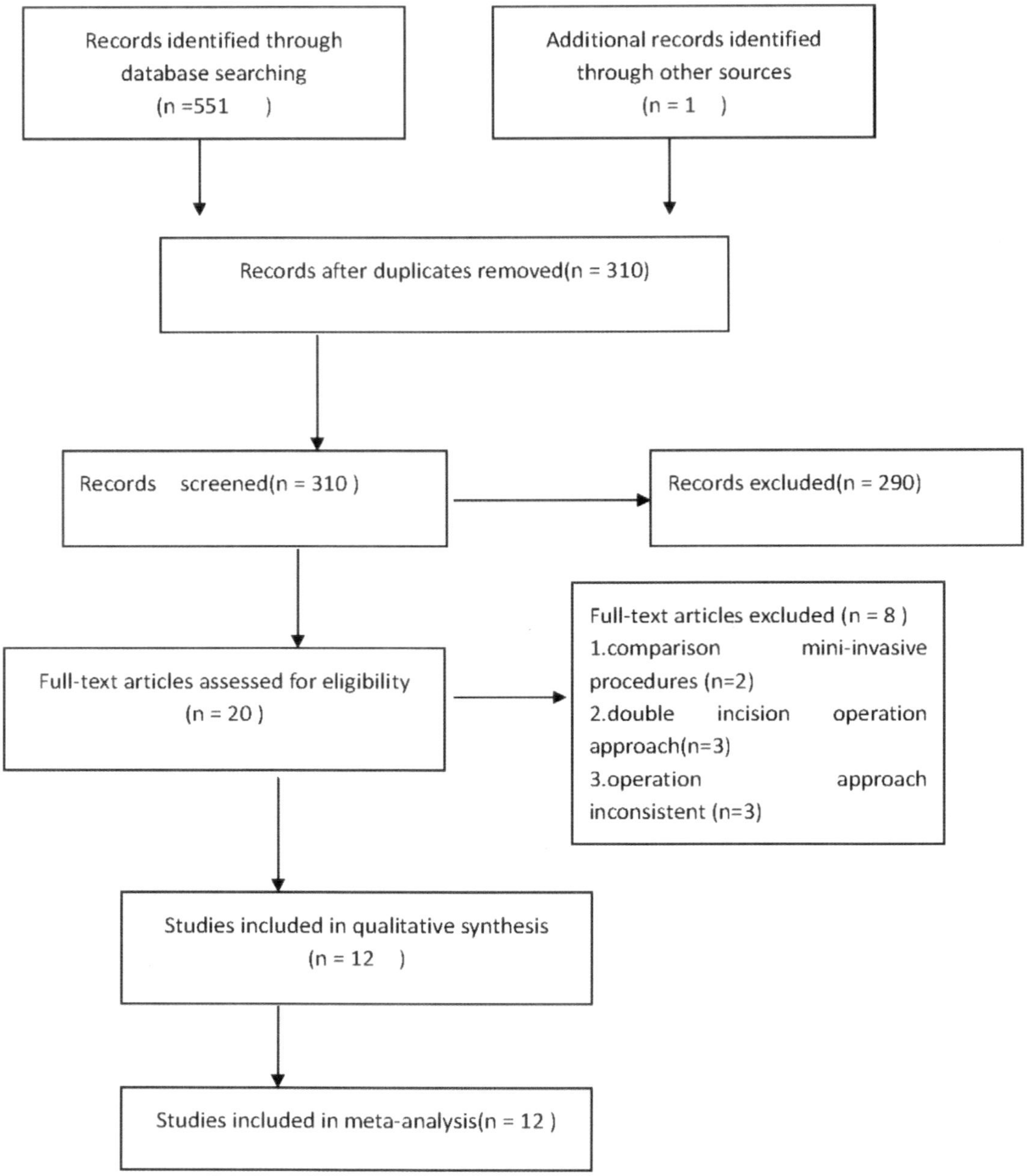

Figure 1. The process of identifying relevant studies is summarized.

The surgical interventions included 4 studies that used the lateral approach [18,19,20,21], 3 studies applied a posterior approach [22,23,24], 6 cases utilized the posterolateral approach [10,11,12,18,25,26], and one case adopted the anterolateral approach [23]. mong them, the study by Goosen et al exercised both, the anterolateral approach and the posterior approach; Shitama et al also employed the posterolateral approach and the lateral approach; and 3 cases make use of the bone cement approach [10,25,23]. Follow-up studies of clinical outcomes and complications ranged between 6 weeks and 80 months.

Risk of bias in included studies

A summary of methodological domain assessment for each study is detailed in figure 2. Overall, the methodological quality of all the trials were found to be of medium risk of bias, The randomization technique was mentioned in 9 trials, which the randomized cohort picked a card, randomization number, or a randomization scheme. Six trials mentioned allocation concealment, 3 studies were single-blinded to the observers [10,11,25], and 2 studies were double-blinded to both the observers and the patients [22,23]. All the studies could result in a potential selection bias. A variety of different THA prostheses were used in the studies reviewed which might result in a performance bias.

Although there were 'lost to follow-up' phenomenon in some studies, missing outcome data balanced in numbers across intervention groups, with similar reasons for missing data across groups, so attrition bias was considered as a low risk of bias.

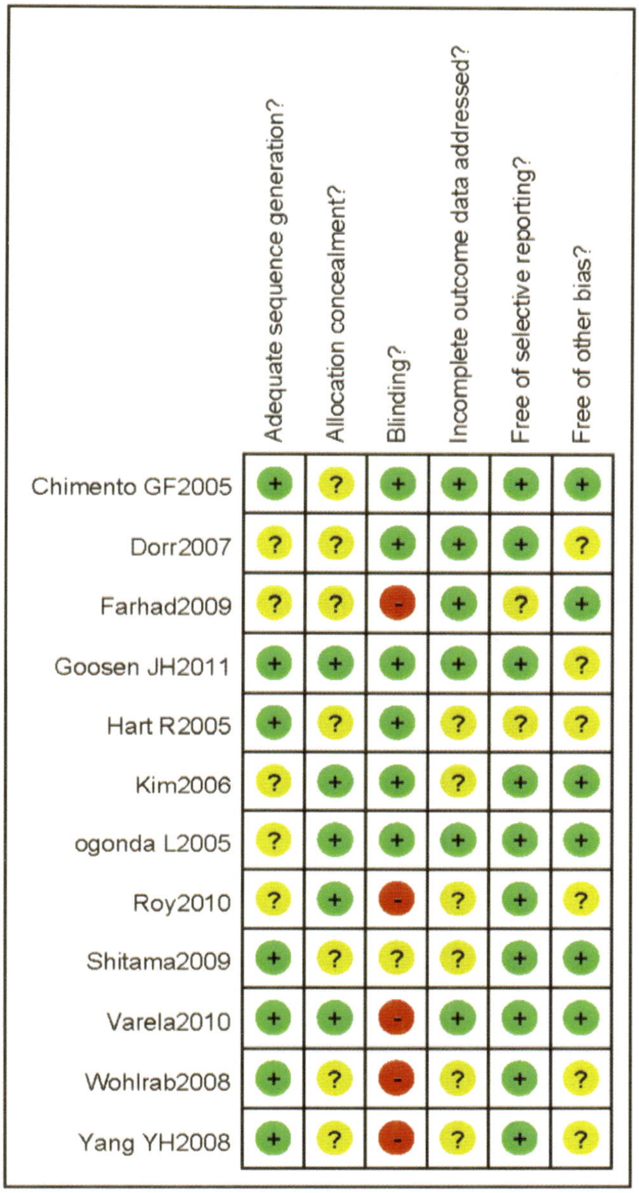

Figure 2. Risk of bias summary. A review of the authors' judgments about each risk of bias item for each included study. + is "yes", − is "no",?is "unclear".

Publication bias analysis

Abduction angle of the acetabular cup was again used for the funnel plot analysis of publication bias (Figure 3), which revealed there was publication bias evident for the primary outcome frequency of the abduction angle.

Primary outcomes: Imaging results

Posterolateral approach. No significant differences were found between the MITHA and the TTHA groups in the imaging data of the acetabular cup abduction angle (p = 0.41), acetabular anteversion (p = 0.96), femoral prosthesis position (p = 0.83). The average femoral offset was significantly increased in the MITHA group than in the TTHA group (WMD = 3.00; 95% CI, 0.40–5.60; p = 0.02) (Tables S3, S4 and Figures 4).

No significant differences were noticed in the complications that occurred [dislocations (p = 0.24), nerve injury (p = 0.57), infection (p = 0.5), deep vein thrombosis (p = 1.00)], and revision rate (p = 0.44) (Tables S3 and S4).

Posterior approach. No significant differences were found between the MITHA and the TTHA groups in the imaging data of the acetabular cup abduction angle (p = 0.46), acetabular anteversion (p = 0.67), femoral prosthesis position (p = 0.25), and femoral offset (p = 0.16) (Tables S3 and S4).

No significant differences were found between the two groups in the complications that occurred [dislocations (p = 0.50), nerve injury (p = 0.50), infection (p = 0.46), deep vein thrombosis (p = 0.10), proximal femoral fracture (p = 0.73)], and revision rate (p = 0.41) (Tables S3 and S4).

Anterolateral approach. No significant differences were found between the two groups in the acetabular cup abduction angle (p = 1.00) and proximal femoral fracture (p = 0.16). However, data on acetabular anteversion, femoral prosthesis position, femoral offset, dislocations, nerve injury, infection, deep vein thrombosis, and revision rate were not adequate for analysis (Tables S3 and S4).

Lateral approach. No significant differences were found in the imaging data of the acetabular cup abduction angle (p = 0.88) and femoral prosthesis position (p = 0.30). Acetabular anteversion and femoral offset were not evaluated (Tables S3 and S4).

No significant differences were found among complications such as dislocations (p = 1.00), infection (p = 1.00), and deep vein thrombosis (p = 0.33). Nerve injury, proximal femoral fracture, and revision rate were not evaluated (Tables S3 and S4).

Discussion

Minimally invasive total hip arthroplasty has often been the subject of debate in recent years. No clear definition exists for what constitutes MITHA, but there is a relative consensus that hip arthroplasties performed with any incision less than 10 centimeters can be included. Proponents of MITHA believe that this approach leads to a faster functional recovery, quicker hospital discharge, and increased patient satisfaction. Opponents believe that compared with TTHA, MITHA leads to increased iatrogenic nerve injury, prosthesis malposition, and revision rate, because of the limited field of vision during the surgery [6–8].

During THAs, the position of prosthesis is directly related to the efficacy of the procedure, and malposition of the prosthesis can cause dislocation, impaction, and pain post-operatively. The bony marks can be clearly visualized in TTHA. In contrast, any approach that is taken in MITHA, is plagued by limited surgical vision and inadequate exposure, thus resulting in difficult, and often, a malpositioning of the prosthesis. Hence, in our study, X-ray assessment of the acetabular abduction angle, anteversion, femoral prosthesis positions were generally considered reliable indicators of successful MITHA.

Total hip arthroplasty -related complications can severely compromise the efficacy of the surgery, such as infection, deep vein thrombosis, fracture adjacent to the prosthesis, and dislocation. The commonly seen complications after THA include dislocation (3.9%), pulmonary embolism (0.9%), and deep infection (0.2%) [27]. Woolson et al [7] described a retrospective cohort study of 135 hip arthroplasties and reported that their mini-incision group had a significantly higher risk of wound complications.

Minimally invasive surgeries for THAs can be divided into five categories: posterior, anterolateral (OCM: a modified Watson-Jones approach) [28], lateral and single anterior minimally

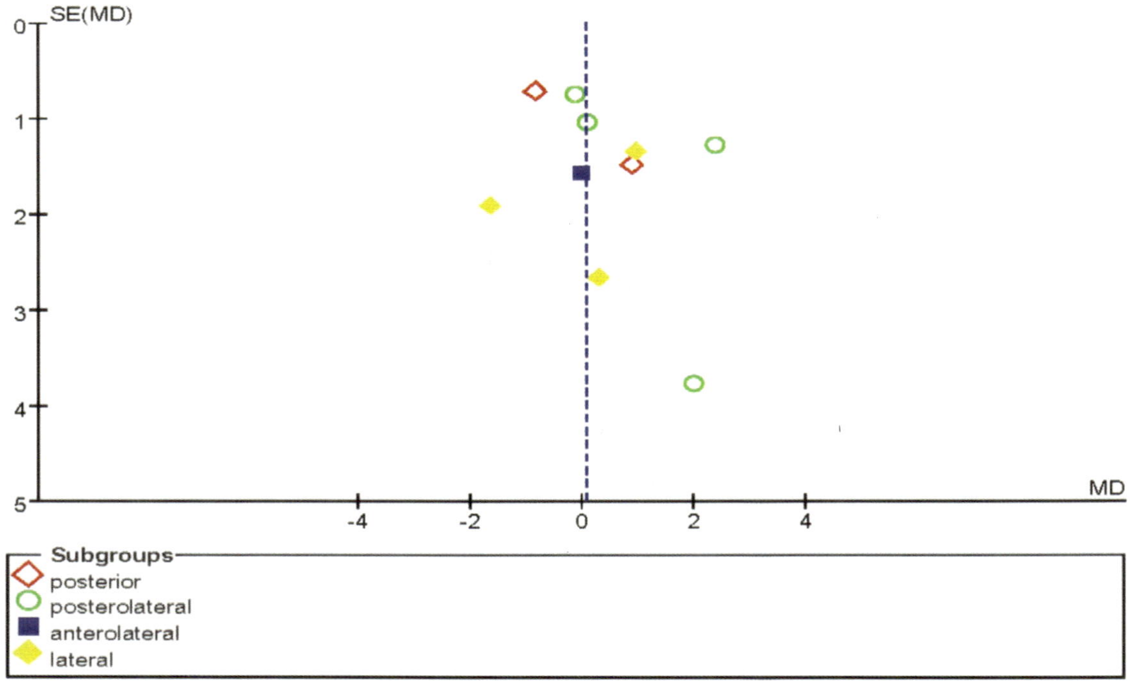

Figure 3. The funnel plot showing the publication bias of the subgroups of different surgical approaches for the most frequently reported outcome—acetabular cup abduction angle. SE (MD) standard error (mean difference).

invasive approach [29], two-incision muscle sparing approach [30] and posterior-lateral minimally invasive approach [31]. Surgical approaches can cause injuries to different soft tissues as they go through different tissue layers. In the past decade, the best surgical approach for THA has been controversially debated. Therefore, previous meta-analyses data of different approaches were not included in our analysis. In contrast, we divided the studies by the surgical approaches to gain a more objective result.

Minimally invasive posterolateral approach

This approach can spare the gluteus medius and the hip flexors. In addition, this approach is a modification of the conventional posterolateral one and is easy for surgeons to master.

In this meta-analysis, no significant differences were found in the acetabular cup abduction angle ($p = 0.41$), acetabular anteversion ($p = 0.96$), and femoral prosthesis position ($p = 0.83$). In addition, there were no significant differences observed with respect to complications. However, one study found that the average femoral offset was significantly increased in the MITHA group (1.6±0.76 cm) than in the TTHA group (1.3±0.81 cm) (WMD = 3.00; 95% CI, 0.40–5.60; $p = 0.02$). Femoral offset is the distance from the center of rotation of the femoral head to a line bisecting the long axis of the femur. A decrease in the femoral offset moves the femur closer to the pelvis, which can result in impingemen at the extremes of movement. Moving the femur medially results in soft tissue laxity. Both of these problems can cause instability and possible dislocation [32,33]. An increase in

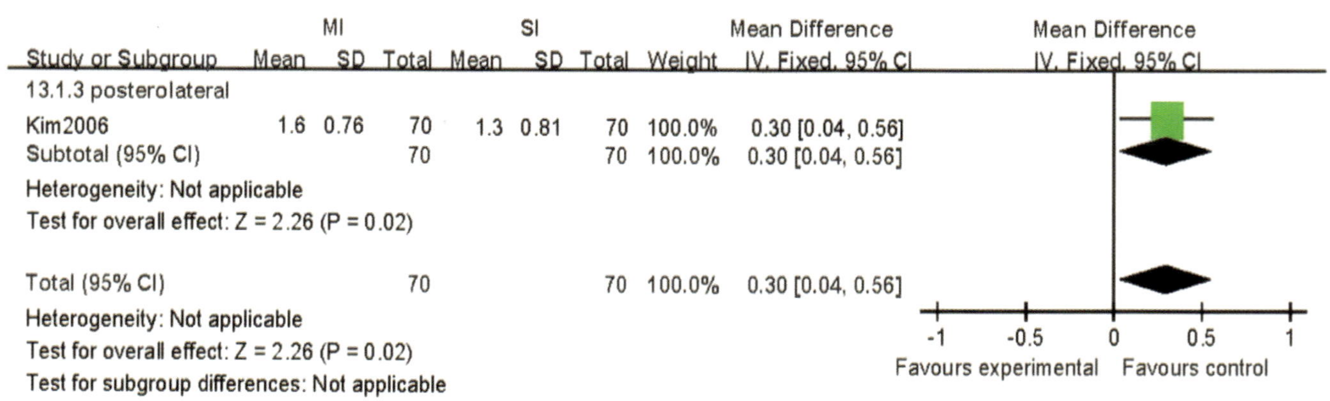

Figure 4. Forest plot of the differences in the increase of post-operative femoral offset in the MITHA and TTHA groups. The MITHA groups had significantly increased femoral offset than the TTHA groups ($p = 0.02$).

the femoral offset will move the femur laterally and will decrease impingement and improve soft tissue tension resulting in better stability without lengthening of the leg. However, excessive femoral offset can result in unevenly distributed stress, increased micromovement, thus increasing the risk of loose, osteolysis, and synovitis [34,35]. This suggests a posterolateral minimally invasive approach may lead to better hip stability. At the same time, it must be pointed out, this result is only a research report with 140 patients and the results still need to be treated with caution.

Minimally invasive posterior approach

In our meta-analysis, the results showed the radiological outcomes [acetabular cup abduction angle ($p = 0.46$), acetabular anteversion ($p = 0.67$), femoral prosthesis position ($p = 0.25$), femoral offset ($p = 0.16$)] and complications [dislocations ($p = 0.50$), nerve injury ($p = 0.50$), infection ($p = 0.46$), deep vein thrombosis ($p = 0.10$), proximal femoral fracture ($p = 0.73$), revision rate ($p = 0.41$)] were not statistically significant between the two treatments by the posterior approach. The possible reason might be that the posterior approach is well-established and the anatomical structures are well understood. The minimally invasive incision can easily be determined in THA through the posterior approach. Additionally, the correct use of retractors can increase the operation field. Particularly, this approach can clearly expose the medullary cavity of the femur at the proximal end of the incision, and expose the acetabulum side at the distal end of the incision. The long-term effects, however, still need further observation.

Minimally invasive anterolateral and lateral approach

The minimally invasive anterolateral and lateral approach was thought to be difficult to perform as the acetabular cup installation was prone to excessive anteversion and abduction, causing postoperative anterior dislocation [36]. Siguier et al. summarized 1037 cases of total hip replacements performed by the anterolateral approach and concluded that this procedure can best spare the external rotators of the hip, fascia lata, great trochanter, and gluteal muscles, thus minimizing the damage to soft tissues adjacent to the hip and maintaining the balance in soft tissues, without increasing the risk of dislocation.

In our meta-analysis, only the acetabular cup abduction angle ($p = 1.00$) and proximal femoral fracture ($p = 0.16$) were analyzed and no statistical significance was found ($p>0.05$). However, no adequate data was available to effectively evaluate the acetabular anteversion, femoral prosthesis position, femoral offset, dislocations, nerve injury, infection, deep vein thrombosis, and revisions. Therefore, no positive conclusion can be drawn from the current study until more high-quality randomized controlled studies are available.

The lateral approach also has a relatively lower risk of postoperative dislocation. he acetabulum can be adequately exposed and the prosthesis can be easily implanted. Nevertheless, the major shortcoming of this procedure is that part of the gluteus medius and gluteus minimus is spliced, causing weakness of the abductor, damage to the superior gluteal nerve, ipsilateral postoperative lameness, and increased risk of heterotopic ossification around the hip [37]. In addition, this procedure has poor exposure when manipulating the prosthesis and the retractor often causes severe damage to the skin. In this study, acetabular anteversion, femoral offset, nerve injury, proximal femoral fracture, and revision were not evaluated and therefore the safety profile is not confirmed yet.

Our findings are mainly limited by the quality and the low number of included studies. This limited our assessment of potential publication bias and unpublished research having negative results that cannot be identified. Therefore, publication bias may exist, which could result in the overestimation of the effectiveness of interventions. Third, the methodological quality of the all trials was found to be medium risk of bias. Due to these limitations, the combined results of this meta-analysis should be cautiously accepted, and more independent high-quality RCTs with effectiveness analyses are needed.

Conclusion

Our meta-analysis indicates that the posterior approach in MITHA is a safe surgical procedure, without increased operative complication rates and component malposition rates. The posterolateral approach may lead to increased femoral offset. No thorough conclusion can be drawn from the lateral or anterolateral approach as the risks of adverse effects and complications are increased at the site of prosthesis. It must be pointed out, that this result is only a research report from140 patients and the results need to be treated with caution. More high-quality studies are needed to assess the best surgical approach in minimally invasive hip arthroplasties.

Author Contributions

Conceived and designed the experiments: HL. Performed the experiments: BY. Analyzed the data: XH. Contributed reagents/materials/analysis tools: GW. Wrote the paper: SX.

References

1. Berry DJ, Berger RA, Callaghan JJ, Dorr LD, Duwelius PJ, et al. (2003) Minimally invasive total hip arthroplasty. Development, early results, and a critical analysis. J Bone Joint Surg Am 85-A(11): 2235–2246.
2. Sculco TP, Jordan LC, Walter WL (2004) Minimally invasive total hip arthroplasty : the Hospital for Special Surgery experience. Orthop Clin North Am 35: 137–142.
3. Szendroi M, Sztrinkai G, Vass R, Kiss J (2006) The impact of minimally invasive total hip arthroplasty on the standard procedure. Int Orthop 30: 160–71.
4. Wall SJ, Mears SC (2008) Analysis of published evidence on minimally invasive total hip arthroplasty. J Arthroplasty 23: 55–58.
5. Pagnano MW, Hebl J, Horlocker T (2006) Assuring a painless total hip arthroplasty: a multimodal approach emphasizing peripheral nerve blocks. J Arthroplasty 21: 80–84.
6. Nakamura S, Matsuda K, Arai N, Wakimoto N, Matsushita T (2004) Mini-incision posterior approach for total hip arthroplasty. Int Orthop 28: 214–217.

7. Woolson ST, Mow CS, Syquia JF, Lannin JV, Schurman DJ, et al. (2004) Comparison of primary total hips replacements performed with standard incision or mini-incision. J Bone Joint Surg 86-A: 1353–8.
8. Bradley P, Graw MD, Steven T, Woolson MD, Heather G, et al. (2010) Minimal Incision Surgery as a Risk Factor for Early Failure of Total Hip Arthroplasty. Clin Orthop Relat Res 468: 2372–6.
9. Bennett D, Ogonda L, Elliot D, Humphreys L, Lawlor M, et al. (2007) Comparison of immediate postoperative walking ability in patients receiving minimally invasive and standard-incision hip arthroplasty: a prospective blinded study. J Arthroplasty 22: 490–495.
10. Chimento GF, Pavone V, Sharrock N, Kahn B, Cahill J, et al. (2005) Minimally invasive total hip arthroplasty: a prospective randomized study. J Arthroplasty 20: 139–144.
11. Kim YH (2006) Comparison of primary total hip arthroplasties performed with a minimally invasive technique or a standard technique: a prospective and randomized study. J Arthroplasty 21: 1092–1098.
12. Ogonda L, Wilson R, Archbold P, Lawlor M, Humphreys P, et al. (2005) A minimal-incision technique in total hip arthroplasty does not improve early postoperative outcomes: a prospective, randomized, controlled trial. J Bone Joint Surg Am 87: 701–710.
13. Cheng T, Feng JG, Liu T, Zhang XL (2009) Minimally invasive total hip arthroplasty: a systematic review. Int Orthop 33: 1473–1481.
14. Smith TO, Blake V, Hing CB (2011) Minimally invasive versus conventional exposure for total hip arthroplasty: a systematic review and meta-analysis of clinical and radiological outcomes. Int Orthop 35: 173–184.
15. Khan RJ (2011) Comments on Smith et al: Comments on Smith et al.: minimally invasive versus conventional exposure for total hip arthroplasty: a systematic review and meta-analysis of clinical and radiological outcomes. Int Orthop 35: 299.
16. Higgins J, Green S (2008) Cochrane Handbook for Systematic Reviews of Interventions Version 5.0.0. The Cochrane Collaboration. Available from www.cochrane-handbook.org.
17. Moher D, Cook DJ, Eastwood S, Olkin I, Rennie D, et al. (1999) Improving the quality of reports of meta-analyses of randomized controlled trials: the QUOROM statement. Quality of reporting of meta-analyses. Lancet 354: 1896.
18. Shitama T, Kiyama T, Naito M, Shiramizu K, Huang G, et al. (2009) Which is more invasive-mini versus standard incisions in total hip arthroplasty? Int Orthop 33: 1543–1547.
19. Varela-Egocheaga J R, Suárez-Suárez M A, Fernandez-Villan M (2010) Minimally invasive lateral approach in total hip replacement: a prospective randomised study. Rev Esp Cir Ortop Traumatol 54: 27–33.
20. Mazoochian F, Weber P, Schramm S, Utzschneider S, Fottner A, et al. (2009) Minimally invasive total hip arthroplasty: a randomized controlled prospective trial. Arch Orthop Trauma Surg 129: 1633–1639.
21. Wohlrab D, Droege JW, Mendel T, Brehme K, Riedl K, et al. (2008) Minimally invasive vs. transgluteal total hip replacement. A 3-month follow-up of a prospective randomized clinical study. Orthopäde 37: 1121–1126.
22. Dorr LD, Maheshwari AV, Long WT, Wan Z, Sirianni LE, et al. (2007) Early pain relief and function after posterior minimally invasive and conventional total hip arthroplasty. A prospective, randomized, blinded study. J Bone Joint Surg Am 89: 1153–1160.
23. Goosen JH, Kollen BJ, Castelein RM, Kuipers BM, Verheyen CC, et al. (2011) Minimally invasive versus classic procedures in total hiparthroplasty: a double-blind randomized controlled trial. Clin Orthop Relat Res 469: 200–208.
24. Roy L, Laflamme GY, Carrier M, Kim PR, Leduc S (2010) A randomised clinical trial comparingminimally invasive surgery to conventional approach for endoprosthesis in elderly patients with hip fractures. Injury 41: 365–369.
25. Hart R, Stipcák V, Janecek M, Visna P (2005) Component position following total hip arthroplasty through a miniinvasive posterolateral approach. Acta Orthop Belg 71: 60–64.
26. Yang YH, Gao ZL, Wang JC (2008) Mini — incision Total Hip Replacement for Femoral Neck Fracture in Senile Patients. Chinese Journal of bone and joint injury 23: 110–112.
27. Phillips CB, Barrett JA, Losina E, Mahomed NN, Lingard EA, et al. (2003) Incidence rates of dislocation, pulmonary embolism, and deep infection during the first six months after elective total hip replacement. J Bone Joint Surg (Am) 85: 20–26.
28. Bertin KC, Röttinger H (2004) Anterolateral mini-incision hip replacement surgery: a modified Watson-Jones approach. Clin Orthop Relat Res 429: 248–255.
29. Siguier T, Siguier M, Brumpt B (2004) Mini-incision anterior approach does not increase dislocation rate: a study of 1037 total hip replacements. Clin Orthop Relat Res 426: 164–173.
30. Berger RA (2004) The technique of minimally invasive total hip arthroplasty using the two-incision approach. Instr Course Lect 53: 149–155.
31. Goldstein WM, Branson JJ (2004) Posterior-lateral approach to minimal incision total hip arthroplasty. Orthop Clin North Am 35: 131–136.
32. Morrey BF (1997) Dificult complications after hip replacem. Clin Orthop 344: 179–187.
33. Dorr LD, Wan Z (1998) Causes of and treatment protocol for instability of total hip replacement. Clin Orthop Relat Res 355: 14–51.
34. Cannestra VP, Berger RA, Quigley LR, Jacobs JJ, Rosenberg AG, et al. (2000) Total hip arthroplasty with a precoated ofset stem. Four to nine — year results. J Bone Joint Surg Am 82: 1291–9.
35. Kleemann RU, Heller MO, Stoeckle U, Taylor WR, Duda GN (2003) THA loading arising from increased femoral an terversion and ofset may lead to critical cement stresses. Onhop Res 21: 767–774.
36. Yang CF, Zhang DW, Niu S, Kong LZ, Zhu JY, et al. (2009) Curative Effect of Minimally-invasive Total Hip Arthroplasty. Chinese Journal of bone and joint injury 24: 385–388.
37. Archibeck MJ, Berger RA, Jacobs JJ, Quigley LR, Gitelis S, et al. (2001) Second-generation cementless total.hip arthroplasty. Eight to eleven- year results 83: 1666–1673.

4

Temperature Modulation of Electric Fields in Biological Matter

Charlotte S. Daniels[1]*, Boris Rubinsky[1,2]

1 Department of Mechanical Engineering, University of California, Berkeley, California, United States of America, **2** Graduate Program in Biophysics, University of California, Berkeley, California, United States of America

Abstract

Pulsed electric fields (PEF) have become an important minimally invasive surgical technology for various applications including genetic engineering, electrochemotherapy and tissue ablation. This study explores the hypothesis that temperature dependent electrical parameters of tissue can be used to modulate the outcome of PEF protocols, providing a new means for controlling and optimizing this minimally invasive surgical procedure. This study investigates two different applications of cooling temperatures applied during PEF. The first case utilizes an electrode which simultaneously delivers pulsed electric fields and cooling temperatures. The subsequent results demonstrate that changes in electrical properties due to temperature produced by this configuration can substantially magnify and confine the electric fields in the cooled regions while almost eliminating electric fields in surrounding regions. This method can be used to increase precision in the PEF procedure, and eliminate muscle contractions and damage to adjacent tissues. The second configuration considered introduces a third probe that is not electrically active and only applies cooling boundary conditions. This second study demonstrates that in this probe configuration the temperature induced changes in electrical properties of tissue substantially reduce the electric fields in the cooled regions. This novel treatment can potentially be used to protect sensitive tissues from the effect of the PEF. Perhaps the most important conclusion of this investigation is that temperature is a powerful and accessible mechanism to modulate and control electric fields in biological tissues and can therefore be used to optimize and control PEF treatments.

Editor: Vladimir N. Uversky, University of South Florida College of Medicine, United States of America

Funding: CSD was supported by a National Foundation (NSF) fellowship. The funders had no role in study design, data collection and analysis, decision to publish, or preparation of the manuscript.

Competing Interests: The authors have declared that no competing interests exist.

* E-mail: daniels.charlotte@gmail.com

Introduction

The current direction of surgical technologies is toward a minimally and non-invasive strategy. In comparison to traditional surgery, minimally and non-invasive surgeries are positioned to transform the field of medicine with shorter hospital stays, reduced surgical trauma, improved immune response and greater precision [1]. These benefits are primarily due to less intrusive procedures and exceptionally targeted tissue treatment.

Pulsed electric fields (PEF) are becoming commonly used in minimally invasive and non-invasive surgery. The PEF technologies utilize electric fields which target the cellular membrane, increasing membrane permeability through the formation of nanoscale defects. The PEFs are usually delivered through electrodes in contact with the tissue. Typical PEF parameters currently used in medicine and biotechnology employ 0.1 to 1E7V/m electric fields, nanosecond to millisecond pulse lengths and one to several hundred pulses. They can be AC or DC. PEFs can have two different effects on the cellular membrane as a function of the electrical parameters: reversible and irreversible electroporation. Reversible electroporation causes the transient permeabilization of the cell membrane. Reversible electroporation is used in genetic engineering for the introduction of genes into targeted cells [2], [3], [4]. It is also used for tissue ablation in electrochemotherapy, which introduces drugs such as bleomycin into PEF treated cells [5], [6], [7]. In irreversible electroporation (IRE), the effect of membrane permeabilization leads to cell death. In the past, it was thought that IRE was produced by microsecond to millisecond pulses only. However, it was recently found that nanosecond pulses also produce IRE when used with appropriate electric field strength [8], [9]. During the last four decades, IRE was used primarily in the food industry for sterilization of micro-organisms [10], [11]. Recently, IRE has emerged as an important minimally invasive technique for tissue ablation, because of its molecular selectivity [12],[13].

Mathematical studies have shown that naturally occurring local heterogeneities in the electrical properties of tissue affect the applied electric fields during PEF and thereby affect the outcome of PEF procedures [14],[15]. It is well established that temperature affects the electrical properties of tissue [16]. It occurred to us that temperature could be used to locally modify electrical tissue properties in a desirable and controlled way and thereby produce greater local control over the outcome of minimally invasive PEF procedures. The goal of this study is, therefore, to explore the hypothesis that local changes in electrical properties of tissue produced by changes in temperature can be used to modulate and control the effect of PEFs on biological matter. This is a mathematical study using the numerical analysis tools described in [14].

Electrical conductivity of tissue is a function of temperature, exhibiting a positive correlation. Consequently, the electrical conductivity of cooled tissues is substantially lower than those at physiological temperatures. In this study, we will focus on an examination of the effect of lowering the temperature locally on

Table 1. Temperature dependent properties used in the Pennes bioheat equation for the purpose of solving the temperature distribution due to the application of the cooling probe.

Thermal Conductivity	Blood Perfusion	Blood Heat Capacity	Metabolic Heat	Tissue Density	Tissue Heat Capacity
0.5 [W/mK]	0.5[kg/m^3 s]	3640 [J/kg K]	33800[W/m^3]	1000 [kg/m^3]	3750 [J/kgK]

the outcome of the PEF protocol. While many methods for cooling tissue locally are possible, this study will simulate the use of cooling probes. Such probes are commonly used in minimally invasive surgery at temperatures below freezing (Rubinsky 2000). Here it is assumed that for this particular application, the probes are cooled to above freezing temperatures and used only as a means for changing tissue electrical properties.

The biophysical effect of temperature on the process of electroporation will be also considered and incorporated into the mathematical model. Several studies have investigated the effects of temperature on electroporation. For instance, Diaz investigated the effect of low temperatures on electroporation efficacy [17]. He accomplished electroporation on kidney epithelial cells at temperatures as low as -2°C [18]. Additionally, Gallo demonstrated the trend between temperature and electroporation; as temperature decreases, initial cell membrane permeabilizing pulse voltage increases [19]. Gallo's study operated on the stratum corneum in the range 0–80°C. The same relationship between temperature and electroporation was found in *alga Valonia*, rye leaf protoplast and mammalian cell lines [20].

As a first order study, the concept introduced here investigated a mathematical analysis of temperature and electric fields produced by the application of PEFs in conjunction with local cooling. The focus of this theoretical study is to examine the effect of changes in temperature on electric fields and the subsequent implications for tissue electroporation. For simplicity and to extract the most salient biophysical aspects of the analysis, we investigate simple two dimensional configurations in cylindrical coordinates in which the electrical and thermal effects are produced by electroporation probes and cooling probes with dimensions typical to commercially available devices. This study focuses on the change in electrical parameters as a result of temperature. It is evident that following this first order analysis, much additional theoretical and experimental work remains to be done.

Methods

The models were generated using numerical analysis executed by Comsol Multiphysics (version 4.1). This initial study utilized 2-dimensional models because these are sufficient to demonstrate the significant effect of temperature induced electrical property heterogeneities. Two equations were solved simultaneously in Comsol. The first of which was the Laplace equation for potential distribution associated with an electric pulse:

$$-\nabla \cdot d(\sigma\nabla - J^e) = dQ_j, \tag{1}$$

where σ is electrical conductivity, V is voltage, $\mathcal{J}^e$ is external current density, d is thickness and Q_j is the current source. For all boundaries, the external current density and the current source

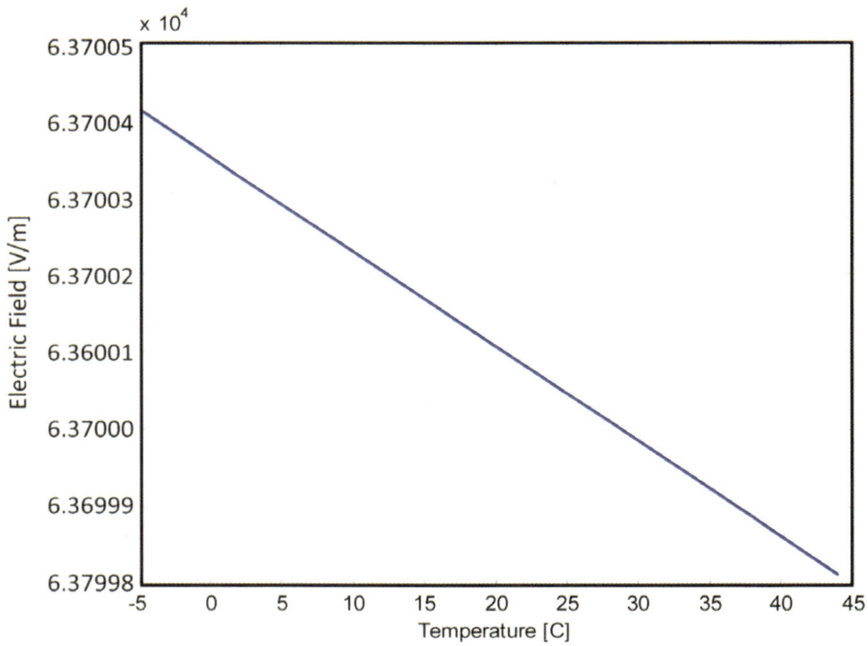

Figure 1. This plot depicts the threshold electric field for irreversible electroporation as a function of temperature. It is clear that as temperature is decreased, the required electric field to achieve electroporation increases. However, the effect of temperature on electric field threshold is very small, on the order of 0.1 V/m.

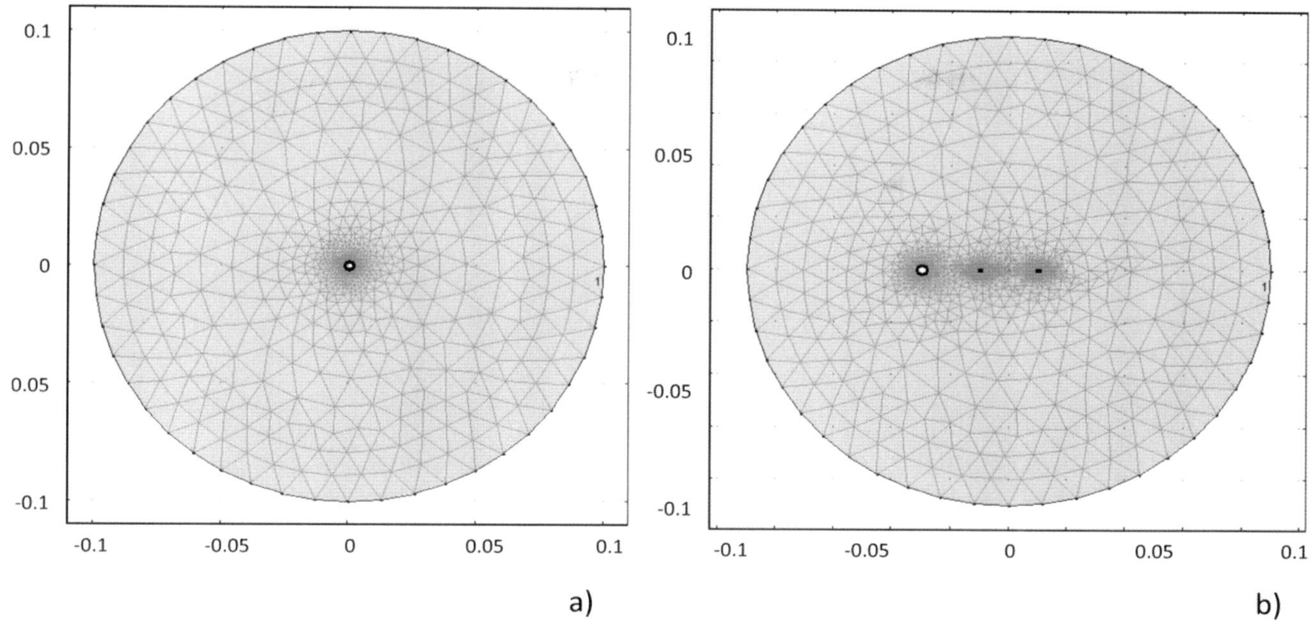

Figure 2. The finite element mesh for the two geometries investigated in this study. a) Mesh for Case 1, in which one cold probe is utilized for both cooling and as a PEF electrode. b) Mesh for Case 2, in which two typical electroporation probes are used to deliver the electric pulses and one cold probe is used to cool the tissue and induce local changes in electric properties. Note that the mesh is extra fine in the vicinity of the probes in order to capture the changes in electric field and temperature that occur due to the effect of the probes.

were set to zero, and thickness was set to one. The electric field was solved in the AC/DC Conductive Media module using a transient analysis to account for electrical pulses.

The electrical conductivity, σ, was determined by the local tissue temperature according to data from the literature. Properties for physiological saline solution were used as a first order simulation for biological tissue, since electrical property data for tissues in the entire range of temperatures of interest is not available. Data from J.J. Arps [21] was curve fitted to calculate the electrical conductivity of the composite medium. The derived electrical conductivity also employed experimental data from [22], resulting in the following function:

$$\sigma(T)=0.03(T-273.15)+0.7, T>272.59. \quad (2)$$

Equation 2 describes the behavior of electrical conductivity in [S/m] as a function of temperature T in [K]. The correlation coefficient of this equation relative to experimental data was tabulated to be $r=0.99989$.

In addition to electrical conductivity, electrical permittivity is also a function of temperature. The following equation [23] was utilized to take into account the temperature dependence of electrical permittivity:

$$\varepsilon(T)=10^{\left(1.94404-1.99\times10^{-3}(T-273.15)\right)}, \quad (3)$$

where ε is electrical permittivity and T is temperature in [K]. This equation is valid for low frequency permittivity, experienced by typical PEF pulse parameters, which are in the range of 0.1-20E-3 seconds [24], [25].

The temperature distribution was obtained from the solution of the Pennes bioheat equation, which was solved simultaneously as the electrical potential equation. The general Pennes bioheat equation to be solved for this case took the following form:

$$\nabla\cdot(k\nabla T)+\rho_b w_b c_b(T_a-T)+q'''=\rho c_p\frac{\partial T}{\partial t}, \quad (4)$$

where k is thermal conductivity, T is temperature, w_b is blood perfusion, c_b is the heat capacity of blood, T_a is arterial temperature, ρ is the tissue density, c_p is the tissue heat capacity and $q'''=Q_{met}+Q_{ext}$. Q_{met} is the metabolic heat generation and $Q_{ext}=\sigma|\nabla\phi|^2$, which accounts for Joule heating, where ϕ is electrical potential and σ is electrical conductivity of the tissue. In this study, the effect of Joule heating on the temperature distribution was considered. The values for biological tissue utilized in the Pennes bioheat equation are listed in Table 1 [26].

Studies on the effect of temperature on electroporation protocols have revealed a negative correlation between temperature and fields. The electric fields required for producing electroporation increase as temperature decreases. The goal of this study is to investigate the ultimate effects of temperature modulation on PEF protocols, such as the fields necessary to induce reversible and irreversible electroporation. To accomplish this, data has been extracted from existing literature to produce a correlation between temperature and the fields required for reversible and irreversible electroporation [27]. The equation used in this study was derived from the experimental data acquired in [17] and is given by:

$$E(T)=\frac{-39}{3200}T+63700.45094, \quad (5)$$

where T is temperature [°C] and E is electric field [V/m]. Equation 5 is plotted in Figure 1. It is clear from both the equation and the graph that temperature dependence of the electric field is very low. However, the data available is very limited and cells in tissue may behave differently from cells in solution. For this

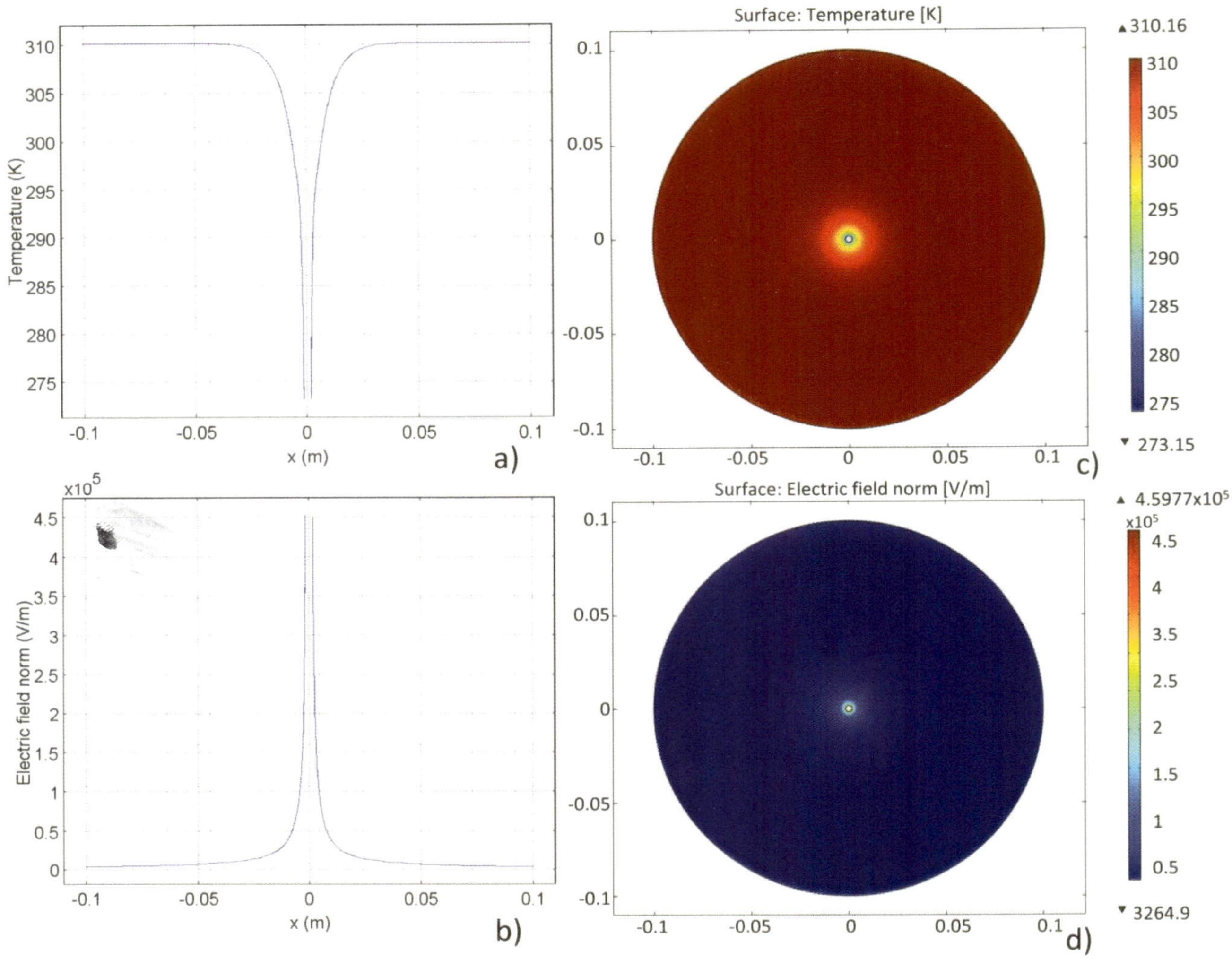

Figure 3. Results for Case 1. a) and b) Temperature and electric field distribution, respectively, at a transection along the diameter of the domain. c) and d) Temperature and electric field surface plots, respectively, in the domain. Plots reflect results after 2000 seconds of cooling at 0°C followed by ten 2500 V pulses (1 Hz, 50 μs) with full bioheat parameters considered.

reason, this equation was used as an approximate correlation for this study. It was used primarily to demonstrate an accurate methodology, but a substantial amount of additional research is needed to generate precise correlations, which currently have not yet been developed.

Models

The primary goal of this study is to examine how local changes in tissue electrical properties due to changes in temperature affect electric fields during PEF protocols. This study will focus in particular on the effects of cold temperatures. The complex volumetric effect of temperature induced changes in tissue electrical properties can be approximated by voltage divider circuits consisting of elements of resistance in series or in parallel. To capture these effects two models were examined. Case 1 includes temperature induced resistance in series with the original tissue impedance. Case 2 includes temperature induced resistance in parallel. These two cases can also be viewed as the difference between an electrically active cooling probe (resistance in series) and an electrically inactive cooling probe (resistance in parallel). These descriptions are only an approximation of the more complex models investigated in this study, and are described here for clarification of the resulting electrical phenomena.

Case 1: Resistors in Series. The first geometry considered was represented in 2D and consisted of a single cryoprobe inserted into the center of a sample of tissue. The cryoprobe simultaneously applied a cold temperature and voltage pulses. In this case, the cooling of tissue simulates the addition of a resistor in series. The cryoprobe, measuring 3.4 mm in diameter [28], was inserted into the center of an infinitely long cylinder of tissue, 6 cm in radius. The outer edge of the cylinder was set to constant deep body temperature, 37°C. The initial temperature of the system was also deep body temperature.

Cryoprobes are designed as hollow conduits through which a coolant flows. Because the probes are made of electrically conductive metal, the same probe can be used to both cool the tissue and apply PEFs as electrodes when connected to a voltage supply. Therefore, the cold probe was modeled as a PEF electrode. A typical PEF voltage of 2500 V was applied between the cold probe and the uniformly grounded outer edge of the tissue cylinder. A typical irreversible electroporation pulse sequence of 50 μs pulse length at a frequency of 1 Hz was used. This geometry

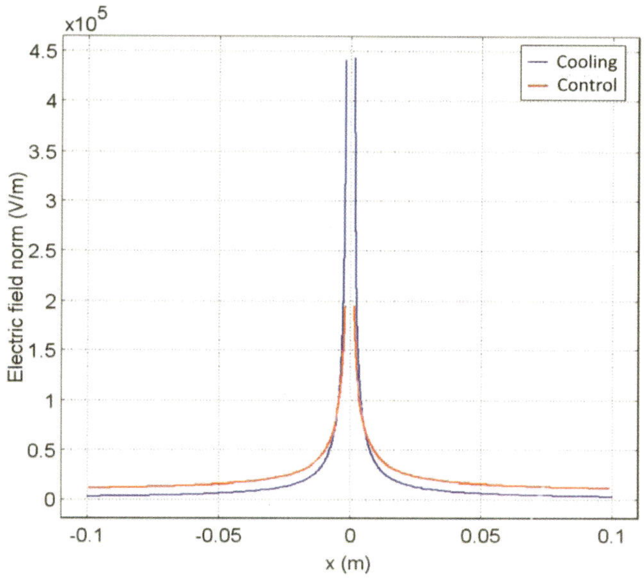

Figure 4. Control results for Case 1. Comparison of electric field distributions along a transection at the diameter of the sample. Blue line: electric field after 2000 seconds of cooling at 0°C followed by ten 2500 V pulses (1 Hz, 50 µs). Red line: control electric field after ten 2500 V pulses (1 Hz, 5 µs), With full bioheat parameters considered. It is clear from this figure that the cooling case achieves a peak electric field of over twice the magnitude of the control case, demonstrating the ability of low temperatures to concentrate and magnify the electric field in this configuration (resistance in series). Additionally, at the outer boundaries of the geometry, it can be seen that the electric field is lower in the cooling case than the control case, which demonstrates the ability of low temperatures to confine the electric field to regions of low temperature in this geometry.

was chosen because it simulates a typical clinical procedure during which a single probe applies a voltage and a grounding pad is placed at a distance, similar to radio-frequency ablation technique.

To understand the implications of temperature induced effects on the electric field, two variations of Case 1 have been modeled. The first applies a temperature of 0°C to the cold probe. The second applies a thermally insulating boundary condition to the probe, which serves as a control.

The finite element mesh for this case utilized triangular elements, as shown in Figure 2a. The element size was smallest adjacent to the cryoprobe, and increased in size as it radiated towards the outer boundary. This was done in order to accurately capture the steep temperature gradient adjacent to the cold probe. The mesh was refined until the solution was no longer affected. Approximately 3800 elements were utilized to cover a 314 cm^2 surface area.

Case 2: Resistors in parallel. The second 2D geometry utilized three probes: two electrodes and a cooling probe at a distance. Because a single probe is not acting as an electrode and a cooling probe simultaneously, this configuration approximates two resistors in parallel. An infinitely long cylinder of tissue 6 cm in radius was set to constant deep body temperature and electrical insulation at the outer margin. The initial temperature of the system was also deep body temperature. The delivery of PEF was applied through two typical irreversible electroporation electrodes [13] of 1 mm in diameter. The leftmost electrode was held at ground and the rightmost probe applied a voltage of 2500 V. A typical irreversible electroporation pulse sequence of 50 µs pulse length at a frequency of 1 Hz was used. As in Case 1, the cold probe was 3.4 mm in diameter. A temperature of 0°C was applied to the cold probe and it was considered electrically insulated. The cold probe was set at various distances from the electrodes, to study the dependence of temperature induced heterogeneities on geometry. The exact geometries are specified in the Results and Discussion section.

To understand the implications of temperature induced effects on the electric field, two variations of Case 2 have been modeled. The first applies a temperature of 0°C to the cold probe. The second applies a thermally insulating boundary condition to the probe, which serves as a control.

The finite element mesh in this study utilized triangular elements, demonstrated by Figure 2b. The element size was smallest in the region surrounding both probes. This was done in order to accurately capture the temperature gradients adjacent to

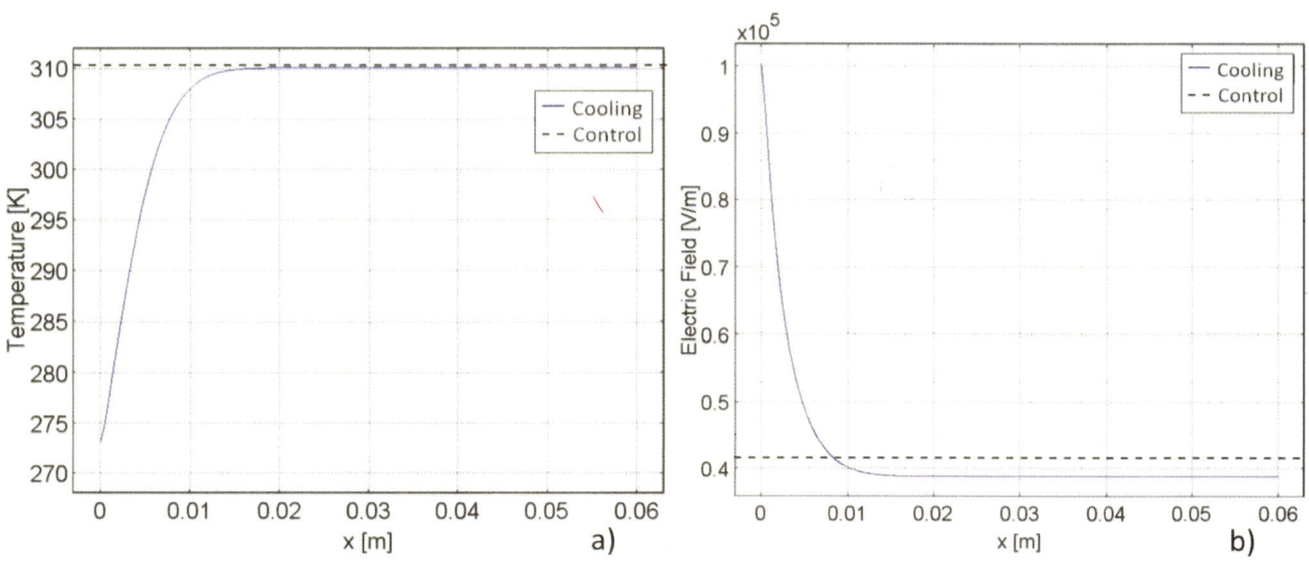

Figure 5. Comparison of cooling and control models for a supplemental one-dimensional study. Graphs illustrate: a) Temperature and b) electric field. Control models are held at constant body temperature.

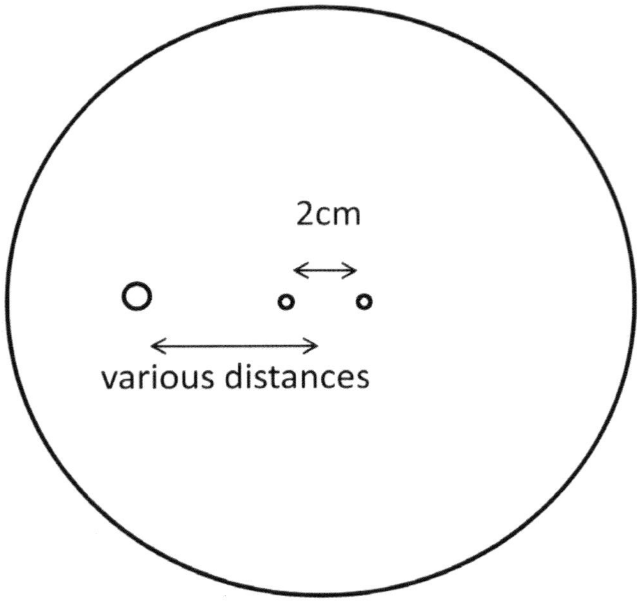

Figure 6. Schematic of the positioning of the cooling probe and electrodes in the different variations of Case 2.

both of the probes. The mesh was refined until the solution was no longer affected. Approximately 5100 elements were utilized to cover a 314 cm^2 surface area.

Results and Discussion

Case 1: Resistance in Series

The first case investigated was a 2D model with the boundary conditions previously specified. The purpose of this model was to illustrate the temperature induced effects on electric field due to a probe simultaneously delivering PEF and cold temperatures.

Cooling. The temperature distribution after the cooling and PEF procedure is illustrated in Figure 3a. The temperature distribution, as expected, increases from the low temperatures at the cold probe surface to body temperature at the outer boundary. The corresponding electric field is demonstrated in Figure 3b. It is clear from these two graphs that the electric field and temperature distribution are inversely proportional. This relationship is a result of the temperature dependence of electrical conductivity, demonstrated by Equation 2. As a result, the highest electric fields occur in the regions of lowest temperature. It can be seen clearly that the electric field is confined within the low temperature region, and reaches zero nearly everywhere else.

Control. It is pertinent that the electric field produced during cooling be compared to a control study. The control study applied the same electrical boundary conditions as the cooling case to tissue held at body temperature. Figure 4 plots the electric field in the control and cooling case on the same axes for comparison purposes. It is evident from this graph that the electric field in the cooled regions is substantially higher than the field produced in the control study in the same region. The peak electric field in the cooling case is, in fact, three times larger than the control case. However, at a distance from the cooled region, in the location of normal body temperatures, the fields for the cooled case are lower than those in the control. This indicates that cold temperatures are capable of both magnifying the electric field and confining it to the cold regions.

The effects of cooling found in Figures 2 and 3 are caused by the change in the electrical properties of tissue due to temperature. Lower temperatures yield a lower ionic conductivity. The electric field distribution (Figure 4), demonstrates the inversely proportional relationship between temperature and electrical conductivity, as described by Equation 2. For the same voltage boundary conditions, from continuity of ionic current, the electric field will be higher in the regions of lower electrical conductivity. Because of the increased electrical resistance in the regions of colder tissue, in a situation in which the cold region acts as a resistor in series with the area of tissue that is not affected by cooling, the highest electric fields are confined to the cold regions. The fields beyond the cooled regions, in tissue at normal temperature, are substantially lower than those in the cooled regions.

This effect is seen best in a supplemental analysis, shown in Figure 5. It consists of a simple one-dimensional Cartesian study of a 6 cm slab of tissue between two parallel plates. The leftmost plate applies a voltage of 2500 V and the rightmost plate applies ground. Figure 5 compares the electric field at constant temperature with the case in which cooling at 0°C is applied on the leftmost plate and body temperature, 37°C, is applied to the rightmost plate for 90 seconds. The effect of temperature induced tissue property heterogeneities is evident. At a constant temperature, the electric field is constant across the slab. For the case of cooling at one plate, the field is substantially higher near the cold surface and it decays to low values away from the cold surface. The difference between the electric field in cold regions and the electric field at body temperature is an order of magnitude. These results, as well as those demonstrated in Figures 2 and 3, suggest that inducing heterogeneity in tissue electrical properties through local cooling, with an analogue circuit of two resistors in series, has the effect of confining and enhancing the electric fields in the colder regions and reducing the field in the higher temperature regions.

The results from Case 1 suggest that it should be possible to design PEF protocols in which the PEF induced effects on cells are confined to the cooled regions of tissue and do not extend beyond the cooled regions. Furthermore, cooling the PEF electrode will yield higher electric fields in the vicinity of the probe. The complementary effect of this observation is that the electric fields beyond the cooled area will be substantially reduced. Several recent studies have shown that stray electric fields beyond the PEF treated areas could have negative effects on other organs, such as the heart [29], or create undesirable muscle contractions. Reducing the electric fields beyond the treated area with cold should also reduce these effects. In addition, it is well established that the electric currents in PEF treatment of tissues are very high, on the order of tens of Amperes. The increased resistance caused by the cooled PEF probes, in a configuration such as the one discussed here, will substantially reduce the currents for the same applied voltage, while, on the other hand increasing the field in the cooled volume.

Note, however, that the effects discussed here, for Case 1, are restricted to situations in which the effect of cooling is that of a resistance in series. The second half of the study will address a situation in which the cooled area is not produced by the PEF probes but rather by a different cooling probe. In that case the effect is that of adding a high resistance in parallel.

Resistance in Parallel

The configuration examined in the second half of this study is illustrated schematically in Figure 6. In Case 2, the effect of cooling delivered by a probe that is not electrically active on a typical irreversible electroporation protocol is investigated. The PEFs were delivered by two electrodes of 1 mm diameter, separated by 2 cm. The 3.4 mm diameter cold probe was placed

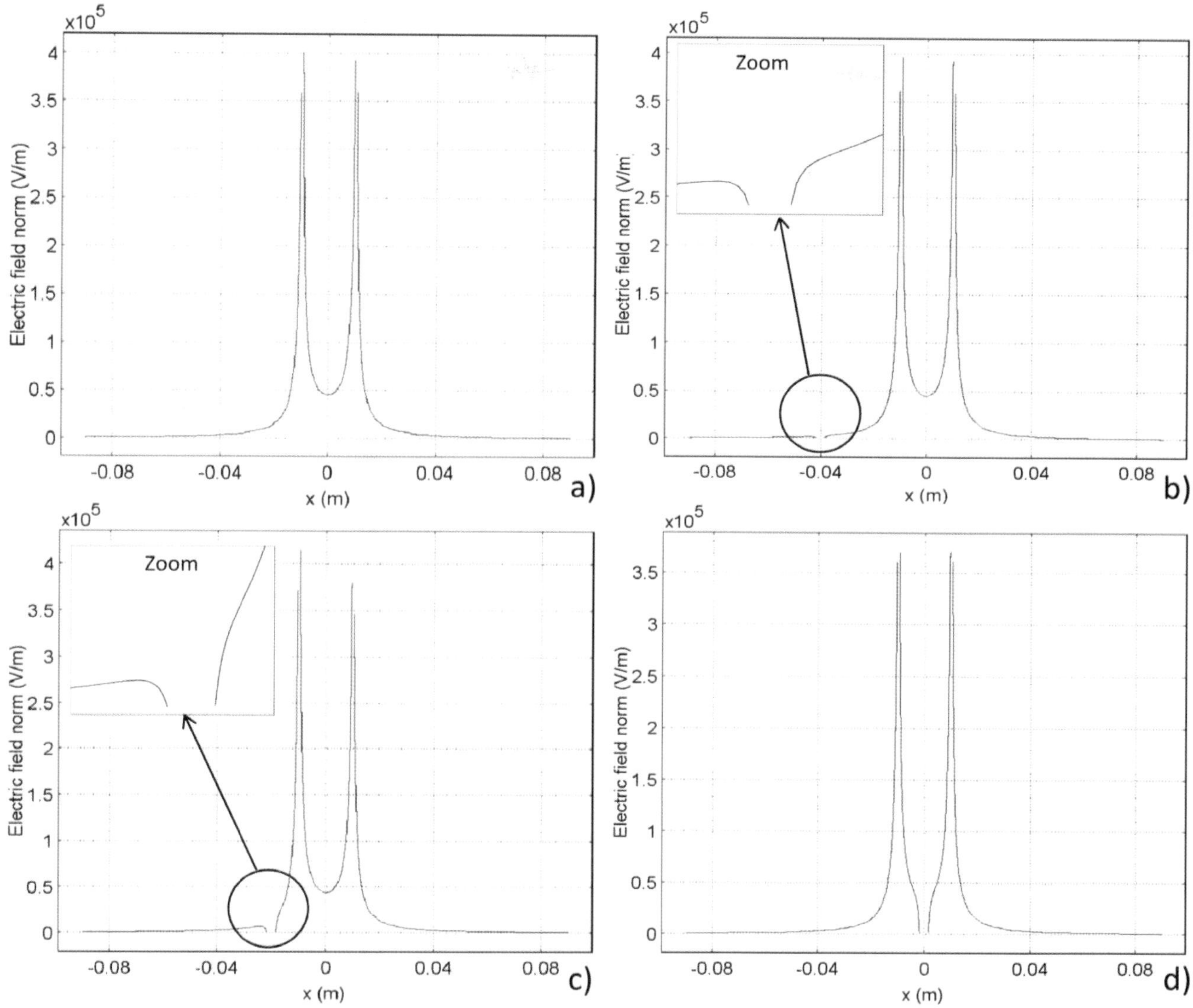

Figure 7. The electric field distributions along a transection at the diameter of the sample for Case 2. a) Control, b) cold probe 4 cm from center, c) cold probe 2 cm from center, and d) cold probe 0 cm from center. These images indicate that in this configuration, resistance in parallel, cooling can be used to protect particular regions in the domain from electric fields. By comparing Figure 7 b, c and d to Figure 7a, it is clear that the cooling temperatures applied lower the electric field in the region of low temperature in this geometry.

at various locations from the center along the axial line connecting the centers of the PEF electrodes. The protocol consisted of 2000 seconds of cooling applied by the cold probe at 0°C, followed by ten, 2500 V pulses (1 Hz, 50 μs length) applied by the PEF electrodes. The cooling probe was electrically insulated. In the control case, ten 2500 V pulses (1 Hz, 50 μs length) applied by the PEF electrodes without using the cooling probe. Full bioheat parameters were utilized to simulate tissue.

Figure 7 illustrates the electric field along a transection through the center of the electrodes and cooling probe for various locations of the cooling probe. Figure 7a shows the control case and Figure 7b shows the cooling case at 4 cm from the center of the domain. It is clear that in the configuration described here the increased electrical resistance due to the cold region acts as a current path of high electrical resistance in parallel to the higher temperature path of lower resistance. This configuration, in contrast to the trends identified in Case 1, results in a substantial decrease in the electric field in the cooled region. In fact, the electric field reaches 0 V/m in the location of the cold probe.

Figure 8 illustrates a potential application of this observation. Equation 5 has been utilized to calculate the regions of tissue that undergo irreversible electroporation. The results are presented as surface plots in Figure 8. Figure 8 demonstrates that a cooling probe can avoid irreversible electroporation damage at a particular location. Figure 8b demonstrates that this can be accomplished outside of the treatment region when the cooling probe is placed at a distance from the electrodes. Figure 8c demonstrates that a cold probe can protect a region between the two electrodes as well.

These results illustrate a potential important application of the use of cooling in PEFs. When comparing Figure 8a and 7b, it is seen that in 7b the temperature induced changes in electrical potential due to the cold probe cause the irreversible electroporation field near the probe to recede (the edge flattens). This suggests that if a sensitive tissue structure is close to the outer edge of the PEF fields of

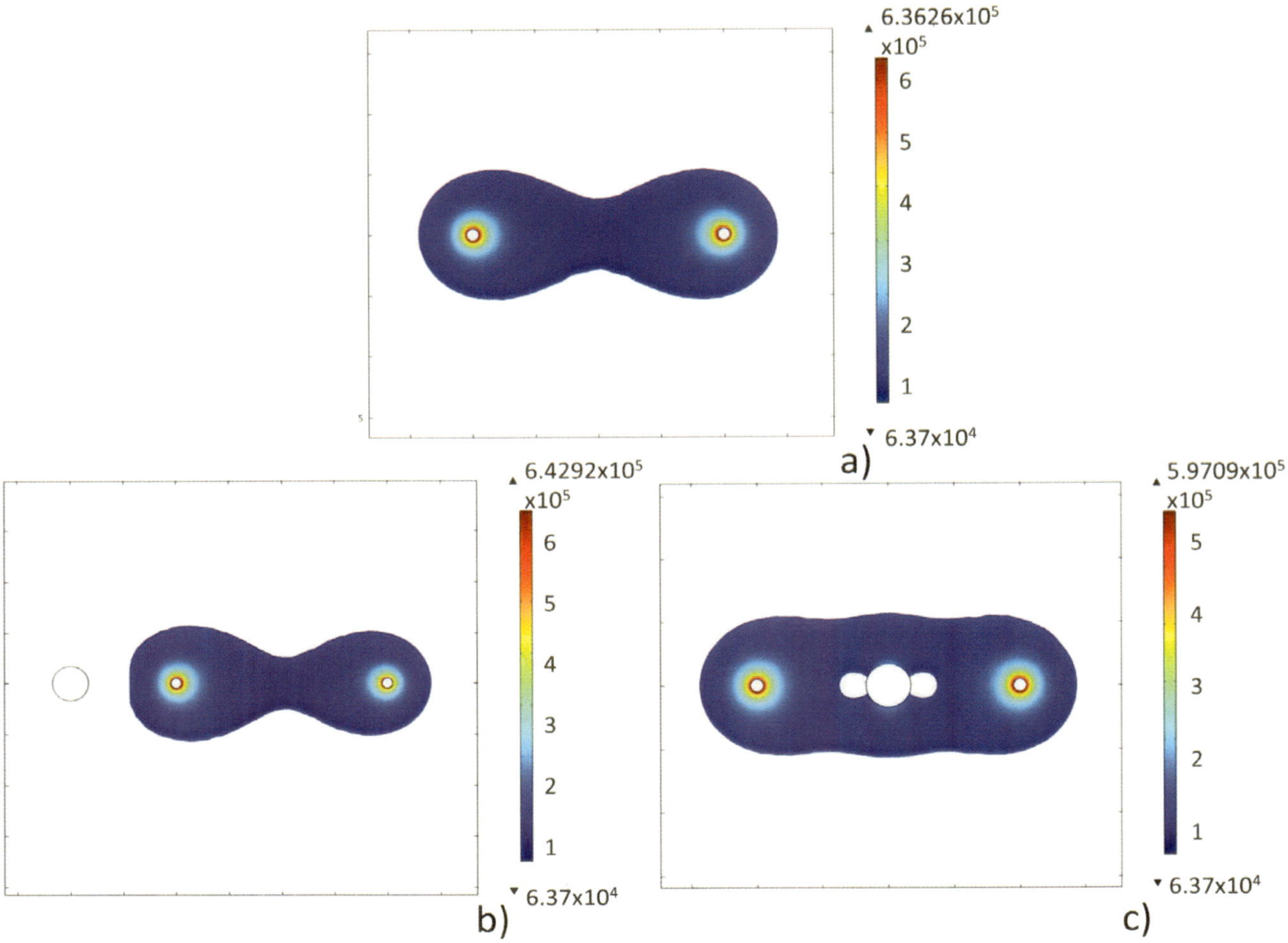

Figure 8. Area of tissue that undergoes irreversible electroporation for Case 2. a) Control case without any cooling applied, b) cooling probe located 2 cm from the center, c) cooling probe located at the center of the tissue.

treatment, the simple application of cold can protect this structure. Figure 8c shows that the use of cold can eliminate PEFs even in the center of the treated area. This suggests that critical tissues, which need protection during a PEF protocol, can be protected by cold. One clinically relevant example is the bladder sphincter, which is particularly vulnerable during the IRE treatment of the prostate. Cooling the sphincter, and thereby increasing its electrical resistance, could protect it from damage during minimally invasive treatment of the prostate with IRE. By increasing the local electrical resistance through the placement of cooling instruments, electric fields can be modulated to obtain desired effects.

Conclusions

The goal of this study was to evaluate the feasibility and the characteristics of a minimally invasive surgical procedure in which changes in electric properties due to local changes in temperature were used to modulate electric fields during PEF procedures. The hope was that control over the outcome of the procedure will improve as a result. This investigation examined two different possible configurations. The first configuration, Case 1, utilizes the PEF electrode also as a cooling probe, with the resulting electrical effect of a resistance in series. In this configuration, the electric fields are confined to the cold region and magnified in that region while the fields at a distance are reduced. The second configuration, Case 2, applies cold with an element that is not electrically active, with the resulting electrical effect of resistances in parallel. In Case 2, the electric field in the cold region is reduced.

Perhaps the most important conclusion from this study is that temperatures can be used to modulate and control electric fields. Through proper placement of cold, various desirable and controlled PEF protocols can be accomplished that could not have been achieved otherwise. It is clear that a variety of configurations of cold and heat could be used to achieve various PEF goals.

Although this is a first order theoretical analysis and additional theoretical and experimental research is needed to further develop this new concept, these primary results act as a promising foundation for future work. For these reasons, this numerical study has indicated the undeveloped potential and the motivation for pursuing the use of temperature to modulate and control PEF.

Acknowledgments

Special thanks to Mary Phillips, Peter Minor, Douglas Daniels and Claudia Vilardy for their support.

Author Contributions

Conceived and designed the experiments: CD. Performed the experiments: CD. Analyzed the data: CD. Contributed reagents/materials/analysis tools: CD BR. Wrote the paper: CD BR.

References

1. Fuch KH (2002) Minimally Invasive Surgery, Endoscopy 34: 154–159.
2. Neumann E, Schaefer-Ridder M, Wang Y, Hofschneider PH (1982) Gene transfer into mouse lyoma cells by electroporation in high electric fields, EMBO 7: 841–845.
3. Jaroszeski MJ, Gilbert R, Nicolau C, Heller R (1999) In vivo gene delivery by electroporation, Advanced Drug Delivery Reviews 35: 131–137.
4. Somiari S, Glasspool-Malone J, Drabick JJ, Gilbert RA, Heller R, et al. (2000) Theory and in vivo application of electroporative gene delivery, Molecular Therapy 3: 178–87.
5. Okino M, Mohri H (1987) Effects of a high-voltage electrical impulse and an anticancer drug on in vivo growing tumors, Jpn J Cancer Re vol. 78, 12: 1319–21.
6. Mir LM, Orlowski S, Belehradek J, Paoletti C (1991) Electrochemotherapy potentiation of antitumour effect of bleomycin by local electric pulses, European Jounal of Cancer 27: 68–72.
7. Mir LM, Glass LF, Sersa G, Teissie J, Domenge C, et al. (1998) Effective treatment of cutaneous and subcutaneous malignant tumours by electrochemotherapy, British Journal of Cancer vol. 77, 12: 2336–42.
8. Joshi RP, Schoenbach KH (2002) Mechanism for membrane electroporation irreversibility under high-intensity, ultrashort electrical pulse conditions, Physical Review E 66.
9. Vernier PT, Sun Y, Chen MT, Gundersen MA, Craviso GL (2008) Nanosecond electric pulse-induced calcium entry into chromaffin cells, Bioelectrochemistry 73: 1–4.
10. Sale AJ, Hamilton WA (1968) Effects of high electric fields on micro-organisms. 3. Lysis of erythrocytes and protoplasts, Biochim Biophys Acta 163: 37–43.
11. Hamilton WA, Sale AJ (1967) Effects of high electric fields on microorganisms: II. Mechanism of action of the lethal effect, Biochim Biophys Acta 148: 789–800.
12. Edd JF, Horowitz L, Davalos RV, Mir LM, Rubinsky B (2006) In vivo results of a new focal tissue ablation technique: irreversible electroporation, IEEE Transactions of Biomedical Engineering 53: 1409–15.
13. Rubinsky B, Onik G, Mikus P (2007) Irreversible electroporation: a new ablation modality - clinical implications, Technology in Cancer Research and Treatment 6: 37–46.
14. Daniels C, Rubinsky B (2009) Electrical field and temperature model of nonthermal irreversible electroporation in heterogeneous tissues, Journal of Biomechanical Engineering 131: 071006-12.
15. Edd JF, Davalos RV (2007) Mathematical Modeling of Irreversible Electroporation for Treatment Planning, Technology in Cancer Research and Treatment 6.
16. Edd JF, Horowitz L, Rubinsky B (2005) Temperature dependence of tissue electrical properties in electrical impedance tomography of cryosurgery, IEEE Transactions of Biomedical Engineering 52.
17. Diaz-Rivera R (2000) Micro and Nano Scale Bioelectronics in Cell Micro-Electroporation, Doctoral Dissertation, UC Berkeley.
18. Diaz-Rivera R, Rubinsky B (2006) Electrical and thermal characterization of nanochannels between a cell and a silicon based micro-pore, Biomedical Microdevices 8: 25–34.
19. Gallo SA, Sen A, Hensen M, Hui SW (2002) Temperature-dependent electrical and ultrastructural characterizations of porcine skin upon electroporation, Biophysics Journal 82: 109–119.
20. Kanduser M, Miklavcic D (2009) Electroporation in biological cell and tissue: an overview, Food Engineering Series. pp 1–37.
21. Arps JJ (1953) The Effect of Temperature on the Density and Electrical Resistivity of Sodium Chloride Solutions, Petroleum Transactions 198: 327–330.
22. Mazzoleni AP, Sisken BF, Kahler RL (1986) Conductivity values of tissue culture medium from 20°C to 40°C, Bioelectromagnetics 7: 95–99.
23. Kaatze U (1989) Complex permittivity of water as a function of frequency and temperature, J Chem Eng Data 34.
24. Granot Y, Rubinsky B (2007) Methods of optimization of electrical impedance tomography, Physiol Meas 28.
25. Ivorra A, Rubinsky B (2007) In vivo electrical impedance measurements during and after electroporation of rat liver, Bioelectrochemistry 70.
26. Davalos RV, Rubinsky B, Mir LM (2003) Theoretical analysis of the thermal effects during in vivo tissue electroporation, Bioelectrochemistry 61: 99–107.
27. Miklavcic D, Semrov D, Mekid H, Mir LM (2000) A validated model of in vivo electric field distribution in tissues for electrochemotherapy and for DNA electrotransfer for gene therapy, Biochim Biophys Acta 1523: 73–83.
28. Edd JF, Ivorra A, Horowitz L, Rubinsky B (2008) Imaging cryosurgery with EIT: tracking the ice front and post-thaw tissue viability, Physiological Measurement 29.
29. Deodhar A, Dickfeld T, Single GW, Hamilton WC, Jr., Thornton RH, et al. (2011) Irreversible Electroporation Near the Heart: Ventricular Arrhythmias Can Be Prevented With ECG Synchronization, American journal of roentgenology 196.

5

Surgeons' Exposure to Radiation in Single- and Multi-Level Minimally Invasive Transforaminal Lumbar Interbody Fusion

Haruki Funao[1,5], Ken Ishii[2,5]*, Suketaka Momoshima[3], Akio Iwanami[2,5], Naobumi Hosogane[2,5], Kota Watanabe[4,5], Masaya Nakamura[2], Yoshiaki Toyama[2], Morio Matsumoto[2]

1 Department of Orthopaedic Surgery, Nerima General Hospital, Tokyo, Japan, **2** Department of Orthopaedic Surgery, School of Medicine, Keio University, Tokyo, Japan, **3** Department of Radiology, School of Medicine, Keio University, Tokyo, Japan, **4** Advanced Therapy for Spine and Spinal Cord Disorders, Keio University, Tokyo, Japan, **5** Society for Minimally invasive spine Stabilization (Clinical research group)

Abstract

Although minimally invasive transforaminal lumbar interbody fusion (MIS-TLIF) has widely been developed in patients with lumbar diseases, surgeons risk exposure to fluoroscopic radiation. However, to date, there is no studies quantifying the effective dose during MIS-TLIF procedure, and the radiation dose distribution is still unclear. In this study, the surgeons' radiation doses at 5 places on the bodies were measured and the effective doses were assessed during 31 consecutive 1- to 3-level MIS-TLIF surgeries. The operating surgeon, assisting surgeon, and radiological technologist wore thermoluminescent dosimeter on the unshielded thyroid, chest, genitals, right middle finger, and on the chest beneath a lead apron. The doses at the lens and the effective doses were also calculated. Mean fluoroscopy times were 38.7, 53.1, and 58.5 seconds for 1, 2, or 3 fusion levels, respectively. The operating surgeon's mean exposures at the lens, thyroid, chest, genitals, finger, and the chest beneath the shield, respectively, were 0.07, 0.07, 0.09, 0.14, 0.32, and 0.05 mSv in 1-level MIS-TLIF; 0.07, 0.08, 0.09, 0.18, 0.34, and 0.05 mSv in 2-level; 0.08, 0.09, 0.14, 0.15, 0.36, and 0.06 mSv in 3-level; and 0.07, 0.08, 0.10, 0.15, 0.33, and 0.05 mSv in all cases. Mean dose at the operating surgeon's right finger was significantly higher than other measurements parts ($P<0.001$). The operating surgeon's effective doses (0.06, 0.06, and 0.07 mSv for 1, 2, and 3 fusion levels) were low, and didn't differ significantly from those of the assisting surgeon or radiological technologist. Revision MIS-TLIF was not associated with higher surgeons' radiation doses compared to primary MIS-TLIF. There were significantly higher surgeons' radiation doses in over-weight than in normal-weight patients. The surgeons' radiation exposure during MIS-TLIF was within the safe level by the International Commission on Radiological Protection's guidelines. The accumulated radiation exposure, especially to surgeon's hands, should be carefully monitored.

Editor: Michael Fehlings, University of Toronto, Canada

Funding: These authors have no support or funding to report.

Competing Interests: The authors have declared that no competing interests exist.

* E-mail: keni8888@z7.keio.jp

Introduction

Open posterior lumbar interbody fusion (PLIF) [1] and transforaminal lumbar interbody fusion (TLIF) [2] have been widely developed in posterior spinal reconstruction surgery and demonstrated significant benefits to patients with various lumbar degenerative diseases. However, one of the drawbacks of both conventional open PLIF and TLIF procedures is the extensive soft tissue dissection and retraction of paraspinal muscles during the surgical approach, because the anatomic landmarks for pedicle screw insertion should be exposed [3,4]. Minimally invasive lumbar spinal fusion using percutaneous pedicle screws was firstly described by Foley *et al* [5]. Khoo *et al* [6] also developed a minimally invasive technique in which PLIF is performed through a tubular retractor by combining a microendoscopic technique with percutaneous instrumentation. Recently, minimally invasive TLIF (MIS-TLIF), which reduces soft tissue dissections through a muscle-dilating approach, has widely developed and shown its advantages in the treatment of degenerative lumbar disease; it reduces blood loss, narcotic use, length of hospital stay, lost work time, and infection rates, and improves postoperative outcomes and cost-effectiveness [7–12]. MIS-TLIF has also shown its feasibility in revision settings [13,14]. Selznick *et al.* reported revision MIS-TLIF was not associated with a higher rate of blood loss, infection or neurologic complication compared to primary MIS-TLIF.

Although MIS-TLIF is advantageous for patients with lumbar degenerative diseases, minimally invasive procedures performed under fluoroscopy have the disadvantage of exposing the surgical team to intraoperative radiation. Radiation doses accumulated by surgeons during MIS-TLIF should be precisely monitored and evaluated, to make sure the level of risk is appropriate. However, only a few studies have prospectively evaluated radiation exposure at multiple points during MIS-TLIF, therefore, the radiation dose distribution of the whole body was still unclear. Furthermore, there have been no studies quantifying the effective dose [15], which represents the radiation dose to the whole body that gives the same risk as the localized exposure, during MIS-TLIF

Table 1. A summary of cases in 1- to 3-level MIS-TLIF.

Case No.	Age	Sex	BMI (kg/m^2)	Level	Disease	Surgical time (min)	Exposure time (min)
1	58	F	31.2	L4-5	DS	184	1.3
2	69	M	23.9	L4-5	MOB (LFC)	218	0.7
3	33	M	24.8	L5-S1	LDH	226	0.5
4	66	M	27	L5-S1	MOB (LDH)	176	0.8
5	75	F	21.8	L5-S1	MOB (ASD)	206	1.2
6	23	M	22.9	L4-5	LDH	153	0.5
7	75	F	22.5	L4-5	DS	190	0.9
8	63	F	23.1	L4-5	DS	240	0.9
9	27	M	21.8	L4-5	LDH	168	0.4
10	53	F	25.2	L4-5	LFC	155	0.3
11	69	F	24.2	L4-5	DS	169	0.4
12	37	M	24.8	L4-5	MOB (LDH)	135	0.4
13	61	F	25.1	L4-5	DS	160	0.5
14	74	F	24.9	L5-S1	DS	168	0.8
15	49	M	22.3	L4-5	LDH	148	0.4
16	33	M	24.9	L4-5	MOB (LDH)	144	0.4
17	62	F	21.1	L2-3	MOB (LDH)	114	0.5
18	56	M	24.5	L3-4	DS	121	0.4
19	73	M	24.6	L4-5	DS	120	0.5
20	58	F	20.3	L4-5	DS	242	1
21	63	M	24.9	L4-5-S1	LDH	249	1.2
22	64	F	20.5	L3-4-5	DS	343	1.6
23	51	F	30.5	L3-4-5	DS	259	0.7
24	61	M	31.6	L3-4-5	LDH	228	0.5
25	76	M	23.9	L3-4-5	MOB (LCS)	272	0.6
26	75	M	25.3	L4-5-S1	MOB (LCS)	271	0.7
27	74	F	26.1	L3-4-5	DS	236	0.9
28	69	F	27	L3-4-5-S1	DLS	411	0.9
29	76	M	22.8	L3-4-5-S1	DLS	263	0.9
30	63	M	23.7	L2-3-4-5	DLS	278	0.8
31	65	F	26.1	L3-4-5-S1	MOB (DLS)	290	1.3

(BMI; body mass index, DS; degenerative spondylolisthesis, LDH; lumbar disc herniation, DLS; degenerative lumbar scoliosis, LFC; lumbar facet cyst, ASD; adjacent segment disease, MOB; multiply-operated back).

procedure. The purpose of the present study was to quantify the radiation doses received by surgeons during single- and multi-level MIS-TLIF procedures. To the best of our knowledge, this is the largest prospective study investigating surgeons' intraoperative radiation exposure during 1- to 3-level MIS-TLIF.

Materials and Methods

This study was approved by the institutional review boards of the participating institutions prior to beginning the study (Keio University, Nerima General Hospital, Tokyo, JAPAN). All patients gave the written informed consent before being included this study. Our study was conducted during 1- to 3-level MIS-TLIF surgeries for 31 consecutive patients, with a total of 46 levels of lumbar spinal fusion. The patients included 16 males and 15 females, with a mean age of 59.7±2.7 years (range 23–76). The mean body mass index (BMI) was 24.6±0.5 kg/m^2 (range 20.3–31.6). MIS-TLIF was performed at 1 level in 20 patients (L2–3, 1; L3–4, 1; L4–5, 14; and L5–S1, 4), at 2 levels in 7 (L3–4–5, 5; L4–5–S1, 2), and at 3 levels in in 4 (L2–3–4–5, 1; L3–4–5–S1, 3). MIS-TLIF was performed on 12 patients with degenerative spondylolisthesis (DS), 6 with lumbar disc herniation (LDH) with Modic changes, 3 with degenerative lumbar scoliosis (DLS), 1 with lumbar facet cyst (LFC), and 9 with multiply-operated back (MOB) (Table 1). Operative indications for LDH with Modic change were severe low back pain which had poor responses to non-surgical treatments for more than 6 months, either Modic type 1 or type 2 change on magnetic resonance imaging, and temporal relief from a low back pain by an intradiscal anesthetic injection and/or a selective nerve root block at the affected level.

All procedures were performed by a single operating surgeon (K.I) and a single assisting surgeon (H.F.). A single C-arm radiographic imaging unit (BV25 Gold6; Philips, Eindhoven, the Netherlands) equipped with 6-inch image intensifier system was used for fluoroscopic imaging. The operating surgeon stood beside the X-ray tube, and the assisting surgeon and radiological

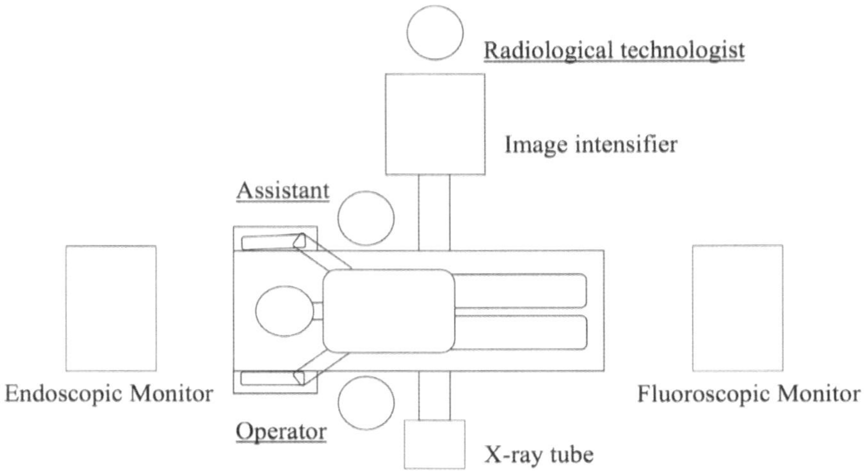

Figure 1. Intraoperative setup of the surgical team and equipment. A single C-arm was used for fluoroscopic imaging. The operating surgeon stood next to the X-ray tube. The assisting surgeon and radiological technologist were stationed at the opposite site, along with the image intensifier.

technologist stood on the opposite site (Figure 1). We wore a lead apron (Hagoromo 0.25 mm Pb; Maeda Co., Japan) that covers the entire torso, and a thyroid collar to protect all of the organs except head. The operating and assisting surgeons and the radiological technologist wore thermoluminescent dosimeter (TLD) badges (Sangyo Kagakų, Co., Japan) at unshielded points—the thyroid, chest, and genitals—and on the chest under a lead apron (Figure 2A). The operating and assisting surgeons wore sterile TLD ring badges on their right hands (middle finger) (Figure 2B). Measurement range of the TLD badges was 0.01 to 10000 mSv. Radiation doses (mSv) were measured from the TLD badges for each MIS-TLIF procedure. The dose at the lens of the eye was calculated as the thyroid dose ×0.905 (conversion factor; 1-cm depth to 0.07-cm depth, 70 keV). The effective dose, defined by the International Commission on Radiation Units and Measurements Inc. (ICRU) [15], was calculated as follows: $E = 0.11\ Ha + 0.89\ Hb$, where Ha was the dose measured at the thyroid (1-cm depth), and Hb was the dose measured on the chest under the apron (1-cm depth). We also recorded the fluoroscopic exposure times and the outputs in kVp and mA.

Fluoroscopy was typically involved at 5 steps during MIS-TLIF: preoperative skin marking (Figure 3A), confirmation of the retractor position (Figure 3B), placement of the cage (Figure 3C and D), insertion of the percutaneous pedicle screws (Figure 3E–I), and placement of the rods (Figure 3J–L). We used one-shot imaging, which provides short exposure times rather than continuous exposure. During the insertion of the percutaneous pedicle screws, we held the Jamshidi needle with a long Kocher clamp to distance the hands from the X-ray tube (Figure 4).

One-way ANOVA followed by Fisher's PLSD post-hoc test were used for statistical comparison in surgical time, estimated blood loss (EBL), and fluoroscopic exposure time between 1-, 2-, and 3-level MIS-TLIF, and in radiation doses between the operating surgeon, assisting surgeon, and radiological technologist. Student t test were used to compare surgical time, EBL, fluoroscopic exposure time, and radiation doses between primary and revision surgery, and between normal- and over-weight patients. SPSS software (14.0 J, SPSS Japan Inc., Tokyo, Japan) was used for analyses, and a P value less than 0.05 was considered significant. All data were expressed as the mean ± standard error.

A

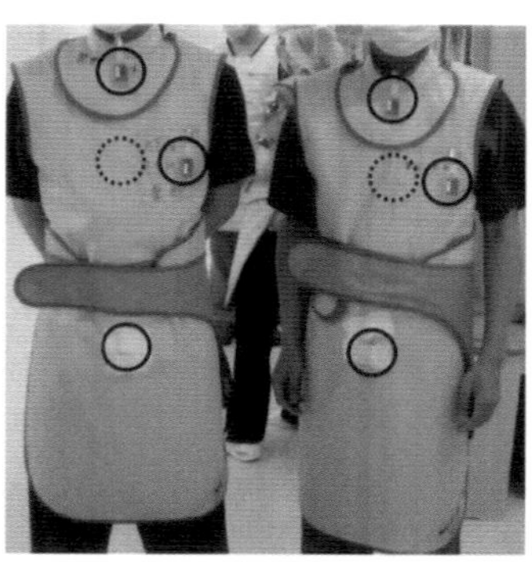

B

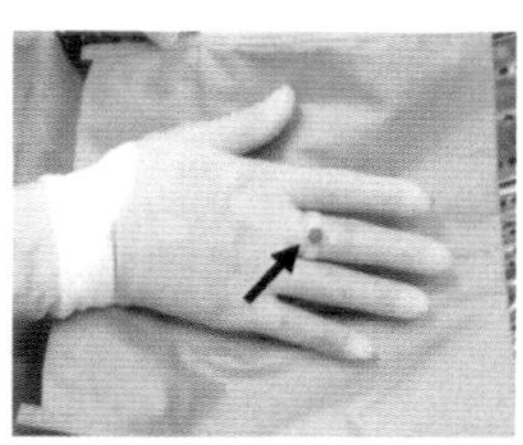

Figure 2. Placement of radiation monitors. The operating and assisting surgeon and radiological technologist wore thermoluminescent dosimeter (TLD) badges at the thyroid, chest, genitals (unshielded; circles in A), and on the chest (shielded; dotted circles in A). The operating and assisting surgeon wore sterile TLD ring badges on their right middle fingers (B).

Results

The mean fluoroscopic exposure times during 1-, 2-, or 3-level MIS-TLIF, respectively, were 38.7±17.1, 53.1±23.3, and 58.5±13.3 seconds. The fluoroscopic exposure time tended to be longer in 2-level than in 1-level MIS-TLIF ($P = 0.092$). The mean fluoroscopic exposure time was significantly longer in 3-level than in 1-level MIS-TLIF ($P = 0.041$). The tube voltage and current were automatically controlled with average readings 99.9±1.1 kVp and 3.3±0.2 mA, respectively. Table 2 shows the mean radiation and effective doses for the operating surgeon, assisting surgeon, and radiological technologist (P values were shown in Figure 5). For all cases, the mean radiation dose at the right middle finger was 0.33±0.06 mSv for the operating surgeon and 0.15±0.02 mSv for the assisting surgeon; for the operating surgeon, this dose was significantly higher than the doses measured elsewhere on the body ($P<0.001$), and significantly higher than the corresponding dose measured for the assisting surgeon ($P<0.001$).

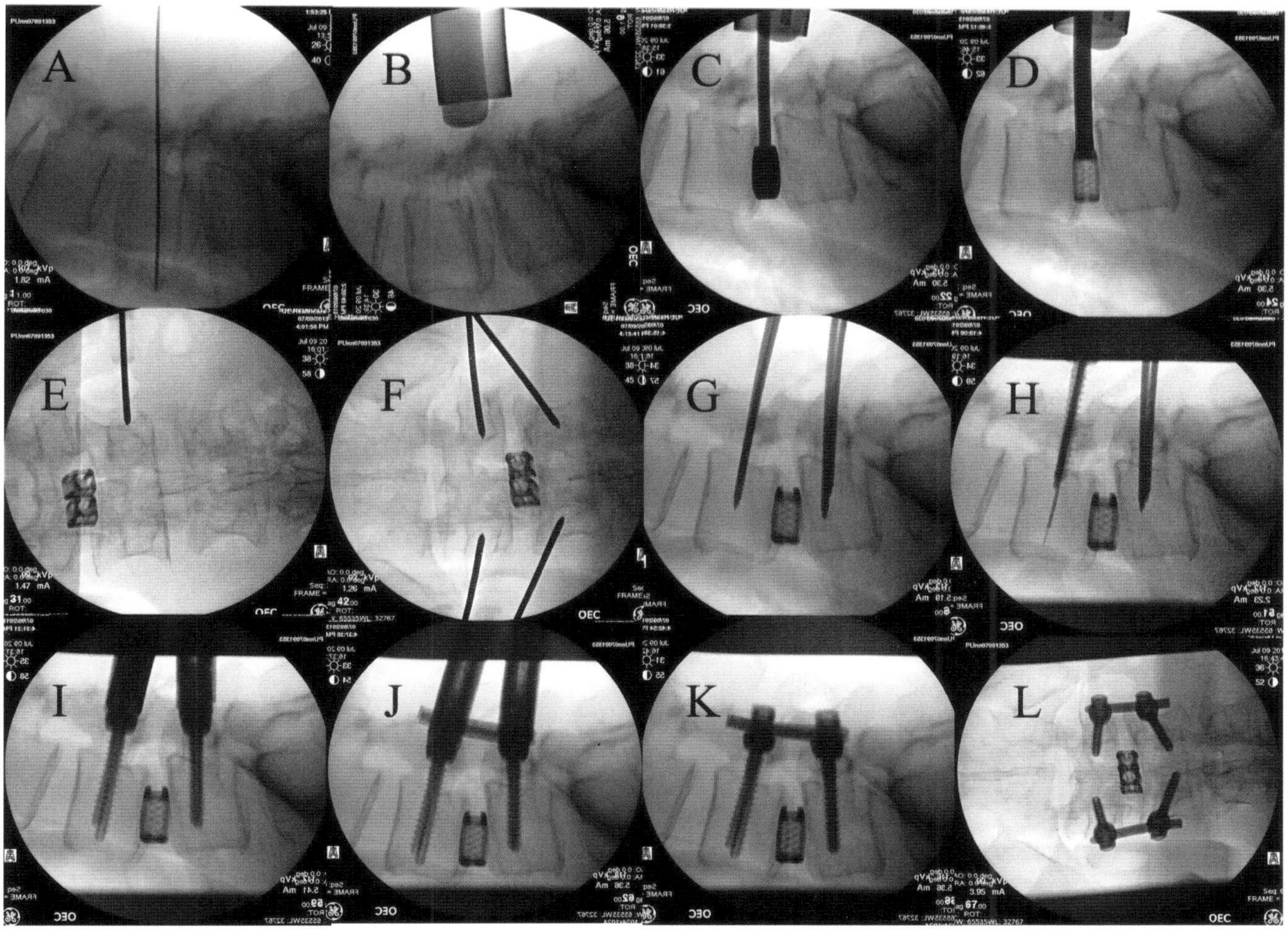

Figure 3. Utilization of fluoroscopy. Fluoroscopy was typically involved at 5 steps during MIS-TLIF: preoperative skin marking (A), confirmation of the retractor position (B), placement of the cage (C, D), insertion of the percutaneous pedicle screws (E–I), and placement of the rods (J–L). We used one-shot imaging, which uses short exposure times rather than continuous exposure.

The assisting surgeon's mean dose at the right finger was also significantly higher than doses at the lens ($P<0.001$), thyroid ($P<0.001$), chest ($P<0.001$), or genitals ($P=0.029$). Interestingly, the operating surgeon's mean radiation dose at the genitals was 0.15 ± 0.01 mSv, which was significantly higher than doses at the lens ($P<0.001$), thyroid ($P<0.001$), and chest ($P=0.012$); this dose was also significantly higher for the operating surgeon than for the assisting surgeon ($P=0.014$) The mean effective doses for the surgeon performing 1-, 2-, or 3-level MIS-TLIF (0.06 ± 0.01, 0.06 ± 0.01, and 0.07 ± 0.02 mSv) were not significantly different from those received by the assisting surgeon (0.04 ± 0.01, 0.06 ± 0.01, and 0.07 ± 0.02 mSv) or the radiological technologist (0.05 ± 0.01, 0.06 ± 0.01, 0.06 ± 0.02 mSv).

The mean surgical time was 171.9 ± 8.6 minutes in 1-level MIS-TLIF, 265.4 ± 14.4 minutes in 2-level MIS-TLIF, and 310.5 ± 34.0 minutes in 3-level MIS-TLIF. There were statistically significant differences in the mean surgical times for single and multi-level MIS-TLIF (1-level *vs.* 2- or 3-level; $P<0.001$). The mean EBL were 178.2 ± 24.1 ml in 1-level MIS-TLIF, 416.1 ± 108.2 ml in 2-level MIS-TLIF, and 360.5 ± 56.4 ml in 3-level MIS-TLIF. There were statistically significant differences in the mean estimated blood loss for single and multi-level MIS-TLIF (1-level *vs.* 2-level; $P=0.003$, 1-level *vs.* 3-level; $P=0.006$). There were no significant differences in surgical time and EBL between 2- and 3-level MIS-TLIF. No major complications were observed during the perioperative period for any patient.

Because our case series included only 2 patients in 2-level MIS-TLIF and 1 in 3-level who had a revision surgery, we compared radiation doses between primary and revision surgery in 1-level MIS-TLIF (primary; $n=14$, revision; $n=6$). There were no significant differences in surgical time (primary; 174.6 ± 10.4 *vs.* revision; 165.5 ± 16.9 minutes), EBL (primary; 191.2 ± 33.4 *vs.* revision; 147.7 ± 17.6 ml), and fluoroscopic exposure time (primary; 38.1 ± 4.6 *vs.* revision; 40.0 ± 7.5 seconds) between the two groups. There were no significant differences in radiation doses at all measurement parts between primary and revision surgery (Table 3).

Normal-weight patients ($BMI<25$, $n=16$) and over-weight patients ($BMI>25$, $n=4$) were also compared in 1-level MIS-TLIF. There were no significant differences in surgical time ($BMI<25$; 172.6 ± 10.8 *vs.* $BMI>25$; 168.8 ± 6.8 minutes), EBL ($BMI<25$; 194.3 ± 28.1 *vs.* $BMI>25$; 113.5 ± 27.8 ml), and fluoroscopic exposure time ($BMI<25$; 37.5 ± 3.8 *vs.* $BMI>25$; 43.5 ± 13.0 seconds) between the two groups. The operating surgeon's mean dose at the chest was significantly higher in over-weight patients (0.14 ± 0.03 mSv) compared to normal-weight

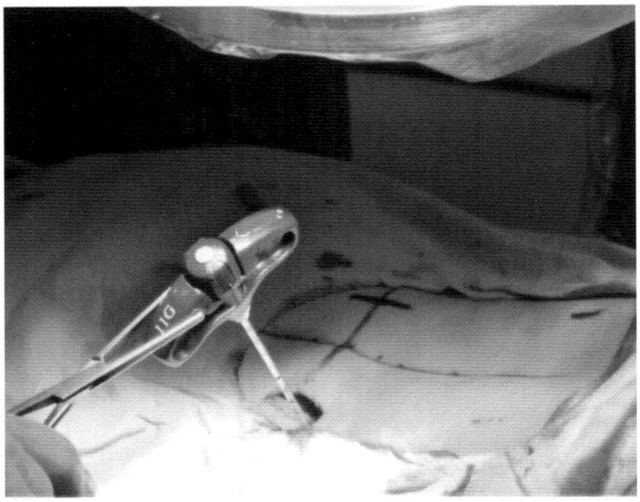

Figure 4. Protective techniques against excessive radiation exposures. Surgeons should always pay attention to the location of their hands at every fluoroscopic shots during MIS-TLIF procedures. The hands are often exposed to the X-ray beam while confirming the insertion point of the Jamshidi needle. A long Kocher clamp can be used to hold the Jamshidi needle for keeping a distance from the X-ray tube.

patients (0.08±0.01 mSv) (P = 0.002). And, the assisting surgeon's mean dose at the genitals was significantly higher in over-weight patients (0.12±0.04 mSv) compared to normal-weight patients (0.06±0.01 mSv) (P = 0.039). There were no significant differences in radiation doses at other measurement parts between the two groups (Table 4).

Discussion

While studies have addressed intraoperative radiation exposures during orthopedic surgeries, the effective doses and doses received at different parts of the body in single- and multi-level MIS-TLIF have not been studied, and the surgeon's intraoperative radiation exposure has not been clarified. In our prospective case-series study, radiation doses at 5 places on the bodies were measured and the effective doses were assessed for the operating surgeon, assisting surgeon, and radiological technologist during 31 consecutive 1- to 3-level MIS-TLIF surgeries. In previous studies reporting that surgeons are exposed to radiation during MIS-TLIF, dosimeters were not worn both inside and outside the protective apron [16–18], and the effective dose was not investigated despite its importance [19]. The surgeon's exposure cannot be accurately gauged without measuring the dose inside the apron and investigating the effective dose. Järvinen *et al* [20] emphasized the usage of two dosimeters, placed outside and underneath the apron. The ICRP also recommends that personnel with a high risk of exposure during interventional radiology use two dosimeters [21,22]; usually, one dosimeter is worn on the chest inside the apron, and the other placed on the neck, outside the apron. The effective dose [15], which is calculated from doses measured both inside and outside the apron, is useful for accurately evaluating occupational limits. However, few studies have investigated the effective dose of fluoroscopic radiation during spine surgeries [23], and there have been no studies quantifying the effective dose during MIS-TLIF procedure. Guidelines from the 1990 International Commission on Radiological Protection (ICRP) allow occupational radiation exposure to accumulate to a maximum annual radiation exposure of 150 mSv to the crystal lens, 500 mSv to the skin or hands, and 20 mSv as the effective dose [21]. In our study, the mean effective doses for the operating surgeon, the assistant, and the radiological technologist of 0.06, 0.05, and 0.05 mSv, respectively. The mean effective dose received by the operating surgeon was well within the safe level, equivalent to 0.3% of the annual occupational limit. One of the reasons for the low radiation exposure is that we typically use a one-shot rather than continuous fluoroscopy exposure technique. Indeed, Goodman *et al* [24] reported pulsed and low-dose fluoroscopy modes reduced exposure times by 56.7% in spinal interventional procedures (e.g. facet injection, lumbar sympathetic block, radiofrequency ablation). In a cadevaric study, Rampersaud *et al* [25] reported a mean dose at the neck of 8.3 mrem (0.083 mSv)/minute, and a mean hand dose of 58.2 mrem (0.582 mSv)/minute during assisted pedicle-screw insertion in spine surgery. Bindal *et al* [19] reported a mean fluoroscopy time of 1.69 minutes per case during 1- or 2-level MIS-TLIF, and a mean exposure to the surgeon per case of 76 mrem (0.76 mSv) to the surgeon's dominant hand, 27 mrem (0.27 mSv) at the waist under a lead apron, and 32 mrem (0.32 mSv) at the level of the unprotected thyroid. In our study, the surgeon's average of the doses measured at the 5 different points were much lower than those reported previously. Therefore, our one-shot fluoroscopic technique would be effective for reduction of radiation exposure.

However, the averaged doses of radiation to the right middle finger of the operating surgeon and assisting surgeon were 0.33 and 0.15 mSv, which were significantly higher than the doses measured at other unshielded areas of the bodies. Previous studies have reported a dose range from 0.08 and 0.2 mSv to the surgeon's hands during routine orthopaedic procedures [26–28]. In femoral or tibial intramedullary nailing, doses of 1.2–1.3 mGy per procedure to the hands have been reported [29]. Jones *et al* [30] reported that in lumbar spine surgery, the surgeon's hands receive a dose of 0.9 mGy per procedure for pedicle screw insertions. The ICRP and the National Radiological Protection Board demonstrated the threshold radiation doses for damage to the skin [21,22,31,32]. Ionizing radiation can cause both acute and chronic skin damage. Although transient erythema caused by acute skin radiation exposure persists for 3 to 9 weeks, repetitive fluoroscopy procedures can also lead to chronic skin damage. Chronic radiodermatitis, which can present from months to several years after irradiation, causes dermal atrophy and telangiectasia. Chronic skin injuries resulting from interventional cardiology procedures have been reported [33]. Moreover, accumulated radiation exposure to the skin is a concern because of the potential of carcinogenesis. Radiation exposure can damage DNA, with cytotoxic and carcinogenic effects [34]. Shan *et al* [35] reported a patient with multiple syringoid eccrine carcinomas in both hands after long-term occupational exposure to X-rays. Radiation exposure to the hands is a long-standing problem; the surgeon or technologist often has to be close to both the X-ray beam and the patient to carry out the procedure [36]. In the orthopedic field, surgeons must maintain the location of instruments under the X-ray beam, and face a risk of high radiation exposure. According to the literature, maintaining a 5–10 cm distance from the patient can reduce exposure by 25–45% [25]. Surgeons should always pay attention to the location of their hands at every fluoroscopic shots during MIS-TLIF procedure. During placement of the percutaneous pedicle screws, surgeons must confirm the position of the Jamshidi needle and pedicle screw under fluoroscopy. At this step, the surgeon's hands often have a

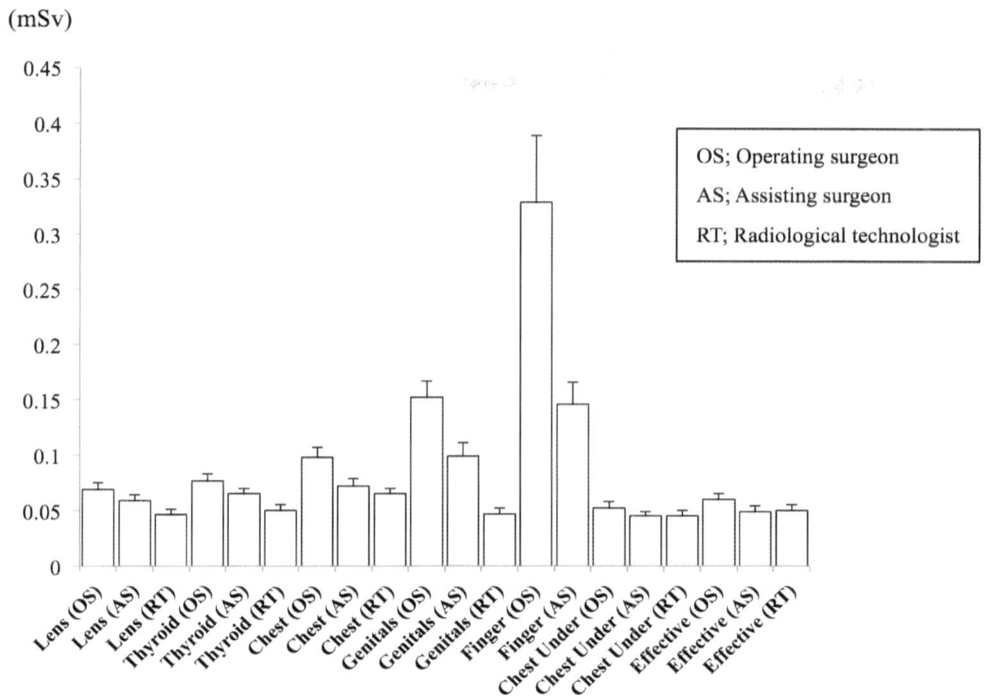

Finger (OS) vs Lens (OS) (P<0.001)
Finger (OS) vs Thyroid (OS) (P<0.001)
Finger (OS) vs Chest (OS) (P<0.001)
Finger (OS) vs Genital (OS) (P<0.001)
Finger (OS) vs Finger (AS) (P<0.001)

Finger (AS) vs Lens (AS) (P<0.001)
Finger (AS) vs Thyroid (AS) (P<0.001)
Finger (AS) vs Chest (AS) (P<0.001)
Finger (AS) vs Genital (AS) (P=0.029)

Genital (OS) vs Lens (OS) (P<0.001)
Genital (OS) vs Thyroid (OS) (P<0.001)
Genital (OS) vs Chest (OS) (P=0.012)
Genital (OS) vs Genital (AS) (P=0.014)

Figure 5. The mean radiation doses measured at different areas, and mean effective doses in all cases. The mean radiation doses and effective doses are shown for all cases. The mean radiation doses measured at the operating and assisting surgeons' right middle fingers were significantly higher than those measured elsewhere on the bodies. The mean radiation dose measured at the operating surgeon's genital area was significantly higher than at the lens, thyroid, or chest. Mean effective doses didn't differ significantly among the operating surgeon, assisting surgeon, and radiological technologist.

high risk of exposure to the X-ray beam. Therefore, we strongly recommend holding the Jamshidi needle with a long Kocher clamp during the fluoroscopic shots to distance the hands from the X-ray tube (Figure 4).

Wearing a lead apron and a thyroid collar is reported to reduce the effective dose [37,38]. Interestingly, our study showed that the mean radiation dose at the genitals was significantly higher than that measured at any other point except the surgeon's hand. We ascertain that the genital area is closer to the X-ray tube (especially in lateral shots) and to the patients, and thus that the genitals are more likely to receive both direct and scattered radiation.

Table 2. Mean surgeons' radiation doses of different measurement parts, and mean effective doses in MIS-TLIF (mSv).

	Overall (n = 31)			1-level (n = 20)			2-level (n = 7)			3-level (n = 4)		
	OS	AS	RT	OS	AS	RT	OS	AS	RT	OS	AS	RT
Crystal lens	0.07±0.01	0.06±0.01	0.05±0.01	0.07±0.01	0.05±0.01	0.04±0.01	0.07±0.01	0.07±0.01	0.05±0.01	0.08±0.02	0.07±0.02	0.06±0.01
Thyroid	0.08±0.01	0.07±0.01	0.05±0.01	0.07±0.01	0.06±0.01	0.05±0.01	0.08±0.01	0.07±0.01	0.05±0.01	0.09±0.02	0.08±0.02	0.06±0.02
Chest 1	0.10±0.01	0.07±0.01	0.07±0.01	0.09±0.01	0.06±0.01	0.06±0.01	0.09±0.02	0.09±0.02	0.07±0.02	0.14±0.04	0.09±0.01	0.07±0.01
Genitals	* 0.15±0.01	0.10±0.02	0.05±0.01	* 0.14±0.01	0.08±0.01	0.05±0.01	* 0.18±0.03	0.15±0.05	0.05±0.01	0.15±0.05	0.13±0.04	0.05±0.01
Finger	* 0.33±0.06	* 0.15±0.02		* 0.32±0.08	* 0.14±0.03		* 0.34±0.10	0.14±0.04		* 0.36±0.10	* 0.20±0.02	
Chest 2	0.05±0.01	0.05±0.01	0.05±0.01	0.05±0.01	0.04±0.01	0.04±0.01	0.05±0.01	0.05±0.01	0.05±0.01	0.06±0.02	0.06±0.02	0.05±0.01
Effective dose	0.06±0.01	0.05±0.01	0.05±0.01	0.06±0.01	0.04±0.01	0.05±0.01	0.06±0.01	0.06±0.01	0.06±0.01	0.07±0.02	0.07±0.02	0.06±0.02

(OS; operating surgeon, AS; assisting surgeon, RT; radiological technologist. Chest 1; a dose at unshielded chest, Chest 2; a dose at chest under a lead apron. *Statistically significant).

Table 3. Comparison of surgeons' radiation doses between primary and revision surgery in 1-level MIS-TLIF.

	OS			AS			RT		
	Primary (n = 14)	**Revision (n = 6)**	**P**	**Primary (n = 14)**	**Revision (n = 6)**	**P**	**Primary (n = 14)**	**Revision (n = 6)**	**P**
Crystal lens	0.07±0.01	0.07±0.01	0.972	0.05±0.01	0.06±0.01	0.952	0.05±0.01	0.04±0.01	0.843
Thyroid	0.07±0.01	0.08±0.02	0.845	0.06±0.01	0.06±0.01	0.912	0.05±0.01	0.04±0.01	0.875
Chest 1	0.09±0.01	0.09±0.02	0.924	0.06±0.01	0.07±0.02	0.912	0.06±0.01	0.07±0.01	0.758
Genitals	0.14±0.02	0.16±0.03	0.717	0.07±0.01	0.09±0.03	0.687	0.05±0.01	0.05±0.01	0.966
Finger	0.32±0.10	0.33±0.16	0.759	0.15±0.04	0.10±0.03	0.317			
Chest 2	0.05±0.01	0.06±0.02	0.759	0.04±0.01	0.04±0.01	0.960	0.04±0.01	0.05±0.02	0.889
Effective dose	0.06±0.01	0.06±0.01	0.980	0.04±0.01	0.04±0.01	0.996	0.04±0.01	0.05±0.01	0.885

(OS; operating surgeon, AS; assisting surgeon, RT; radiological technologist. Chest 1; a dose at unshielded chest, Chest 2; a dose at chest under a lead apron.).

Therefore, it is also important to wear a lead apron that covers the entire torso.

In this study, primary and revision surgery were compared in 1-level MIS-TLIF. Our study showed no significant differences in surgical time, EBL, and fluoroscopic exposure time between the two groups. Selznick *et al.* [13] reported blood loss was slightly higher in revision MIS-TLIF, however, it was not significantly high. They also found there was no significant higher rate of infection or neurologic complication between primary and revision MIS-TLIF. Our results also showed there were no significant differences in radiation doses at all measurement parts between primary and revision MIS-TLIF. Wang *et al.* [14] reported their 52 revision TLIF case series, and they found the mean fluoroscopic exposure time in revision MIS-TLIF (72 seconds) was significantly longer than that in revision open-TLIF (39 seconds). Our results showed the mean fluoroscopic exposure time in revision MIS-TLIF was 44.0 seconds. Therefore, one-shot fluoroscopic technique was considered as a key factor for reduction of fluoroscopic exposure time. In this study, most of MOB patients already had previous decompression surgery and they showed one-side lateral recess stenosis or intervertebral instability. For this reason, decompression and interbody fusion were completely performed from one-side lateral approach. Because we didn't have to remove all the scar tissues from the dura when we decompressed a nerve root and approached to the disc, it seemed not to be related to a time-consuming procedure due to previous surgeries.

We also compared normal- and over-weight patients. The operating surgeon's mean dose at the chest and the assisting surgeon's mean dose at the genitals were significantly higher, and the fluoroscopy also tended to have a longer exposure time in over-weight patients. It is sometimes difficult to get a good fluoroscopic resolution, and the tube voltage and current are automatically adjusted for signal-to-noise in over-weight patients. Kuon *et al.* [39] reported that higher BMI and larger body surface area were associated with higher radiation exposures in their invasive cardiac procedures. Ector *et al.* [40] also found that BMI was more determinant of radiation dose than a total fluoroscopic exposure time in their catheter ablation case series. Although there were no significant differences in surgical time, EBL, and fluoroscopic exposure time between normal- and over-weight patients in our study, higher scatter radiation caused by higher radiation outputs and larger body surface areas might increase the surgeons' radiation doses in over-weight patients. Ideally, surgeons should distance their bodies from the X-ray tube and the patient during a floroscopy shot.

Our study found considerably less intraoperative radiation exposure than has previously been reported [16,17,19]. Our findings suggested that careful fluoroscopy techniques, such as avoiding continuous exposure and keeping a distance from the X-ray tube, can effectively reduce radiation exposure times and doses. Our data emphasize the importance of taking basic precautions against excessive radiation exposure. Additionally,

Table 4. Comparison of surgeons' radiation doses between normal-weight (BMI<25) and over-weight patients (BMI>25) in 1-level MIS-TLIF.

	OS			AS			RT		
	BMI<25 (n = 16)	**BMI>25 (n = 4)**	**P**	**BMI<25 (n = 16)**	**BMI>25 (n = 4)**	**P**	**BMI<25 (n = 16)**	**BMI>25 (n = 4)**	**P**
Crystal lens	0.06±0.01	0.08±0.02	0.198	0.05±0.01	0.08±0.02	0.053	0.05±0.01	0.03±0.01	0.106
Thyroid	0.07±0.01	0.09±0.02	0.288	0.05±0.01	0.08±0.02	0.066	0.05±0.01	0.03±0.01	0.142
Chest 1	0.08±0.01	*0.14±0.03	0.002	0.06±0.01	0.09±0.03	0.095	0.07±0.01	0.05±0.02	0.253
Genitals	0.15±0.02	0.13±0.02	0.623	0.06±0.01	*0.12 ±0.04	0.039	0.05±0.01	0.04±0.02	0.714
Finger	0.32±0.11	0.33±0.06	0.963	0.13±0.03	0.18±0.08	0.722			
Chest 2	0.05±0.01	0.07±0.01	0.225	0.04±0.01	0.06±0.02	0.185	0.05±0.01	0.02±0.00	0.136
Effective dose	0.05±0.01	0.07±0.01	0.170	0.04±0.01	0.06±0.02	0.057	0.05±0.01	0.03±0.01	0.103

(OS; operating surgeon, AS; assisting surgeon, RT; radiological technologist. Chest 1; a dose at unshielded chest, Chest 2; a dose at chest under a lead apron. *Statistically significant).

several authors reported that protective gloves [41,42] and a navigation system [17] may also reduce radiation exposure. Our goal on the development of MIS-TLIF is to seek how to carry out procedures safely with low radiation exposure or without any radiation exposures. In this study, we demonstrated the importance of taking basic precautions during MIS-TLIF procedure. We also expect that either new lower-radiation alternative or protective equipment would be developed for MIS-TLIF near future.

Conclusions

The present study demonstrated that radiation doses to surgeons during single- and multi-level MIS-TLIF were well within the level of safe occupational exposure risk outlined by ICRP 1990. Appropriate fluoroscopy techniques, such as avoiding continuous fluoroscopy and keeping an adequate distance from the X-ray tube, can effectively reduce excessive radiation exposure. Revision MIS-TLIF was not associated with higher surgeons' radiation doses compared to primary MIS-TLIF. Surgeons' radiation doses were higher in over-weight patients than in normal-weight patient during MIS-TLIF procedure. The accumulated radiation exposure, especially to the surgeon's hands, should be carefully monitored.

Acknowledgments

The authors appreciate the radiological advice and cooperation of Munechika Otani, R.T. and Minoru Sasaki, R.T. of Nerima General Hospital, Tokyo, for their help with this study.

Author Contributions

Conceived and designed the experiments: HF KI. Performed the experiments: HF KI. Analyzed the data: HF KI. Contributed reagents/materials/analysis tools: HF KI SM AI NH KW MN YT MM. Wrote the paper: HF KI MM.

References

1. Cloward RB (1953) The treatment of ruptured intervertebral discs by vertebral body fusion. I. Indications, operative technique, after care. J Neurosurg 10(2): 154–168.
2. Harms J, Rolinger H (1982) A one-stager procedure in operative treatment of spondylolithesis: dorsal traction-reposition and anterior fusion (author's transl). Z Orthop Ihre Grenzgeb 120(3): 343–347.
3. Rosenberg WS, Mummaneni PV (2001) Transforaminal lumbar interbody fusion: technique, complications, and early results. Neurosurg 48(3): 569–574.
4. Lowe TG, Tahernia AD, O'Brien MF, Smith DA (2002) Unilateral transforaminal posterior lumbar interbody fusion (TLIF): indications, technique, and 2-year results. J Spinal Disord Tech 15(1): 31–38.
5. Foley KT, Gupta SK, Justis JR, Sherman MC (2001) Percutaneous pedicle screw fixation of the lumbar spine. Neurosurg Focus 10(4): E10.
6. Khoo LT, Palmer S, Laich DT, Fessler RG (2002) Minimally invasive percutaneous posterior lumbar interbody fusion. Neurosurg 51(5 Suppl): S166–1.
7. Schwender JD, Holly LT, Rouben DP, Foley KT (2005) Minimally invasive transforaminal lumbar interbody fusion (TLIF): technical feasibility and initial results. J Spinal Disord Tech 18 (suppl): S1–6.
8. Ozgur BM, Yoo K, Rodriguez G, Taylor WR (2005) Minimally-invasivetechnique for transforaminal lumbar interbody fusion (TLIF). Eur Spine J 14(9): 887–894.
9. Parker SL, Adogwa O, Witham TF, Aaronson OS, Cheng J, et al. (2011) Postoperative infection after minimally invasive versus open transforaminal lumbar interbody fusion (TLIF): literature review and cost analysis. Minim Invasive Neurosurg 54(1): 33–37.
10. Adogwa O, Parker SL, Bydon A, Cheng J, McGirt MJ (2011) Comparative effectiveness of minimally invasive versus open transforaminal lumbar interbody fusion: 2-year assessment of narcotic use, return to work, disability, and quality of life. J Spinal Disord Tech 24(8): 479–484.
11. Lee KH, Yue WM, Yeo W, Soeharno H, Tan SB (2012) Clinical and radiological outcomes of open versus minimally invasive transforaminal lumbar interbody fusion. Eur Spine J 21(11): 2265–2270.
12. Parker SL, Adogwa O, Bydon A, Cheng J, McGirt MJ (2012) Cost-Effectiveness of Minimally Invasive Versus Open Transforaminal Lumbar Interbody Fusion for Degenerative Spondylolisthesis Associated Low-Back and Leg pain over two years. World Neurosurg 78(1–2): 178–184.
13. Selznick LA, Shamji MF, Isaacs RE (2009) Minimally invasive interbody fusion for revision lumbar surgery: technical feasibility and safety. J Spinal Disord Tech 22(3): 207–213.
14. Wang J, Zhou Y, Zhang ZF, Li CQ, Zheng WJ, et al. (2011) Minimally invasive or open transforaminal lumbar interbody fusion as revision surgery for patients previously treated by open discectomy and decompression of the lumbar spine. Eur Spine J 20(4): 623–628.
15. International Commission on Radiation Units and Measurements (1985) Determination of Dose Equivalents Resulting from External Radiation Sources, Part 1. ICRU Report 39.
16. Mariscalco MW, Yamashita T, Steinmetz MP, Krishnaney AA, Lieberman IH, et al. (2011) Radiation exposure to the surgeon during open lumbar microdiscectomy and minimally invasive microdiscectomy: a prospective, controlled trial. Spine 36(3): 255–260.
17. Kim CW, Lee YP, Taylor W, Oygar A, Kim WK (2008) Use of navigation-assisted fluoroscopy to decrease radiation exposure during minimally invasive spine surgery. Spine J 8(4): 584–590.
18. Clark JC, Jasmer G, Marciano FF, Tumialán LM (2013) Minimally invasive transforaminal lumbar interbody fusions and fluoroscopy: a low-dose protocol to minimize ionizing radiation. Neurosurg Focus 35(2): E8.
19. Bindal RK, Glaze S, Ognoskie M, Tunner V, Malone R, et al. (2008) Surgeon and patient radiation exposure in minimally invasive transforaminal lumbar interbody fusion. J Neurosurg Spine 9(6): 570–573.
20. Järvinen H, Buls N, Clerinx P, Jansen J, Miljanic' S, et al. (2008) Overview of double dosimetry procedures for the determination of the effective dose to the interventional radiology staff. Rad Prot Dosim 129: 333–339.
21. International Commission on Radiological Protection (1991) 1990 Recommendations of the International Commission on Radiological Protection. ICRP publication 60. Ann ICRP 21(1–3): 1–201.
22. International Commission on Radiological Protection (2007) The 2007 Recommendations of the International Commission on Radiological Protection. ICRP publication 103. Ann ICRP 37(2–4): 1–332.
23. Theocharopoulos N, Perisinakis K, Damilakis J, Papadokostakis G, Hadjipavlou A, et al. (2003) Occupational exposure from common fluoroscopic projections used in orthopaedic surgery. J Bone Joint Surg Am 85A(9): 1698–1703.
24. Goodman BS, Carnel CT, Mallempati S, Agarwal P (2011) Reduction in average fluoroscopic exposure times for interventional spinal procedures through the use of pulsed and low-dose image settings. Am J Phys Med Rehabil 90(11): 908–912.
25. Rampersaud YR, Foley KT, Shen AC, Williams S, Solomito M (2000) Radiation exposure to the spine surgeon during fluoroscopically assisted pedicle screw insertion. Spine 25: 2637–2645.
26. Goldstone KE, Wright IH, Cohen B (1993) Radiation exposure to the hands of orthopaedic surgeons during procedures under fluoroscopic X-ray control. Brit J Radiol 66(790): 899–901.
27. Singer G (2005) Occupational radiation exposure to the surgeon. J Am Acad Orthop Surg 13(1): 69–76.
28. Blachut P (2008) Radiation exposure in orthopaedic trauma surgery. J Bone Joint Surg Br. (Suppl 1): 139.
29. Muller LP, Suffner J, Wenda K, Mohr W, Rommens PM (1998) Radiation exposure to the hands and the thyroid of the surgeon during intramedullary nailing. Injury 29(6): 461–468.
30. Jones DP, Robertson PA, Lunt B, Jackson SA (2000) Radiation exposure during fluoroscopically assisted pedicle screw insertion in the lumbar spine. Spine 25(12): 1538–1541.
31. Edwards AA, Lloyd DC (1996) National Radiological Protection Board. Risk from deterministic effects of ionising radiation. Documents of the NRPB 7(3). London: HMSO.
32. Little MP, Charles MW, Hopewell JW, Mayall A, Lloyd DC, et al. (1997) National Radiological Protection Board. Assessment of skin doses, Documents of the NRPB 8(3). London: HMSO.
33. Lichtenstein DA, Klapholtz L, Vardy DA, Leichter I, Mosseri M, et al. (1996) Chronic radiodermatitis following cardiac catheterisation. Arch Dermatol 32: 663–667.
34. Baskar R. (2010) Emerging role of radiation induced bystander effects: Cell communications and carcinogenesis. Genome Integr 1(1): 13.
35. Shan SJ, Chen J, Xu X, Guo Y, Wei H, et al. (2011) Multiple syringoid eccrine carcinomas with a long-term exposure to X-rays. Eur J Dermatol 21(5): 821–822.
36. Mould RF (1993) A century of X-rays and radioactivity in medicine: with emphasis on photographic records of the early years (Bristol: Institute of Physics Publishing); Chapter 23.
37. Martin CJ (2009) A review of radiology staff doses and dose monitoring requirements. Radiat Prot Dosimetry 136(3): 140–157.
38. Theocharopoulos N, Damilakis J, Perisinakis K, Manios E, Vardas P, et al. (2006) Occupational exposure in the electrophysiology laboratory quantifying and minimising radiation burden. Brit J Radiol 79(944): 644–651.

39. Kuon E, Glaser C, Dahm JB (2003) Effective techniques for reduction of radiation dosage to patients undergoing invasive cardiac procedures. Br J Radiol 76(906): 406–413.
40. Ector J, Dragusin O, Adriaenssens B, Huybrechts W, Willems R, et al. (2007) Obesity is a major determinant of radiation dose in patients undergoing pulmonary vein isolation for atrial fibrillation. J Am Coll Cardiol 50(3): 234–242.
41. Marx MV, Ellis JH (1996) Radiation protection of the hand in interventional radiology: should it fit like a glove? Radiology 200(1): 24–25.
42. Wagner LK, Mulhern OR (1996) Radiation-attenuating surgical gloves: effects of scatter and secondary electron production. Radiology 200(1): 45–48.

6

Automated Objective Routine Examination of Optical Quality of Rigid Endoscopes in a Clinical Setting

Rens Wientjes*, Herke J. Noordmans, Jerine A. J. van der Eijk, Henk van den Brink

University Medical Centre Utrecht, Utrecht, The Netherlands

Abstract

Rigid endoscopes degrade during clinical use due to sterilization, ionizing radiation and mechanical forces. Despite visual checks on functionality at the department of sterilization, surgeons are still confronted with suboptimal instruments as it is difficult to assess this degradation in an objective manner. To guarantee that endoscopes have sufficient optical quality for minimal invasive surgery, an experimental opto-electronic test bench has been developed in order to be used at the department of sterilization. Transmission of illumination fibres and lens contrast values are stored in a database to enable empirical criteria to reject endoscope for further clinical usage or to accept endoscopes after repair. Results of the test bench are given for an eight month period, where a trained operator performed 1599 measurements on 46 different types. Stability of the system, trends in quality of clinical endoscopes, and effect of repair or replacement were assessed. Although the period was too short to draw firm conclusions, a slow downwards trend in quality of clinically used endoscopes could be observed. Also, endoscopes generally improve in quality after repair or replacement, while endoscope replacement seems to slightly outperform endoscope repair. To optimize the measurement process, a new system is being developed requiring less user interaction and measuring more optical parameters of an endoscope. By commercializing this system, we hope that measurements at different hospitals will give improved insight which acceptance and rejection criteria to use and which factors (usage, cleaning protocol, and brands) determine the economic lifetime of endoscopes.

Editor: James P. Brody, University of California Irvine, United States of America

Funding: This work is funded by University Medical Center Utrecht. The funders had no role in study design, data collection and analysis, decision to publish, or preparation of the manuscript.

Competing Interests: The authors have the following interests. The described results are derived from the authors' own test system that was developed before they started the collaboration with DOVIDEQ Medical B.V., Deventer, The Netherlands. A new system called 'Scope Control' is being developed in collaboration with DOVIDEQ Medical. There are no further patents, products in development or marketed products to declare.

* E-mail: r.wientjes@umcutrecht.nl

Introduction

Since 1990 endoscopic surgery has become a commonly used technique in a wide range of applications [1]. Two types of endoscopes exist: rigid or flexible. Flexible endoscopes are used to examine the interior of organs (such as oesophagus, stomach, duodenum, colon, lung, etc.). Compared to flexible endoscopes, rigid endoscopes generally provide better image quality for the same diameter and can be sterilized in an autoclave to enable usage in artificially created body cavities. Rigid endoscopes are applied for diagnoses and surgical interventions through small incisions or natural orifices. Although the optical quality of both types of endoscopes is important, we will focus on the optical quality of rigid endoscopes in this paper.

Endoscopic surgery requires more complex and fragile instruments than conventional open surgery. A typical system for endoscopic surgery consists of a bright light source, a light cable, endoscope, a camera, a video processor and a monitor. In this chain, the endoscope is the most complex and fragile critical part as it is can be easily damaged but still is being re-used after cleaning and sterilization (figure 1). Being a small tubular telescope it offers two pathways for light transport. First, the illumination pathway consisting of a fibre bundle transmitting the light into the body cavity illuminating the surgical area. Second, the viewing pathway where several lenses transport the image of the surgical area back to the eyepiece.

Rigid endoscopes degrade during clinical use due to sterilization, ionizing radiation and mechanical forces. The endoscope is fragile and therefore at high risk of damage. The degradation is often difficult to assess by the naked eye [2] [3]. The image as observed by the surgeon is used for diagnosis and Intervention guidance. Poor image quality may increase the risk of wrong diagnosis and treatment. Trouble shooting a defective endoscopic system is a time-consuming and frustrating process. Expensive OR time is lost when parts of the system have to be exchanged to determine which component is malfunctioning [4]. There is a need for a practical quantitative testing method to assure the optical quality of an endoscope for clinical use [2] [3].

Current Situation

Dutch regulations require a quality control of endoscopes before every reuse [2] [5]. The quality check is performed at the department of central sterilization after the endoscopes have been cleaned and before they are packed for sterilization [2] [4]. Often the examination of the endoscope is limited to a visual check of the endoscope; sometimes cold spray is applied to detect moisture or an additional lens is used to detect impurities at the individual lens surfaces [2] [4]. When endoscopes are found with bad optical

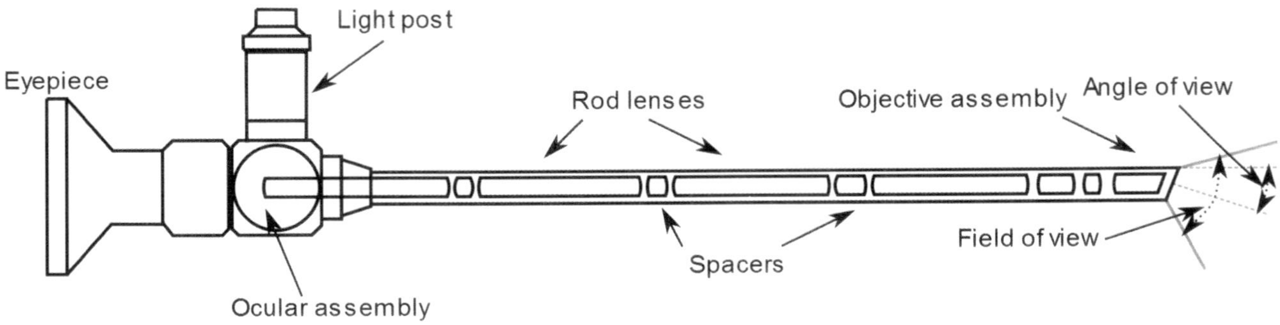

Figure 1. Schematic of a rigid endoscope.

quality during surgery or quality control at the department of central sterilization, they are typically sent to the original manufacturer to be replaced by new or refurbished endoscopes. For many years, the original manufacturer was the sole source of endoscope refurbishment. With the growth of minimal invasive surgery, third-party repair companies have been established during the past decades [4], in general offering repairments at lower costs.

A problem with these manual tests at the department of central sterilization is that it is difficult to assess the quality of an endoscope objectively. This makes it hard to maintain clear and uniform acceptance and rejection criteria. Also, for a human observer it is almost impossible to detect gradual changes in optical quality over time, especially for a large number of different types of endoscopes. Some manufacturers of endoscopes do specify acceptance and rejection criteria, like maximum number of dark illumination fibres and check on dents and lens cracks. It is however, unclear what the relation is with visibility problems in the OR and whether these criteria are under- or overestimations.

There are several possibilities to measure the optical quality of endoscopes. The company Karl Storz sells a test bench (type 499T) with one single circular target and a fibre transmission measurement. The result of the image quality is assessed visually. Reference levels for Karl Storz endoscopes are given on a printed paper. This instrument is intended to be used by repair companies and other specialised users. EndoLume from Lighthouse Imaging can measure the light transmission of the illumination fibres. The result is displayed and has to be compared with the values that can be looked up per type of endoscope. The EndoBench, also from Lighthouse Imaging, is capable to measure the optical quality of endoscopes. This system uses slides as targets and is intended for use at the department of medical technology or repair firms. These products require experienced users. Comparison between endoscopes of the same type is not implemented in the software. Unfortunately none of these test instruments are intended for routine use at the department of central sterilization.

Experimental Test Bench

Our aim was to create a device that is capable of objectively measuring the optical quality at the department of central sterilisation. To minimize workflow disturbance, the quality control(s) should preferably be automatic, quick and easy to perform. Also, it should provide unambiguous outcomes (pass/fail indication) and have an intuitive user interface. In addition to the regular quality-control check, the device should facilitate the acceptance of new or repaired endoscopes.

In the year 2005 we started the design of our first experimental test bench [6]. Based on clinical measurements, several problems were addressed in the years after: Stability of the \LCD display, reproducibility of measurements (electronic ruler, camera focus) and switch to serial number identification, because endoscopes were exchanged between baskets during surgery [7] [8].

To overcome these problems, we started a new measurement period from 2011-07-07 to 2012-3-06, where a trained operator from the technical department performed the measurements. Identification was performed on the serial number of an endoscope and repaired and new endoscopes were registered carefully. This paper describes the results of the measurements during this period. In this period, the measurements were performed two times a week, due to the limited availability of the trained operator.

Methods

Technical Approach

To assure the optical quality of rigid endoscopes in clinical practice, a test bench was developed. Dedicated software was developed to instruct the operator, generate test patterns, capture images, analyse and store these results.

The endoscope was mounted in the endoscope test bench (figure 2) and attached to the camera. Based on the type of endoscope the camera was set to the correct position, within 0.1 mm, measured on an electronic ruler. The screen angle was set in discrete steps to match the angel of view of the type of endoscope under test. The illumination pathway was measured using a white power LED and a photocell. The current output is converted to a voltage and amplified by a low noise differential operational amplifier. The output is sampled by an AD converter and fed back to the PC. The measurement started with a calibration with the light source attached directly to the photocell. Then the amount of transmitted light was measured with the light source coupled to the endoscope's light-coupling connector and the distal end of the endoscope pointed at the photocell.

The viewing pathway was assessed using a computer generated test pattern displayed on a LCD display. The test patterns consisted of alternating lines of black and white with seven different spatial frequencies. The test patterns were captured by a high-resolution camera fitted on the eyepiece of the endoscope. The pixels in the region of interest were binned in grey level. The contrast was defined as the distance in grey levels between 25% and 75% of the accumulated counts of pixels with ascending grey levels. The method is illustrated in figure 3. To allow comparison between successive measurements, the contrast value was averages over the seven line frequencies. After testing the endoscope on the test bench, cold spray is applied to the eye piece of the endoscope

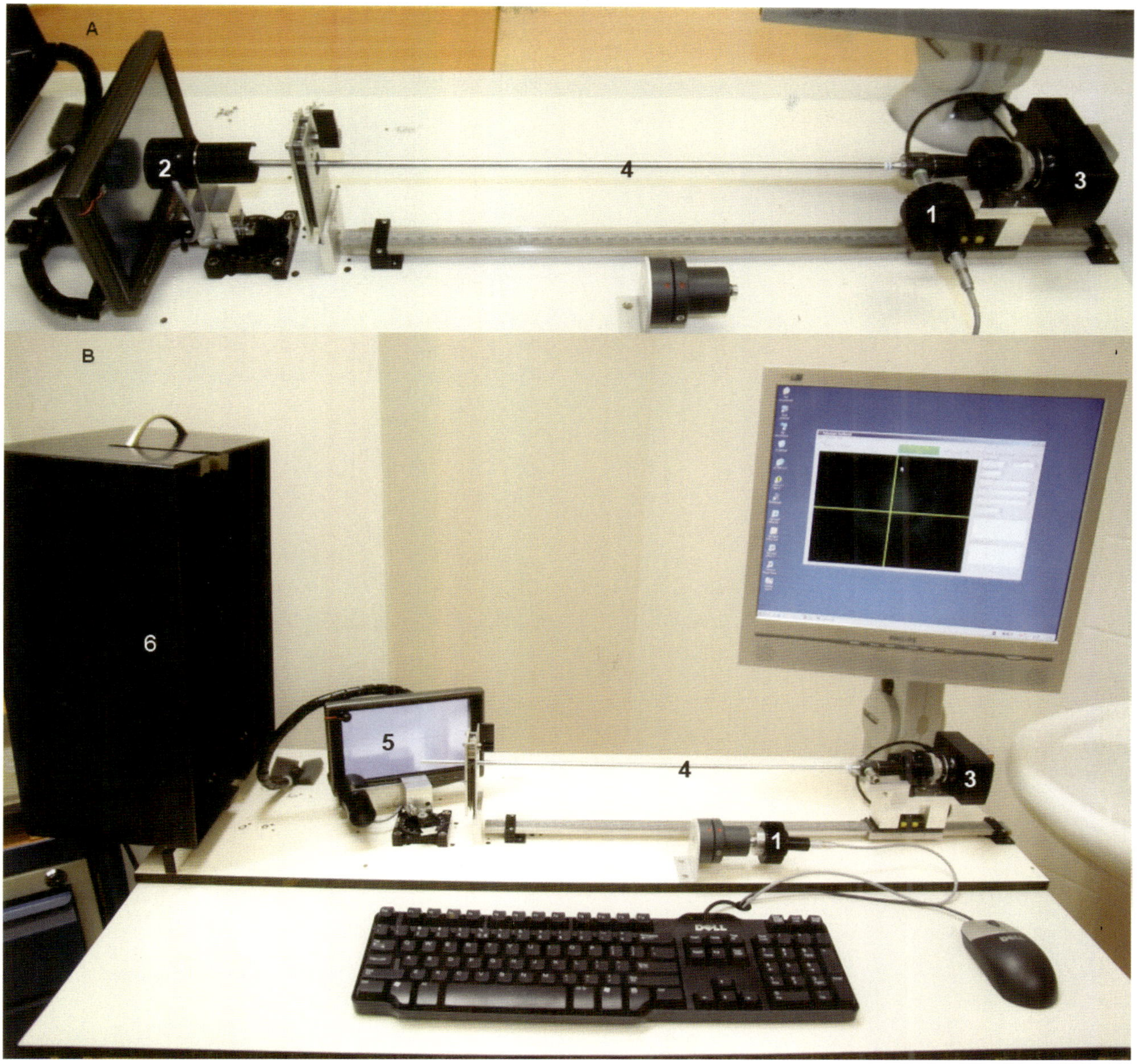

Figure 2. Illustration of measuring the two optical pathways of an endoscope. (A) The transmission of the illumination fibres is measured using a power LED (1) and a photo cell (2). (B) The camera (3) captures a line pattern trough the endoscope (4). The LCD-screen (5) is placed at a 70° angle for this particular endoscope. Surrounding light is blocked with a light cover (6) (open in this picture).

te detect moisture. All measurement results were stored in a custom database.

Acceptance and Rejection Levels

To give the user insight when to accept or reject an endoscope for clinical use, we set acceptance levels before accepting new, refurbished or repaired endoscopes and rejection levels for rejecting clinical used endoscopes before re-use. We decided to base acceptance and rejection levels on the results stored in the test bench's database: New, refurbished or repaired endoscopes were accepted when their measurement values were at least 40% of the measurement values of the best endoscopes of the same type found in the database. The rejection level was set to 20% of the best endoscope of the same type. Both values were chosen conservatively, in order not to challenge the hospital with high replacement costs in this experimental phase.

Reference Endoscope

To assess the stability of the system the illumination-fibre transmission and contrast were determined for the reference endoscope. In every measurement session the reference endoscope (a Storz 10320 A bronchoscope) was measured once. The reference endoscope is used only to verify the stability of the system. It is not used, washed or sterilized.

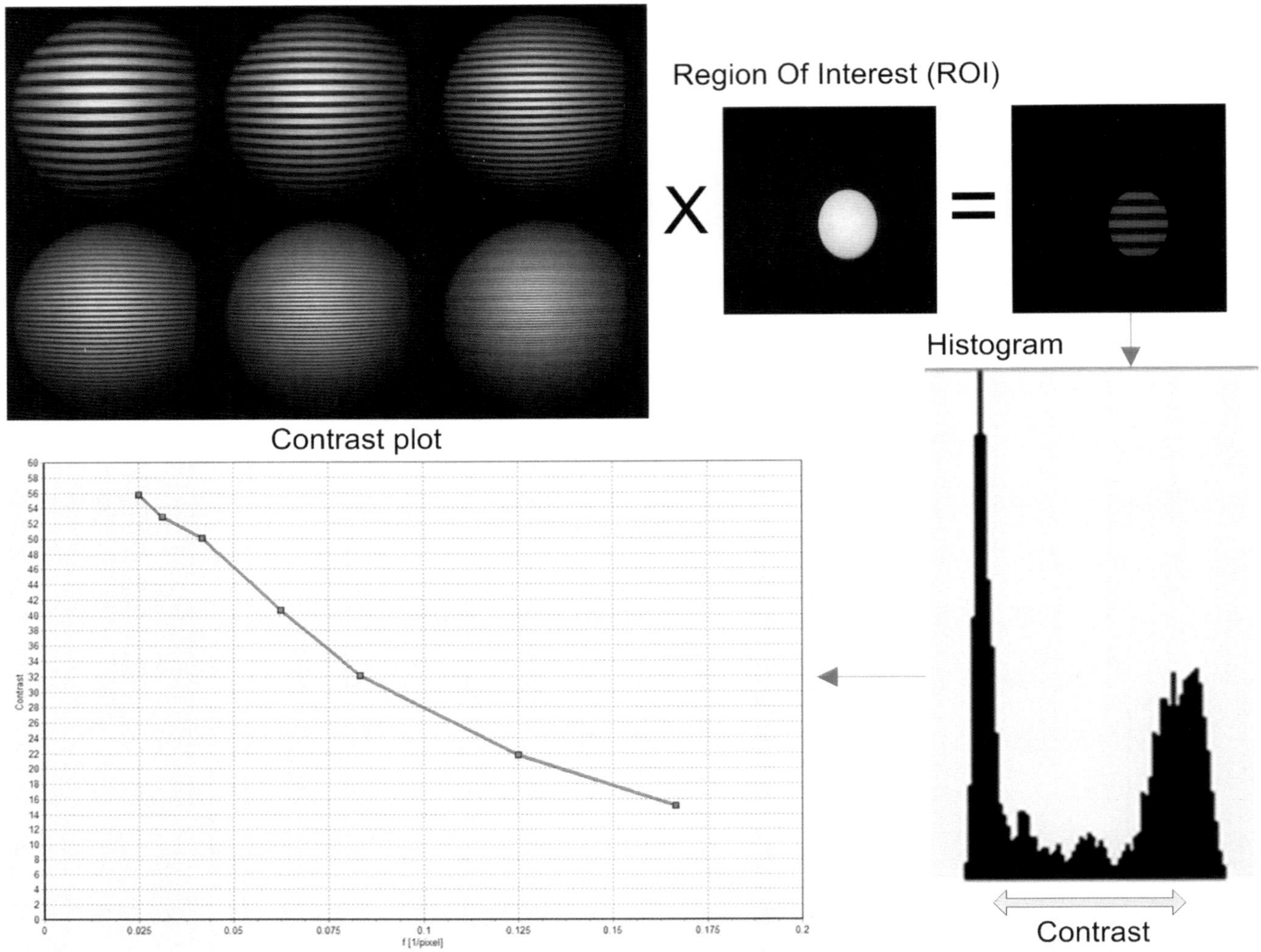

Figure 3. Overview of contrast calculation (clockwise). Test patterns are generated on the LCD display and pictures are captured by a camera through the endoscope. One of the test patterns is a circle in the centre of the LCD display, defining the region of interest where the endoscope image should be sharp. The contrast for a specific line pattern is determined by calculating the distance between the light and dark peak in the histogram for this region of interest.

Results

Over the measurement period, 1599 measurements were performed in the department of central sterilization on 288 rigid endoscopes of 46 different types. Forty-nine of these measurements where performed on the reference endoscope.

System Stability

The illumination-fibre transmission and contrast value of the reference endoscope are shown in figure 4. Ninety-five per cent of the transmission data points are within two per cent of the mean value. The transmission data show no evidence of a drift in this period (figure 4, left). The average contrast value is displayed in figure 4, right. Ninety-five per cent of the contrast data points are within three per cent of the mean value. We therefore considered differences larger than five per cent to be significant for the rest of the measurements.

Performance Tracking Over Time

The system allowed us to track the performance of an individual endoscope or a group of endoscopes of the same type over time. Figure 5 shows a typical example of a group of three endoscope of the same type. A slight downwards trend over time was observed, for endoscope C this trend was significant for both the transmission and the contrast. The transmission of one endoscope (C) reached the rejection level and was sent in to be repaired.

New and Repaired Endoscopes

In the measurement period, 68 endoscopes were sent in to be repaired or replaced. In sixteen cases the endoscope has been measured before repair, in eighteen cases this was done immediately after repair. In fourteen cases the same endoscope was measured before and after repair. Seven new endoscopes were measured in this period. Six out of seven new endoscopes measured more than 80% compared to the best performing endoscope of the same type. The contrast of one new endoscope was measured at 67% (see figure 6).

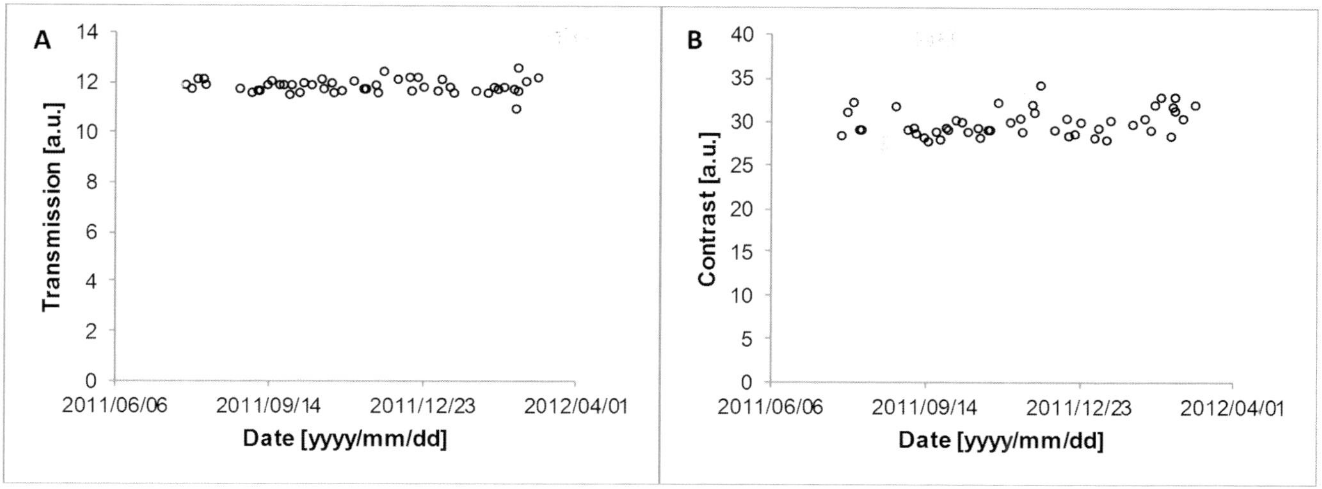

Figure 4. Scatter plot of measurements of the reference endoscope over the measuring period. (A) The illumination fibre transmission is shown. Full scale (100 units) transmission is defined by the value that is measured with the light source directly fitted on the photo cell. (B) The measured contrast is shown.

A typical example of defects and their frequency of occurrence is shown table 1. Most of the time, more than one deficiency was reported per endoscope. Most repairs were on the lens system. Replacing the illumination fibres is relatively expensive and rarely opted for.

In general the performance of a repaired endoscope was better after than before repair. The transmission increased with more than five per cent in nine cases, the remaining five cases stayed within five per cent of the value before repair. In ten cases the contrast improved by more than five per cent, in two cases the contrast decreased more than five per cent. The 100 per cent reference level is set by the best performing endoscope of the same type. In general the performance of a repaired endoscope seems to be somewhat below that of a similar, new endoscope, see figure 6. Figure 7 shows an example of the quality of a repaired endoscope. The transmission and the contrast were improved by the repair. Both measures were above the acceptance level. The transmission drops rapidly in the period after repair.

Discussion

In this paper we have presented the results of measuring the quality of rigid endoscopes at the department of central sterilization by a trained person from the technical department in an eight months period. Based on the measurements of the reference endoscope, we considered changes above 5% to be significant. We investigated whether the test bench can be used for quality control of clinically used endoscopes by measuring the illumination-fibre transmission and the transferred contrast of line patterns by the lens system.

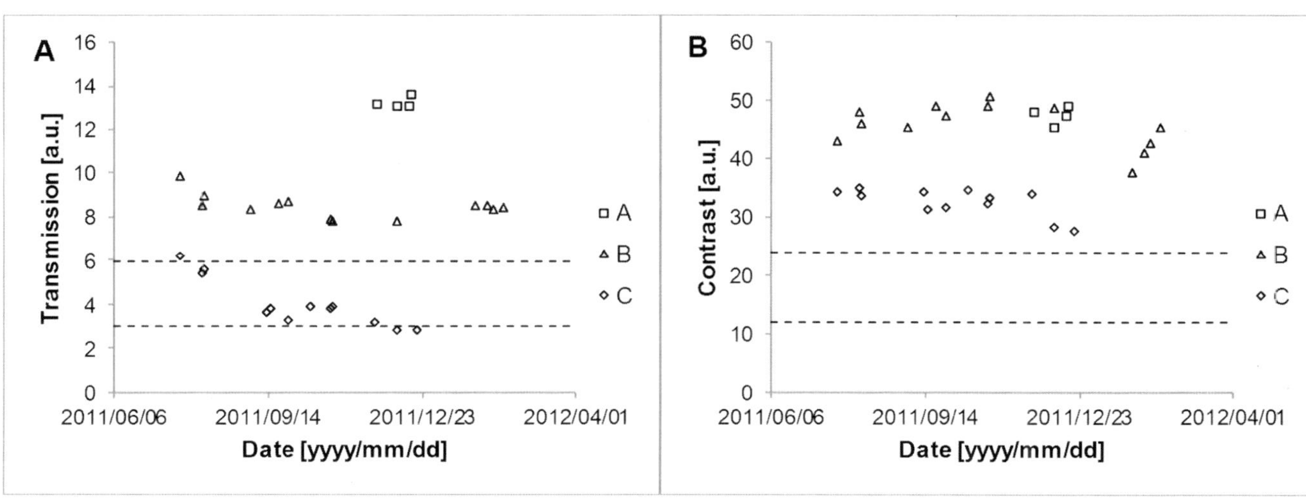

Figure 5. Measurements of illumination fibre transmission (A) and contrast (B) over time for three endoscopes of the same type. Examples of a good (A), moderate (B) and low-performing (C) endoscope are shown. The upper dashed line is the acceptance level for new or repaired endoscopes, the lower dotted line is the rejection level for clinically used endoscopes.

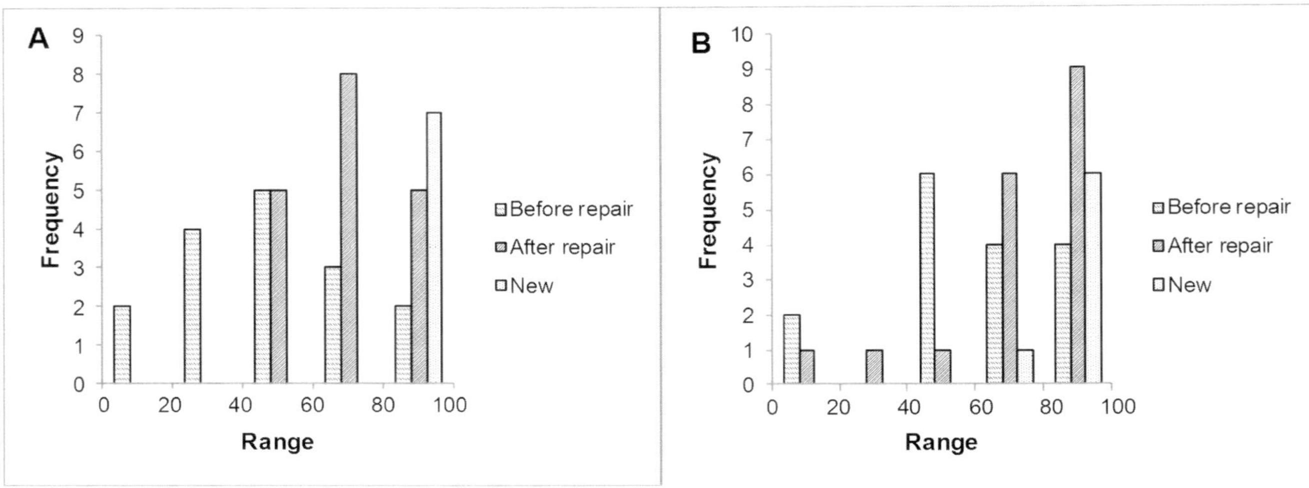

Figure 6. Histogram of relative illumination fibre transmission (A) and contrast (B) of repaired and new endoscopes. The relative performance is calculated. The 100% reference level is set by the best performing endoscope of the same type. The contrast of two endoscopes was below 40% after repair, those two were sent back to the repair company.

Track Performance Over Time

The endoscope test bench is able to track the optical quality of endoscopes which are used clinically. During the endoscope's lifecycle gradual deterioration is expected. Our measurements seem to agree with that, as a gradual deterioration in both the fibre transmission and the quality of the lens system can be observed. From the current measurements it is difficult to draw firm conclusions. As measurements were performed two times a week, endoscopes could be re-sterilized several times in-between. It is therefore hard to determine which factors cause the fibre transmission to drop rapidly after repair (figure 7). Our hypothesis is that although the fibres at the light post are cleaned and polished at the repair firm, debris from cleaning in combination with a high power light source is probably responsible for these burning-in effects. We expect that, when all endoscopes are measured in every re-use cycle, we can distinguish between a normal and an abnormal slope of deterioration.

During this phase of development we have set the levels for rejection of endoscopes at 20% of the best endoscope of the same type. This value is chosen conservatively as during implementation we did not want to reject large numbers of endoscopes at once, given the fact that repairing or replacing an endoscope takes about four weeks and most departments only have 4–6 endoscopes of the same type. Therefore we started with rejecting the poorest performing endoscopes combined with severe moisture inside. Moisture was detected in 43 out of 288 endoscopes. We detected moisture 150 times, but some surgical departments kept using the leaking endoscopes up to 10 times after we reported the issue. At the time of writing it is not clear whether the procedure to report these defects to the operating room is insufficient, or the severity of the defect is subordinate to the need of the use.

Table 1. Identified deficiencies, as reported by repair firm in the eight-month measurement period based on 68 endoscopes that were sent in.

Defect	Counts
Dusty, particles are visible on the lens surface	54
Mechanical damage, dents, scratches, bended shaft or damaged tip	46
Broken rod lens(es)	41
Sapphire window at the tip needs to be replaced	27
Objective assembly needs to be replaced	17
Moisture condenses inside the endoscope	11
Eye piece loose, torn or adhesive damaged	9
Fibre transmission low	5
Other	3

Measurement Setup

The camera has to be accurately focused and the endoscope has to be positioned within 0.1 mm of the position stored for that type in the database. This requires attentiveness of the operator and can best be performed by technically trained staff. We learned that the next version of an endoscopic test bench should have a more robust user interface and should be less dependent on manually performed actions. The identification of the tested endoscope should be robust and automated to avoid measurement results stored under the wrong identity. During the measurement period reported here, we used a single operator instructed to use serial numbers to minimize this effect.

Future Development

Based on the experience with our experimental test bench in clinical practice, we believe that there is a clear need for objective quality control of endoscopes. To enable robust quality control of endoscopes, we envision a next generation test bench in which endoscopes are identified automatically, which is easy to use by quick and robust mounting of the endoscope and has a simple user interface with no more than one start button. It should also be connected to the hospital's track and trace system. A test bench that meets these requirements will bring 100% functional control of rigid endoscopes one step closer.

To get closer to these goals, we started collaborating with DOVIDEQ Medical B.V. (Deventer, The Netherlands) to develop the "Scope Control". It has been designed for quick and easy use

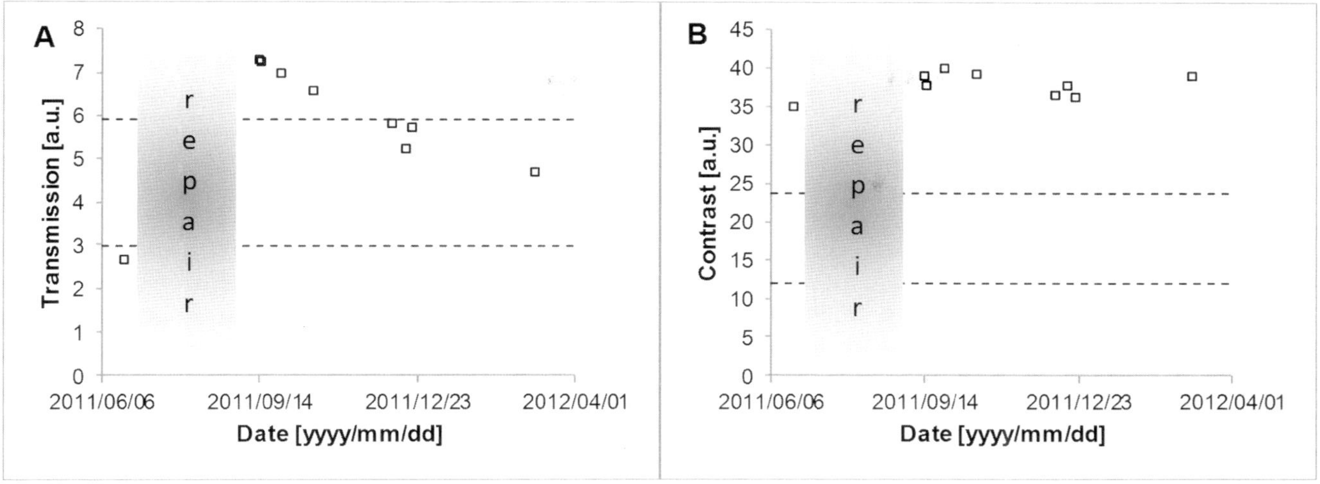

Figure 7. Measurements of illumination fibre transmission (A) and contrast (B) before and after repair for a single endoscope. The endoscope showed mechanical damage at the distal end. The sapphire window was replaced by the repair firm. The upper dashed line is the acceptance level, the lower dashed line is the rejection level. The acceptance and rejection levels were set at respectively 40% and 20% of the measurement values of the best endoscopes of the same type.

at the department of sterilization. It offers quick mounting of endoscope followed by automatic measurements of transmission of the illumination pathway, and transmission, colour, dust, moisture and view angle of the viewing pathway. Measurements are compared with reference values in a database for objective acceptance or rejection. As the database will be shared among hospitals, deterioration trends and endoscope brands may be compared.

Conclusions

The opto-electronic test bench has been proven in clinical practice. It is possible to record the performance of rigid endoscopes in a quantitative way. It provides useful information about the current state of the endoscopes in use. Endoscopes can be rejected in time, based on quantitative measurements. Repaired or new endoscopes can be assessed and compared to other endoscopes of the same type before they are accepted.

To optimize the measurement process at the department of sterilization, a new system called 'Scope Control' is being developed in collaboration with DOVIDEQ Medical requiring less user interaction and measuring more optical parameters of an endoscope. By commercializing this system, we hope that measurements at different hospitals will give improved insight which acceptance and rejection criteria to use and which factors (usage, cleaning protocol, and brands) determine the economic lifetime of endoscopes.

Author Contributions

Conceived and designed the experiments: RW HJN. Performed the experiments: JE. Analyzed the data: RW HJN. Contributed reagents/materials/analysis tools: RW HJN. Wrote the paper: RW HJN.

References

1. Darzi A, Munz Y (2004) The impact of minimal invasive surgical techniques. Annual review of medicine 55: 223–237 DOI: 10.1146/annurev.med.55.091902.105248.
2. Boer I de, Noordmans HJ, Brink H van den, Gips R, Janssen MJH, et al. (2008) Kwaliteitsborging van Instrumenten en Apparatuur gebruikt bij Minimaal Invasieve Chirurgie, rapport van de projectgroep MICADO. WIBAZ/NVKF Available: http://www.wibaz.nl/media/download_gallery/W2008-579.pdf accessed 14 November 2012.
3. Ayliffe GAJ, Babb JR, Bradley CR (1992) 'Sterilization' of arthroscopes and laparoscopes. Journal of Hospital Infection 22: 265–269.
4. Spry C, Leiner DC (2004) Rigid endoscopes – ensuring quality before use and after repair. AORN Journal vol 80 no 1: 103–109.
5. Health Care Inspectorate (2009) Toetsingskader Follow-up Minimaal invasieve chirurgie ten behoeve van het tweede-faseonderzoek vanaf september 2009. (Dutch) Available: www.medischetechnologie.nl/download.php?refid=740&ei=j9-sUKHpNsTS0QWju4HwBg&usg=AFQjCNGIOfy-cRfbHaV2jHSFrHnSlXJq5w. Accessed 2012 Nov 21.
6. Noordmans HJ, Mil I, Daoudi S, Kruit S, Brink H van den, Verdaasdonk R (2006) Optical quality assessment of rigid endoscopes during clinical lifetime. San Francisco: SPIE Photonics West. SPIE - Design and Quality for Biomedical Technologies.
7. Noordmans HJ, Kruit S, Stroosnijder P, Brink H van den, Verdaasdonk R (2008) Quantitative assessment of degradation of the optical quality of rigid endoscopes in clinical practice. San Francisco: SPIE Photonics West. SPIE - Design and Quality for Biomedical Technologies.
8. Karl Storz - Endoscope. Manual Telescopes and [HOPKINS]® Telescopes. Version 2.5_04/2002.

Combined Minimally Invasive Percutaneous Nephrolithotomy and Retrograde Intrarenal Surgery for Staghorn Calculi in Patients with Solitary Kidney

Dehui Lai[1], Yongzhong He[2], Yuping Dai[1], Xun Li[2]*

1 Department of Urology, The First Affiliated Hospital of Sun Yat-sen University, Guangzhou, Guangdong, China, 2 Department of Urology, The Fifth Affiliated Hospital of Guangzhou Medical University, Guangzhou, Guangdong, China

Abstract

Background: To present our experience with simultaneous combined minimally invasive percutaneous nephrolithotomy (MPCNL) and retrograde intrarenal surgery (RIRS) to manage patients with staghorn calculi in solitary kidney, and evaluate the safety, efficiency and feasibility of this approach.

Methodology/Principal Findings: The study included 20 patients with staghorn calculi in solitary kidney. Demographic characteristics, stone location and surface area were recorded. After informed consent, the patients underwent one stage MPCNL firstly. Combined second stage MPCNL and RIRS simultaneously were performed at postoperative 5–7 days. Operative parameters, stone-free rate (SFR), stone analyses and complications were evaluated. Serum creatinine (Scr), glomerular filtration rate (GFR) and chronic kidney disease (CKD) were measured preoperatively, postoperatively at 1 month, and each follow-up visit. All patients had staghorn stones involving multiple calyces. The mean stone burden was 1099.9±843.95 mm^2. All patients had only one percutaneous access tract. The mean whole operative duration was 154.37±32.45 min. The mean blood loss was 64 (12–140) ml. The final SFR was 90%. During the 1-month follow-up study period, four patients improved in CKD stage. Two patients who had CKD (stage 5) still needed dialysis postoperatively. Mean Scr of the rest patients preoperatively was 187.16±94.12 compared to 140.99±57.92 umol/L by the end of 1-month follow-up period ($p = 0.019$). The same findings were observed in GFR in that preoperatively it was 43.80±24.74 ml/min and by the end of the 1-month follow-up it was 49.55±21.18 ml/min ($p = 0.05$).

Conclusions/Significance: Combined MPCNL and RIRS management effectively decrease the number and size of percutaneous access tracts, which is safe, feasible, and efficient for managing staghorn calculi in solitary kidney with satisfactory SFR and reducing blood loss, potential morbidity associated with multiple tracts. The approach did not adversely affect renal function at both short-term and long-term follow-up.

Editor: Utpal Sen, University of Louisville, United States of America

Funding: No current external funding sources for this study.

Competing Interests: The authors have declared that no competing interests exist.

* E-mail: 157773933@qq.com

Introduction

Staghorn calculi are branched stones that occupy the renal pelvis contain one or more caliceal extensions [1]. A heightened risk of chronic renal failure and life-threatening urosepsis are well-known risks of untreated staghorn calculi, especially for patients with solitary kidney [2].Percutaneous nephrolithotomy (PCNL) has evolved into widely accepted and primary recommended management for staghorn calculi since its first described in 1976 [3].However, The stone-free rate (SFR) of staghorn calculi following PCNL monotherapy is only 74% to 83% [4]. Furthermore, PCNL among the staghorn patients is associated with potential risk, such as significant hemorrhage, urosepsis, urine leakage, uncontrolled hemorrhage, embolization, nephrectomy, or even death [5]. In patients with solitary kidney, staghorn calculi occupying several calyces had to require multiple access tracts to achieve complete stone-free. It may be associated with greater potential risk. Performing PCNL with a small size tract (12–20 F), named minimally invasive percutaneous nephrolithotomy (MPCNL), may decrease the injured of the kidney and operative morbidity, comparing to the standard PCNL with (26–30 F) tract [6,7,8]. But the disadvantages of MPCNL are relatively low efficiency to fragment large stones and high intrapelvic pressure than the standard PCNL.

Retrograde intrarenal surgery (RIRS) is become popular, benefited from the advance in flexible ureteroscopic (FU) instrumentation and holmium laser lithotripsy. It allows retrograde access to the entire intrarenal collecting system in treating renal calculi to achieve complete stone-free, and it is safer than PCNL. However, RIRS is burdened with high rates of fiber breakage and lower efficiency in larger stone [9]. Less ideal for manage the whole staghorn calculi, RIRS can be used as an auxiliary procedure of MPCNL to reach peripheral renal residual calculi in patients with solitary kidney, on the purpose of stone-free and keeping the maximum renal function.

In this study, we evaluated the safety, efficiency and feasibility of combined MPCNL and RIRS on management of staghorn calculi in patients with solitary kidney and determined long-term renal functional results.

Materials and Methods

We obtained approval for this study from the ethics committee of the fifth affiliated hospital of Guangzhou Medical College. Written informed consent was obtained for all the participants in our study. We performed a retrospective analysis of 20 patients (staghorn calculi involving multiple calyces) who underwent single-tract MPCNL and RIRS combination for staghorn calculi in a solitary kidney between July 2009 and March 2011 at the Urology Department of the 5th affiliated hospital of Guangzhou Medical College. Stones was divided into complete [7 cases, 35%, (occupying all calyces and renal pelvis, or filled >80% of the renal collecting system)] and partial [13 cases, 65%, (occupying renal pelvis, or at least 2 or more calyces)] staghorn calculi [10]. Stone burden was assessed as the surface area and calculated according to the European Association of Urology guidelines [11].The causes of solitary kidney were congenital in three cases (15%), previous contra lateral nephrectomy in 10 cases (50%), and nonperfused contra lateral in 7 cases (35%).

Patient characteristics analyzed were age, sex, BMI, causes of solitary kidney, previous renal intervention history, hypertension and diabetes. Preoperative tests, such as blood routine tests, coagulation tests, serum biochemistry, urinalysis, urine culture, ultrasonography and plain X-ray were recorded. Computerized tomography (CT) was done routinely, in order to analyze the size and location of the stone, the thickness of renal parenchyma, the anatomical structure and plan the target percutaneous tract and calyx. Preoperative antibiotics were administered to the results of urine culture.

For each patient, serum creatinine (Scr) and glomerular filtration rate (GFR) were measured before and after the whole procedure, and each follow-up visit. GFR was calculated using the Cockroft and Gault formula by Scr [12,13]. Chronic kidney disease (CKD) was classified by the National Kidney Foundation Kidney Disease Outcome Quality Initiative (NKFK/DOQI) classification system [14]. CKD stages 1 to 5 were classified as a GFR that was normal, mildly, moderately, severely decreased and a requirement for dialysis or kidney transplantation (greater than 90, 60 to 89, 30 to 59, 15 to 29 and less than 15 ml/minute, respectively). The Scr, GFR and CKD stage during preoperative period were compared with those at the follow-up visit.

Surgical Technique

One-stage single-tract MPCNL. All procedures were performed under continual epidural anesthesia. Patients were inserted a 5 F ureteral catheter into the target ureter and placed a 16 F Foley catheter in the bladder under lithotomy position. Then, patients were placed in the prone position with a pillow under the abdomen. MPCNL was performed under C-arm fluoroscopic guidance using an 18 gauge needle for access to the target calyx. A posterior middle calyx puncture via the 11th intercostal space between the posterior axillary line and scapula line was preferred. The needle was directed into the papilla of the intended posterior calyx using the "bull's-eye" technique [15]. Once the needle was properly placed into the calyx, a 0.035-inch guidewire was inserted through the needle into the intrarenal collecting system. Tract dilatation was serially accomplished using Amplatz dilators from 8 F to 20 F.A matched diameter working sheath was advanced into the collecting system. The stones were fragmented with a holmium laser or pneumatic lithotripter through an 8.5/12 F rigid nephroscope (designed by Li Xun, Richard Wolf, German)(Figure 1), and with Cyberwand® dual probe ultrasonic intracorporeal lithotripter through 18 F rigid nephroscope (designed by Li Xun, Richard Wolf, German) (Figure 1).

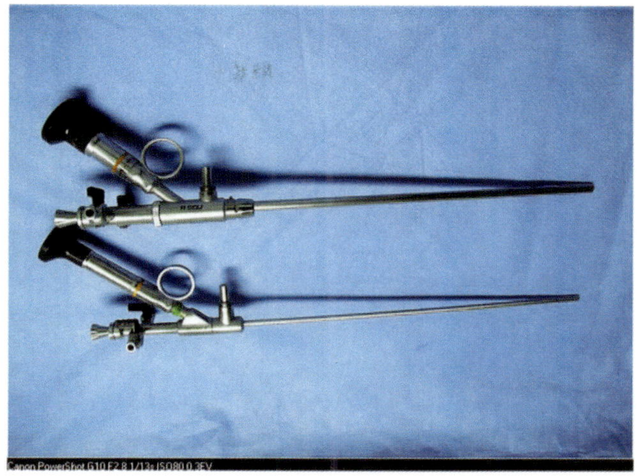

Figure 1. The 8.5/12 F rigid nephroscope and 18 F rigid nephroscope (designed by Li Xun, Richard Wolf, German).

The left valve of nephroscope was connected with an endoscopic pulsed perfusion pump, and the right valve was connected with Suction. The big fragments were removed with a forceps, and small fragments were pushed out with an endoscopic pulsed perfusion pump and suck out with suction. During the procedure, remove the stone in the renal pelvis and the low calyces, as for as possible. Meanwhile, rudely inserting the nephroscope to arrive the peripheral calyx is not supported. Finally, a 6 F modified Double-J stent, which had two open tails, was inserted via the percutaneous tract with the assistance of guidewire, and a matched size balloon nephrostomy tube was inserted in the involved calyx. The operative duration was calculated from the time of percutaneous puncture to the completion of nephrostomy tube placement.

On postoperative day 1 or 2, routine KUB and retrograde nephrostogram were done in all patients to assess for residual stone fragments, urinary leakage and infrarenal obstruction. On postoperative day 5~7, second stage procedure was done for the patients.

Combination of Single-tract MPCNL and RIRS

The procedures were performed under continual epidural anesthesia. Patients were prepared for Galdakao-modified supine Valdivia (GMSV) position [16] (Figure 2). Two groups of doctors were needed. MPCNL group was doing second stage MPCNL using the former single-tract access. Briefly, a 0.035 guidewire is inserted into the renal calyx though the nephrostomy tube. Tract dilatation was serially accomplished using Amplatz dilators up to the match size, and working sheath was advanced into the renal collecting system. Nephroscope was inserted into the renal collecting system. Simultaneously, RIRS was performed by another group. (Figure 2). After retrograde pyelography and placing a safety guidewire, a 12/14 ureteric access sheath was advanced into the proximal ureter, allowing easy passage of the 7.5 F flexible ureteroscope into the collecting system. The renal stones and collecting system were carefully inspected. Residual stones in the peripheral calyces, which would have required a second or third nephrostomy access, were fragmented with a 200 μm holmium laser fiber. Alternatively, a stone basket or grasping devices was used to transfer calyceal stones into the renal pelvis, where the MPCNL group can use concomitant lithotripsy and remove the fragments efficiency. At the end of procedure, the collecting system accessible to the rigid and flexible nephroscope was examined for potential fragments. Patients were discharged home 2 days after second stage procedure, following removal of their nephrostomy tube, provided no significant residual stone was seen on the KUB.

Follow-up

One month after the final procedure, all patients were assessed by CT to confirm the final SFR. Complete stone-free was defined as the absence of any fragments in kidney or had clinically insignificant residual fragments (CIRFs), defined as 4 mm or smaller, nonsymptomatic, nonobstructive and noninfectious residual fragments [17]. The Double-J stent would be removed in the complete stone-free patients.

After the first follow-up evaluation, patients returned for an assessment with urinalysis, serum creatinine, KUB and urinary ultrasound was used every 3 months during the first year and every 6 months thereafter. When stones appeared in stone-free patients or the size of residual stones increased, patients were reevaluated by CT to guide the appropriate treatment modality.

Statistical analysis was done with SPSS 16.0® for Windows®. Continuous variables were compared with student t test and Wilcoxon test, and Proportions of categorical variables were analyzed for statistical significance using the Fisher exact test. Differences resulting in $p<0.05$ were considered significant.

Results

The study identified 20 patients, including 8(40%) men and 12(60%) women. Mean age was 52.75±13.13 years (range 21 to 77) and mean BMI was 22.98±3.51 kg/m^2 (range 17.76 to 31.99). Mean stone burden was 1099.9±843.95 mm^2 (range 291 to 2925).Five patients had a previous renal intervention history in the procedure side. Six staghorn calculi were in the right side, and 14 were in the left. All patients were suffered from medical comorbidities (1 cardiac; 2 diabetes; 5 hypertension; 12 renal failure).15(75%) patients were identified as hydronephrosis, including 8(40%) mild, 4(20%) moderate and 3(15%) severe. Preoperative urine cultures were positive in 10 (50%) patients. All these infections were administrated with culture-specific antibiotics. Demographic and clinical preoperative characteristics of patients were shown in Table 1. During the preoperative period, one (5%) patient had CKD stage 1, four (20%) had stage 2, eight (40%) had stage 3, five (25%) had stage 4 and two (10%) had stage 5. Two patients required dialysis preoperatively.

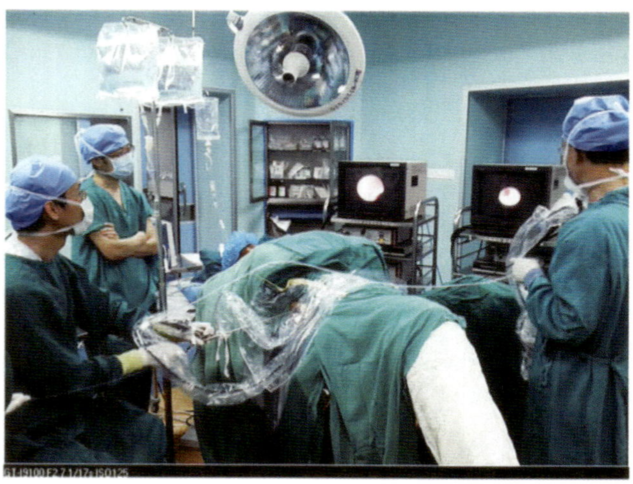

Figure 2. Sigle-tract minimally invasive percutaneous nephrolithotomy and retrograde intrarenal surgery were performed simultaneously in Galdakao-modified supine Valdivia (GMSV) position by two urological groups.

Table 1. Demographic and clinical preoperative characteristics of patients.

Age, year, mean(SD), range	52.75(13.13), 21–77
Sex, no.(%)	
Male	8(40)
Female	12(60)
BMI, kg/m^2, mean (SD)	22.98(3.51)
Cause of solitary kidney, no. (%)	
Congential	3(15)
Previous nephrectomy	10(50)
Nonperfused kidney	7(35)
Stone side, no. (%)	
Left	14(70)
Right	6(30)
Staghorn Stone type, no. (%)	
Complete	7(35)
Partial	13(65)
Stone burden, mean (SD), range (mm^2)	1099.9(843.95), 291–2925
Previous renal intervention history, no, (%)	
Open surgery	2(10)
ESWL	2(10)
PCNL	1(5)
Grade of hydronephrosis, no. (%)	
None	5(25)
Mild	8(40)
Moderate	4(20)
Severe	3(15)
Medical Comorbidities, no. (%)	
Hypertension	5(25)
Diabetes	2(10)
Cardiac	1(5)
Renal failure	12(60)
Positive preoperative urine culture, no. (%)	10(50)
E. coli	3(15)
Enterococcus faecalis	1(5)
Acinetobacter	1(5)
Pseudomonas aeruginosa	1(5)
Enterobacter cloacae	2(10)
Proteus mirabilis	2(10)

All patients had only one percutaneous access tract. Access to calices through an 11th intercostal route was established in 17 renal units, and sub-12th costal approach was in three renal units. The mean operative duration was 96.88±30.42 min in one stage and 87.86±34.90 min in second stage. The mean whole operative duration was 154.37±32.45 min, which was not significantly different from previous experience with standard multiple accesses PCNL had reported [18,19]. The mean blood loss was 64 (12–140) ml, which was less than multiple-puncture PCNL had reported [18,19]. There was no intraoperative complications in all cases. Postoperative complications noted in 5(25%) patents according to the Clavien classification. Four patients had fever on the day 1 after MPCNL, which resolved spontaneously in two, while the remaining two patients required antibiotic treatment because of positive urine cultures suggested urinary tract infection, and positive blood cultures. Two patients were treated with a complete culture-specific antibiotics until body temperature, urinalysis and urine culture were normal. One patient was prolonged tract leakage because of diabetes. No patients required blood transfusion. Mean hospitalization time was 12.11±2.77 days, two patients prolonged hospitalization time because of poor wound healing induced by diabetes. The Initial SFR after the procedure was 95%. One patient had small asymptomatic residual calculi (largest 6 mm) in the lower pole. Three patients had CIRFs. The final SFR was 90%, confirmed by CT 1 month after the final operation. Stone recurred in one patient in the lower pole (diameter<6 mm, asymptomatic). Operative characteristics and stone composition were shown in Table 2. During the whole follow-up period, another patient had recurred stone (diameter<12 mm, in the upper pole) in postoperative 6 months, who was treated with RIRS. Stone recurred was not found in the rest patients.

CKD stage was compared in Table 3 before and after the treatment. During the 1-month follow-up study period, 4 patients improved to be CKD (stage 3) postoperatively, who were identified as CKD (stage 4) preoperatively. Two patients who had CKD (stage 5) still needed dialysis postoperatively. No more patients progressed to end-stage renal disease requiring dialysis. Mean Scr of the rest patients before operation was 187.16±94.12 umol/L compared to 140.99±57.92 umol/L by the end of 1-month follow-up period with statistical significance ($p = 0.019$). The same findings were observed in GFR in that before operation it was 43.80±24.74 ml/min and by the end of the 1-month follow-up it was 49.55±21.18 ml/min with statistical significance ($p = 0.05$). However, there were no statistically significant differences between these parameters from 1 month to 1-year follow-up ($p>0.05$). Table 3 also compared Scr and calculated GFR of 18 patients before and after the treatment.

Discussion

In patients with solitary kidney, an untreated staghorn calculus is likely to destroy the renal function and cause life-threatening urosepsis. Complete removal of the stone is crucial aim to eradicate any causative organisms, relieve obstruction, prevent further stone recurrence and preserve the renal function as far as possible [20]. PCNL is currently the recommended treatment for patients with staghorn calculi based on the superior outcomes and acceptable low morbidity, with the advent of endourologic instruments, lithotripsy devices, and surgical techniques [1,21]. Although rare, PCNL is associated with significant complications, especially in patients with solitary kidney. One of the most common and worrisome complications following PCNL is renal hemorrhage [22]. Because of physiological compensatory hypertrophy of the renal parenchyma in the solitary kidney, it is more likely to increase the risk of hemorrhage owe to damaging more renal tissue and blood vessel in puncturing and dilating the thick renal parenchyma [23]. Previous study has demonstrated that compared with the tract of standard PCNL (26–30 F), the small tract (12–20 F) of MPCNL obviously reduced the damage of renal parenchyma and vessel. Although, previous literature has proved that mean intrapelvic pressures of the minimum tract (14 F) in MPCNL was still lower than the causing backflow (30 mmHg) [24], performing PCNL in lower intrapelvic pressures is effective to reduce the absorption of toxinum and pyrogen. In this study, 17(85%) MPCNL was performed with 20 F because each effective lithotripsy can be placed through the nephroscope in this size of working sheath. Accessing the collecting system through the posterior middle calyx provided the most direct and shortest tract from skin to renal collecting system, and may enable to access the majority of the collecting system. Performing MPCNL by an 8/9.8 F rigid ureteroscope was usual in the past, with the advantage of its slender body, which can access to more calyces to acquire a higher SRF and a lower complication in a single tract [8,25]. However, urologists often complained of fatigue, bad visual fields, and low efficiency in stone removal, when using ureteroscope. With the development of endourology, an 8.5/12 F rigid nephroscope was designed to overcome the disadvantage of ureteroscope in MPCNL procedure. It not only has a relative suitable body (12 F), which can access to most calyces, but also had a wider working channel (8.5 F), which is to facilitate stone removal with a forceps. Addition, because front mouth of the nephroscope is flat, the small fragments were pushed out with an endoscopic pulsed perfusion pump and suck out with suction easily. The valves of the nephroscope were connected with pulsed perfusion pump and suction, which can be regulated by the urologist. This convenient regulated system was used so that irrigation fluid could escape easily with no increase in the intrapelvic pressure. An 18 F rigid nephroscope was designed specially for dual probe ultrasonic intracorporeal lithotripter, which was a high effective lithotripter in managing large bulk stone with low intra-pelvic pressure through a single tract.

Access to all the calyces through one percutaneous tract may be difficult due to the peculiar anatomical structure of the collecting system. Meanwhile, solitary kidney with large burden stone, branched stone and satellite stone or residual stone in parallel calyces of the access often requires multiple access tracts during PCNL. Furthermore, multiple access tracts may be associated with greater risk of renal hemorrhage [26,27]. RIRS has been used successfully to access and treat complex renal calculi smaller than 2 cm with high reported stone-free rates [9]. RIRS has fewer overall complications compared to PCNL, even absence of renal injure. However, the small working channels of RIRS had limited the usefulness of effective instrumentation that allows concurrent stone fragmentation and removal [18]. Multiple procedures or combined approach may be required to clear a large stone. Although, Wong et al [28] in their study could achieve clearance rates of 95% in 45 renal units with a single puncture followed by flexible nephroscopy in a staged manner, SRF after the first stage was only 51.4%, and flexible nephroscopy with a large diameter was not easy to access to the narrow calyces. Perhaps, the same group of patients would have been rendered completely stone free with the addition of multiple tracts even at the cost of extending the hospital stay. Landman et al [29] use simultaneously ureteroscopy and lower calix single-tract PCNL for single-access of six complete and three partial staghorn calculi with no major complication. But SRF was only 78%. Marguet et al [18] applied the same concept, albeit with the difference that ureterorenoscopy

Table 2. operative characteristics and stone composition of patients.

Puncture (one staged MPCNL), no. (%)	
Posterior middle calyx via 11th intercostal	17(85)
Posterior lower pole below 12th costal	3(15)
No. of tracts, no. (%)	
Single	20(100)
Access tract Size, no. (%)	
18 F	17(85)
20 F	3(15)
Time to access the collecting system, mean, (SD), range (min)	14.3(11–23)
Residual calculi characteristics after one staged MPCNL	
Stone size, mean, (SD), range (mm^2)	743.12(312.34), 112–1831
Stone position, no. (%)	
Upper pole	6(30)
Middle calyx	2(10)
Lower pole	1(5)
Mix	11(55)
Operative duration, mean (SD), range(min)	
One stage	96.88(30.42), 65–175
Second stage	87.86(34.90), 30–165
The whole	154.37(32.45), 99–224
Mean blood loss, mean (SD), range(ml)	64(13.2), 12–140
Stone-free rate, no. (%)	
Initial SFR	19(95%), lower pole residual small fragments largest 6 mm diameter.
Final SFR	18(90%), two patients with largest 6 mm fragments in lower pole.
Nephrostomy removal time, Mean, (SD), range (days)	6.3(0.5), 5–11
Hospitalization time, Mean, (SD), range (days)	12.11(2.77), 8–22
Lithotripsy, no. (%)	
Holmium laser	20(100)
Pneumatic lithotripter	14(70)
Cyberwand® dual probe ultrasonic	10(50)
Complications of operation, no. (%)	
Postoperative fever (>38.5°C)	4(20)
Prolonged tract leakage	1(5)
Urinary tract infection	2(10)
Stone analysis	
Calcium oxalate	5(25)
Calcium oxalate and phosphate	6(30)
Uric acid	2(10)
Struvite	3(15)
Mix	4(20)

was performed firstly to clear the stones in the peripheral calices, which would have needed a second or third nephrostomy access. Then the patient was placed in the prone position and single access PCNL performed to remove the residual stone.

In this study, combination of single-tract MPCNL and RIRS was performed in the second stage, when the drainage was clear and the visual fields were well. Take the advantage of single tract one-stage MPCNL, the residual stone burden can be fragmented by holmium laser or translocated into the renal pelvis, using a basket or grasp by RIRS doctor group. Simultaneously, MPCNL doctor group can manage the stone with effective intracorporeal lithotripsy or removed them with a forceps easier for previous access. Despite retrograde irrigation, stone fragments often fail to clear completely after intracorporeal lithotripsy. Combination of single-tract MPCNL and RIRS offers a larger bore access that can allow efficient removal of these remaining fragments. The mean whole operative duration was not significantly different from previous experience with standard multiple accesses PCNL had

Table 3. Serum creatinine, GFR of 18 patients and CKD stage of all patients before and after operation.

	Preoperative	Postoperative, 1 month	p value
Serum creatinine (umol/L)			
Mean(SD)	187.16(94.12)	140.99(57.92)	0.019
Range	77–580	77–420	
GFR (ml/min)			
Mean (SD)	43.80(24.74)	49.55(21.18)	0.05
Range	15.12–104.36	22.46–104.36	
CKD stage, no. (%)			0.48
1	1(5)	1(5)	
2	4(20)	4(20)	
3	8(40)	12(60)	
4	5(25)	1(5)	
5	2(10)	2(10)	

reported. The mean blood loss was 64 (12–140) ml, which was less than multiple-puncture PCNL had reported by other urologist [18,19]. The initial and final SFR were 95% and 90%, which was higher than the PCNL monotherapy (74% - 83%) [4] and Landman's study [29].

Previous study has demonstrated that no significant change in estimated Scr and GFR under PCNL with solitary kidney [28,30]. However there are at present no available well-constructed trials comparing the long-term renal effects of multiple-tract PCNL with single-tract PCNL. According to our surgical approach, regardless of 2 dialysis patients, a significant improvement in Scr and GFR was demonstrated. Mean Scr before operation was 187.16±94.12 umol/L compared to 140.99±57.92 umol/L by the end of 1-month follow-up period with statistical significance ($p = 0.019$). The same findings were observed in GFR in that before operation it was 43.80±24.74 ml/min and by the end of the 1-month follow-up it was 49.55±21.18 ml/min with statistical significance ($p = 0.05$). Four patients improved by CKD stage. However, there were no statistically significant differences between these parameters from 1 month to 1-year follow-up ($p > 0.05$). As is known, the most deleterious effect on renal function is neglected obstruction. If obstruction in a solitary kidney is rapidly relieved the kidney will regain basal function. It seems that our surgical approach did not adversely affect renal function.

In conclusion, our surgical approach modified here effectively decreases the number and size of percutaneous access tracts, which combines the advantages of both MPCNL and RIRS. It is safe, feasible, and efficient for managing staghorn calculi in solitary kidney with satisfactory SFR and reducing blood loss, potential morbidity associated with multiple tracts. The approach did not adversely affect renal function at both short-term and long-term follow-up.

Statement

The subjects included in figure 2 have given written informed consent, as outlined in the PLoS consent form, to publication of their photograph.

Author Contributions

Conceived and designed the experiments: DL YH YD XL. Performed the experiments: DL YH XL. Analyzed the data: DL YD. Contributed reagents/materials/analysis tools: DL YD. Wrote the paper: DL.

References

1. Preminger GM, Assimos DG, Lingeman JE, Nakada SY, Pearle MS, et al. (2005) AUA Nephrolithiasis Guideline Panel. Chapter 1: AUA guideline on management of staghorn calculi: Diagnosis and treatment recommendations. J Urol 173: 1991–2000.
2. Koga S, Arakaki Y, Matsuoka M, Ohyama C (1991) Staghorn calculi–long-term results of management. Br J Urol 68: 122–124.
3. Fernstrom I, Johansson B (1976) Percutaneous pyelolithotomy: a new extraction technique. Scand J Urol Nephrol 10: 257–259.
4. Singla M, Srivastava A, Kapoor R, Gupta N, Ansari MS, et al. (2008) Aggressive approach to staghorn calculi safety and efficacy of multiple tracts percutaneous nephrolithotomy. Urology 71: 1039–1042.
5. Michel MS, Trojan L, Rassweiler JJ (2007) Complications in percutaneous nephrolithotomy. Eur Urol 51: 899–906.
6. Jackman SV, Docimo SG, Cadeddu JA, Bishoff JT, Kavoussi LR, et al. (1998) The "mini-perc" technique: a less invasive alternative to percutaneous nephrolithotomy. World J Urol 16: 371–374.
7. Monga M, Oglevie S (2000) Minipercutaneous nephrolithotomy. J Endourol 14: 419–421.
8. Lahme S, Bichler KH, Strohmaier WL, Goetz T (2001) Minimally invasive PCNL in patients with renal pelvic and calyceal stones. Eur Urol 40: 619–624.
9. Bryniarski P, Paradysz A, Zyczkowski M, Kupilas A, Nowakowski K, et al. (2012) A randomized controlled study to analyze the safety and efficacy of percutaneous nephrolithotripsy and retrograde intrarenal surgery in the management of renal stones more than 2 cm in diameter. J Endourol 26(1): 52–7.
10. Soucy F, Ko R, Duvdevani M, Nott L, Denstedt JD, et al.(2009) Percutaneous nephrolithotomy for staghorn calculi: a single center's experience over 15 years. J Endourol 23(10): 1669–73.
11. Tiselius HG, Alken P, Buck C (2008) Guidelines on Urolithiasis. Arnhem: European Association of Urology.
12. Cockcroft DW, Gault MH (1976) Prdiction of creatinine clearance from serum creatinine. Nephron 16: 31.
13. El-Assmy A, El-Nahas AR, Hekal IA, Badran M, Youssef RF, et al. (2008) Long-term effects of extracorporeal shock wave lithotripsy on renal function:our experience with 156 patients with solitary kidney. J Urol 179: 2229–2232.
14. Levey AS, Coresh J, Balk E, Kausz AT, Levin A, et al. (2003) National Kidney Foundation practice guidelines for chronic kidney disease: evaluation, classification, and stratification. National Kidney Foundation. Ann Intern Med 139: 137.
15. Lazarus J, Williams J (2011) The Locator: novel percutaneous nephrolithotomy apparatus to aid collecting system puncture–a preliminary report. J Endourol. 25(5): 747–50.
16. Ibarluzea G, Scoffone CM, Cracco CM, Poggio M, Porpiglia F, et al. (2007) Supine Valdivia and modified lithotomy position for simultaneous anterograde and retrograde endourological access. BJU Int 100: 233–236.
17. Rassweiler JJ, Renner C, Eisenberger F (2000) The management of complex renal stones. BJU Int 86: 919–928.
18. Marguet CG, Springhart WP, Tan YH, Patel A, Undre S, et.al. (2005) Simultaneous combined use of flexible ureteroscopy and percutaneous nephrolithotomy to reduce the number of access tracts in the management of complex renal calculi. BJU Int 96(7): 1097–100.
19. Pietrow PK, Auge BK, Zhong P, Preminger GM (2003) Clinical efficacy of a combination pneumatic and ultrasonic lithotrite. J Urol 169: 1247–9.
20. Desai M, Ganpule AP (2008) Management of the staghorn calculus: multiple-tract versus single-tract percutaneous nephrolithotomy. Curr Opin Urol 18: 220–223.
21. Falahatkar S, Khosropanah I, Roshani A, Neiroomand H, Nikpour S, et al. (2008) Tubeless pecutaneous nephrolithotomy for staghorn stones. J Endouro 22: 1447–1451.
22. Williams SK, Leveillee RJ (2008) Management of staghorn calculus: single puncture with judicious use of the Xexible nephroscope. Curr Opin Urol 18: 224–228.
23. El-Nahas AR, Shokeir AA, El-Assmy AM, Mohsen T, Shoma AM, et al. (2007) Post-percutaneous nephrolithotomy extensive hemorrhage: a study of risk actors. J Urol 177: 576–579.
24. Zhong W, Zeng G, WU K, Li X, Chen W, et al. (2008) Does a smaller tract in percutaneous nephrolithotomy contribute to high renal pelvic pressure and postoperative fever? J Endourol 22: 2147–2151.
25. Xun LI, Zhaohui HE, Kaijun WU, Li SK, Zeng G, et al. (2009) Chinese Minimally Invasive Percutaneous Nephrolithotomy: The Guangzhou Experience. J Endourol 23: 1693–1697.

26. Auge BK, Dahm P, Bach T (2001) Critical analysis of multiple access PNL in managing complex renal calculi. J Endourol 15: A60.
27. Stoller ML, Wolf JS Jr, St Lezin MA (1994) Estimated blood loss and transfusion rates associated with percutaneous nephrolithotomy. J Urol 152: 1977–81.
28. Wong C, Leveillee RJ (2002) Single upper-pole percutaneous access for treatment of > or =5 cm complex branched staghorn calculi: is shockwave lithotripsy necessary? J Endourol 16: 477–481.
29. Landman J, Venkatesh R, Lee DI, Rehman J, Ragab M, et al. (2003) Combined percutaneous and retrograde approach to staghorn calculi with application of the ureteral access sheath to facilitate percutaneous nephrolithotomy. J Urol 169(1): 64–7.
30. Streem SB, Zelch MG, Risius B, Geisinger MA (1986) Percutaneous extraction of renal calculi in patients with solitary kidneys. Urology 27: 247.

8

Pure Laparoscopic and Robot-Assisted Laparoscopic Reconstructive Surgery in Congenital Megaureter: A Single Institution Experience

Weijun Fu[1*¶], Xu Zhang[1*¶], Xiaoyi Zhang[2¶], Peng Zhang[1], Jiangping Gao[1], Jun Dong[1], Guangfu Chen[1], Axiang Xu[1], Xin Ma[1], Hongzhao Li[1], Lixin Shi[1]

1 Department of Urology, PLA General Hospital/Medical school, Beijing, China, **2** Department of Urology, The Second Artillery General Hospital of PLA, Beijing, China

Abstract

To report our experience of pure laparoscopic and robot-assisted laparoscopic reconstructive surgery in congenital megaureter, seven patients (one bilateral) with symptomatic congenital megaureter underwent pure laparoscopic or robot-assisted laparoscopic surgery. The megaureter was exposed at the level of the blood vessel and was isolated to the bladder narrow area. Extreme ureter trim and submucosal tunnel encapsulation or papillary implantations and anti-reflux ureter bladder anastomosis were performed intraperitoneally by pure laparoscopic or robot-assisted laparoscopic surgery. The clinical data of seven patients after operation were analyzed, including the operation time, intraoperative complications, intraoperative bleeding volumes, postoperative complications, postoperative hospitalization time and pathological results. All of the patients were followed. The operation was successfully performed in seven patients. The mean operation times for pure laparoscopic surgery and robotic-assistant laparoscopic surgery were 175 (range: 150–220) and 187 (range: 170–205) min, respectively, and the mean operative blood loss volumes were 20 (range: 10–30) and 28.75 (range: 15–20) ml, respectively. There were no intraoperative complications. The postoperative drainage time was 5 (range: 4–6) and 5.75 (range: 5–6) d, respectively, and the indwelling catheter time was 6.33 (range: 4–8) d and 7 (range: 7–7) d, respectively. The postoperative hospitalization time was 7.67 (range: 7–8) d and 8 (range: 7–10) d, respectively. There was no obvious pain, no secondary bleeding and no urine leakage after the operation. Postoperative pathology reports revealed chronic urothelial mucosa inflammation. The follow-up results confirmed that all patients were relieved of their symptoms. Both pure laparoscopic and robot-assisted laparoscopic surgery using different anti-reflux ureter bladder anastomoses are safe and effective approaches in the minimally invasive treatment of congenital megaureter.

Editor: Lorna Marson, Centre for Inflammation Research, United Kingdom

Funding: This work was supported by the National High Technology Research and Development Program ("863"Program) of China (NO. 2012AA021100). The funder had no role in study design, data collection and analysis, decision to publish, or preparation of the manuscript.

Competing Interests: The authors have declared that no competing interests exist.

* E-mail: fuweijun68@hotmail.com (WF); xuzhang@foxmail.com (XZ)

¶ These authors contributed equally to this work.

Introduction

Congenital megaureter is a rare adult urinary tract anomaly that is due to distal ureteral muscle abnormalities, the loss of peristalsis from the vesicoureteral connection and vesicoureteral obstruction. Therefore, excision of the diseased segment plus with reimplantation of the distal ureter is often required.[1] Traditionally, open ureteral reparation and reimplantation is the gold standard therapy for primary symptomatic obstructive megaureter. Within the past decade, however, laparoscopic surgery has become popular in urology and has resulted in improved outcomes compared with open surgery, even in reconstruction procedures.[2] Today, the Da Vinci robot-assisted laparoscopic surgery platform (Intuitive Surgical, Sunnyvale, CA), which is characterized by stereoscopic vision and a flexible operating arm, provides us with the distinct advantages of minimally invasive reconstruction of the urinary tract, particularly in intracorporeal reparation and suturing. Particularly, for lower urinary tract reconstruction surgery, which is likely to be delayed by the narrow pelvic space, the robot-assisted laparoscopic surgery platform can be advantageous.[3] Here, we present our experience in the treatment of primary symptomatic obstructive megaureter by intracorporeal ureteral reparation, suturing and different anti-reflux methods using traditional pure laparoscopic surgery and robot-assisted laparoscopic surgery. To the best of our knowledge, this is the first time that ureteroneocystostomy has been reported to be performed by pure robotic repair followed by different anti-reflux strategies with a reasonable follow-up time.

Materials and Methods

The study was reviewed and approved by an institutional review board (IRB) of the Chinese PLA Medical School. Written informed consent was obtained from all participants before the initiation of study procedures. The stored specimen and database analysis was approved by the IRB and ethics committee at Chinese PLA Medical School.

We retrospectively reviewed seven patients (one of these patients exhibited bilateral megaureters) undergoing traditional pure laparoscopic surgery or robot-assisted laparoscopic surgery for primary symptomatic obstructive megaureter from December 2009 to August 2013 at PLA General Hospital (Beijing, China) (**Table 1**). There were two male patients and five female patients with a mean age of 28.14 years. All patients were evaluated by urinalysis, urine culture and assays of serum urea and creatinine levels as well as by imaging with ultrasonography, intravenous urography, computed tomography and emission computer tomography (ECT) renography. All surgeries were performed by experienced surgeons. (**Figure 1**)

For traditional pure laparoscopic surgery, the patient was placed in a supine position. The primary 10-mm port for the camera was placed along the lower lip of the umbilicus in the midline, and 2 secondary ports (5 mm and 12 mm) were placed in the mid clavicular lines on either side 2 fingers lower than the camera port. An additional 5 port mm for the assistant was placed 2 cm above the iliac crest if necessary.

For robot-assisted laparoscopic surgery, a low dorsal lithotomy with a steep Trendelenburg position was used. Trocar placement was distributed to 5 points. A 12 mm port for the camera was placed three fingers superior to the umbilicus. Two 8-mm robotic ports for arm 1 and 2 were placed 8 cm lateral to umbilicus. A port for arm 3 was placed 8 cm contralaterally parallel to arm 1 or 2. An additional 12-mm port for the assistant was placed in the anterior axillary line 2 cm above the iliac crest on the ipsilateral surgical side of the ureter.

Monopolar scissors and bipolar grasping forceps were used to cut the Toldt line. The colon was reflected medially to expose the megaureter at the bifurcation of the common iliac vessels. The reproductive vessels were protected, and the megaureter was gently grasped with a latex band by robotic arm 3. The megaureter was isolated down to the distal ureteral stricture segment with attention to the preservation of the ureteral adventitia. The bladder was then filled with 150 ml normal saline and isolated fully along the Retzius space. The lateral top of the free bladder was fixed to the on psoas muscle by suturing, if necessary.

The ureter was partially amputated at the junction of the stricture and the dilated section of the ureter. To facilitated trimming and suturing, the ureter was drafted by a rubber belt or robot arm 3. The ureter was longitudinally sharply incised in a 3–4 cm extension over a 7-Fr plastic urethral catheter and, for heavy dilated in megaureter, intracorporeally tailored using a 4-zero absorbed polyglactin running suture. The ureteral stricture specimen was mobilized and excised for histopathological examination.

We applied two methods to achieve anti-reflux, submucosal tunnel reimplantation or ureteral nipple implantation according to the degree of dilated in megaureter of patients to avoid the post-operative stricture. For those seriously dilated megaureter we chose ureteral nipple implantation; however, for those slightly dilated megaureter we chose submucosal tunnel reimplantation. For submucosal tunnel reimplantation, the bladder was filled with normal saline and longitudinally opened in the posterolateral aspect to expose the mucosa of the bladder. A submucosal tunnel was created with blunt dissection at the lowest part of the bladder with a ratio of 5:1 between the tunnel length and the diameter of the ureteral orifice. The ureter was positioned through the submucosal tunnel and a mucosa-to-mucosa ureterovesical anastomosis was completed with 4-zero absorbed polyglactin interrupted sutures. During this procedure, a 7Fr double J stent was passed into the ureter and advanced to the renal pelvis, and its

Table 1. Patient general information.

Patient	Sex	Age	Magaureter Side	Method	Operating Time(min)	Bleeding (mL)	Follow-up Time (mo)	Result
1	F	24	Right	Laparoscopic	150	10	46	Relieved
2	M	20	Left	Laparoscopic	155	20	38	Relieved
3	F	37	Bilateral	Laparoscopic/Right	220	30	17	Relieved/Right
				Laparoscopic/Left				Relieved/Left
4	M	25	Left	Robot-assisted	190	20	3	Relieved
5	F	35	Left	Robot-assisted	170	15	57	Relieved
6	F	32	Left	Robot-assisted	205	30	4	Relieved
7	F	24	Left	Robot-assisted	185	50	3	Relieved

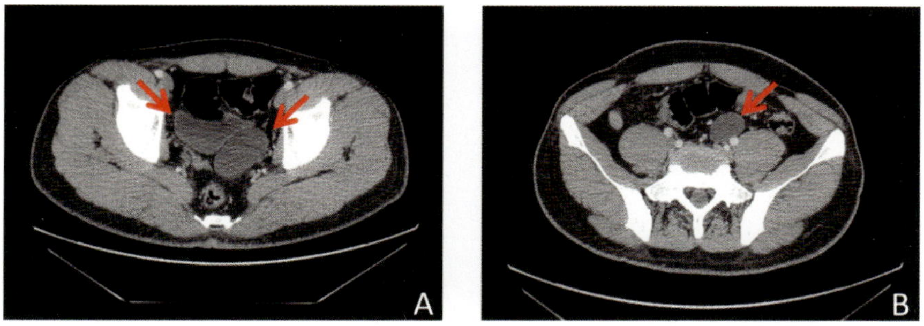

Figure 1. Preoperative CT scan of two patients. (A) The megaureter and bladder could be identified by CT scan. (B) The megaureter could be identified by CT scan.

distal end was fixed in the bladder. Subsequently, a running single layer suture with 2-zero polyglactin closed the bladder muscle. For this method, the ureter was covered with bladder detrusor muscle by suturing to form an anti-reflux submucosal tunnel (**Figure 2 A–C**).

For ureteral nipple implantation, the distal ureter was tailored and formed into a nipple structure. Subsequently, the bladder detrusor and mucosa were dissected laterally. At the position 6 o'clock to the anastomotic stoma, the bladder was sutured full-thickness with the seromuscular layer to the ureter at a distance of 1.5 cm to the end. Subsequently, a 7-Fr double J stent was indwelled. After the fixation at 12 o'clock position of the anastomotic stoma, an additional 4 interrupted sutures were performed bilaterally to complete the anastomosis (**Figure 2 D–F**, **Figure 3**).

A 14-Fr Nelaton drain was indwelled within the 5-mm port. Intravenous pyelography for the evaluation of residual obstruction and voiding cystourethrography for the evaluation of residual vesicoureteral reflux were performed postoperatively in all of the patients. Urinalysis, urine culture, assays of serum urea and creatinine levels and renal ultrasonography were also performed to evaluate renal function after the operation. The 7-Fr double J stent placed in operation was removed 4 weeks after operation by cystoscope.

Results

All of the operations were successfully completed. The mean operation time of pure laparoscopic surgery and robotic-assisted laparoscopic surgery were 175 (range: 150–220) min and 187 (range: 170–205) min, with an average intraoperative estimated blood loss of 20 (range: 10–30) ml and 28.75 (range: 15–20) ml, respectively. No major complications occurred during the two surgeries. Drainage times were 5 (range: 4–6) d and 5.75 (range: 5–6) d, respectively, and indwelling catheter times were 6.33 (range: 4–8) d and 7 (range: 7–7) d, respectively. The mean lengths of the postoperative hospital stay were 7.67 (range: 7–8) d and 8 (range: 7–10) d for the two groups, respectively. No significant postoperative pain, secondary bleeding, incontinence or other complications were observed after the operation. Histopathological reports for all of the patients revealed chronic inflammation of the urothelial mucosa (**Figure 4**). The double J ureteral stent was removed at 4 weeks after the operation.

The mean follow-up was 24 (range: 3–57) months. All patients experienced symptomatic relief. Follow-up ultrasonography and intravenous urography confirmed good drainage combined with a reduction of hydronephrosis. A statistically significant reduction was also achieved in the follow-up ureteral diameter compared with the preoperative ureteral diameter (**Figure 5**). The function of the salvaged kidney was preserved when compared with preoperative function. Nonobstructed clearance was also documented on diuretic renogram in all patients. The results retrograde cystogram also ensured that both of our two anti-reflux anastomses methods for reimplantation gained approving results. (Table 1).

Discussion

Congenital megaureter is caused by a short or absent intravesical ureter, congenital para-ureteric diverticulum or other derangements of the vesico-ureteric junction (VUJ). According to the international classification, congenital megaureter can be classified as obstructed, refluxing or unobstructed and unrefluxing.[1] Congenital megaureter is most frequently observed in males of 30–40 years old. Most patients report lower back pain, and 1/3 present with stones. For clinical treatment, surgery of megaureter tailoring plus ureteroneocystostomy is recommended.[4]

Patients with congenital megaureter can undergo a variety of surgical treatment, including endoincision with stent indwelling, trimmed or not trimmed VUJ anastomosis or nephroureterectomy, on the basis of the ureter state and residual renal function. In situations of competent renal function, one commonly used surgical approach is to remove the non-functioning ureter followed by distal ureter bladder anastomosis. With traditional technical limitations, the open space of the narrow pelvis must be exposed during surgery, which requires for a large abdominal incision. This approach leads to increased complications and delayed postoperative recovery.[5]

To reduce complications and shorten recovery time, minimally invasive surgery, including endoscopic incision and laparoscopic ureteral reimplantation, has been proposed in recent years. Although transurethral endoscopic laser or electronic ureteral resection provided good short-term results, further observation of its long-term effects are needed. [6,7] In recent years, laparoscopic ureteral reimplantation has been widely recommended in the treatment of congenital megaureter as a minimally invasive therapy. Pure laparoscopic reconstructive surgery requires extensive experience in laparoscopic surgery. Even for skilled surgeon, pure laparoscopic reconstructive surgery is a challenging technique.

The robot-assisted laparoscopic platform provides a new opportunity for complex urinary tract reconstruction surgery. The use of this approach in upper urinary tract reconstruction surgery has been widely reported and has proven to exhibit good

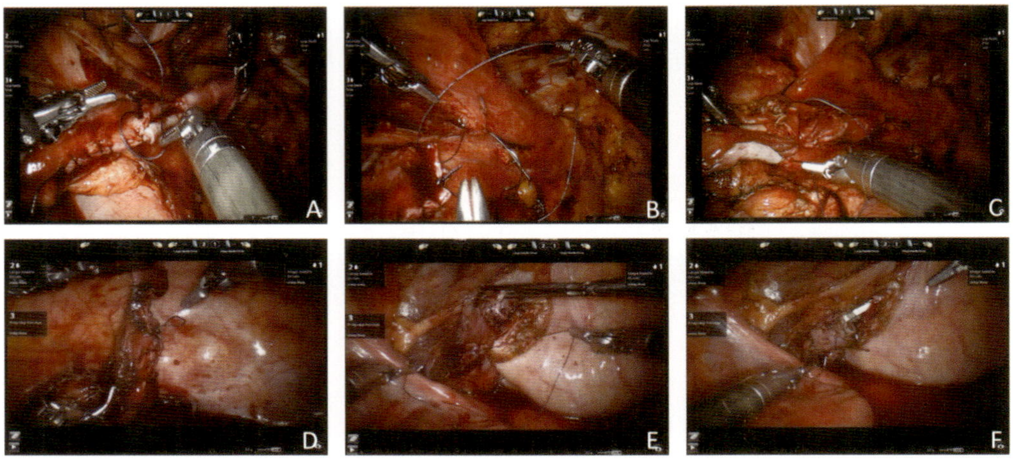

Figure 2. Robot-assisted laparoscopic surgery in congenital megaureter (A–C,submucosal tunnel reimplantation; D–E, direct ureteral nipple implantation). (A) The megaureter was intracorporeally tailored using a 4-zero absorbed polyglactin running suture. (B) The ureter was positioned through the submucosal tunnel and a mucosa-to-mucosa ureterovesical anastomosis was completed with 4-zero absorbed polyglactin interrupted sutures. (C) A running single layer suture with 2-zero polyglactin closed the bladder muscle. (D) The distal ureter was tailored and formed into a nipple. (E) The bladder was sutured full-thickness with the seromuscular layer to the ureter at a distance of 1.5 cm to the end at the 6 o'clock position to the anastomotic stoma. (F) After the fixation 4 interrupted sutures were made bilaterally to complete the anastomosis at the 12 o'clock position.

long-term results.[8] Robot-assisted laparoscopic ureteral reimplantation, vesico-ureteric anastomosis, psoas muscle fixation and bladder valvuloplasty have also been reported, which have provided us with new approaches to the minimally invasive treatment of distal ureteral reconstruction.[9,10] The robot-assisted surgery system has better dimensional vision and a more flexible operating arm and is therefore more suitable for narrow space reconstruction surgery.[11] In the lower urinary tract (lower ureter, the bladder and prostate) robot-assisted laparoscopic surgery, patients are placed in the low lithotomy position to facilitate the placement of the robot arm. Trocar placement for distal ureteral operations aims to provide the best operating space in the pelvic. During our surgery, robot arm 3 was used to hold the tissue dynamically. These alterations provide advantages by narrowing the necessary operating compared with pure laparoscopic surgeries.

In our single-institution study, we applied both pure laparoscopic and robot-assisted laparoscopic surgeries to patients with primary symptomatic obstructive megaureter. In both approaches, we tailored and sutured the megaureter intracorporeally to reduce the invasion of the ureter. In addition, we applied the vesico-ureteric anastomosis using two different methods, submucosal tunnel reimplantation or ureteral nipple implantation, to achieve an anti-reflux effect. To our knowledge, ureteral nipple implantation is not conventional according to the previous reports.

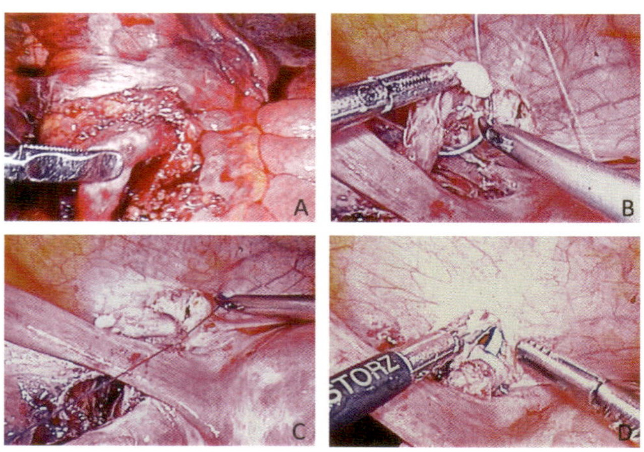

Figure 3. Pure laparoscopic surgery in congenital megaureter. (A) The megaureter was exposed at the bifurcation of the common iliac vessels. (B–C) The bladder was sutured full-thickness with the seromuscular layer to the ureter at a distance of 1.5 cm to the 6 o'clock position to the anastomotic stoma. (D) A 7-Fr double J stent was indwelled.

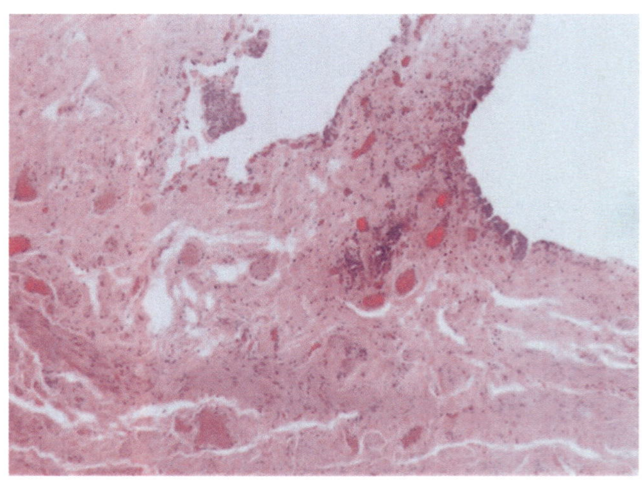

Figure 4. Histopathological reports for all the patients revealed chronic inflammation of the urothelial mucosa.

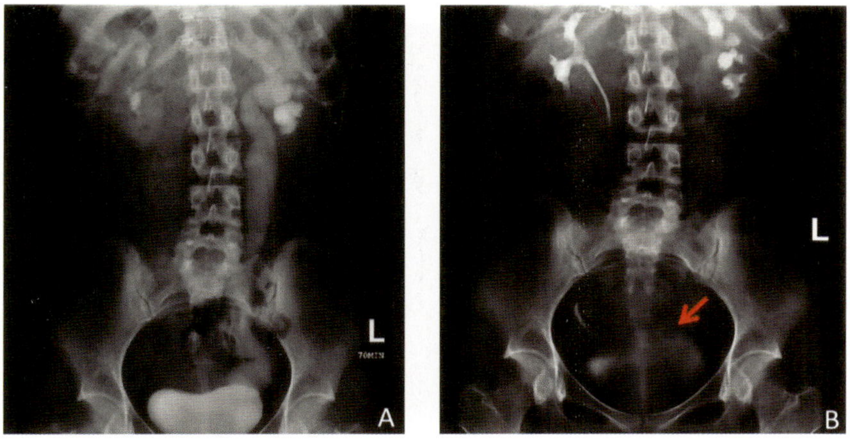

Figure 5. Preoperative and postoperative intravenous pyelography of one patient. (A) Preoperative intravenous pyelography of one megaureter patient. (B) Forty-months postoperative intravenous pyelography of one megaureter patient. The megaureter and hydronephrosis were relieved. The appearance of a filling defect due to the left nipple was identified.

[12,13] Al-Shukri and Alwan first reported direct nipple ureteroneocystostomy in patients with ureteral stricture.[14] Here, we approved several cases of ureteral nipple implantation, including pure laparoscopic and robot-assisted laparoscopic surgery. In both pure laparoscopic and robot-assisted laparoscopic surgery, we perform direct nipple ureteroneocystostomy by suturing the bladder full-thickness with the seromuscular layer of the ureter at a distance of 1.5 cm to the end at the 6 and 12 o'clock positions of the anastomotic stoma. Subsequently, 4 additional interrupted sutures are made bilaterally to complete the anastomosis. During this procedure, the double J stent is placed. According to the postoperative examinations, the anti-reflux effect of this strategy has demonstrated that it is a simple, safe and feasible means of vesico-ureteric anastomosis. In particular, the ureteral nipple implantation shortens the operative time.

These groups of patients in our center have been treated with pure laparoscopic surgery or robotic-assisted laparoscopic surgery. Both approaches have reasonable and similar operating times and blood loss, but robotic ureteroneocystostomy is easier and takes less time than pure laparoscopic ureteroneocystostomy. However, robotic surgery is new to China, and with the accumulation of experiences, the operation time will be shortened further in the future. There were no major complications occurred during or after the operations. The drainage time, indwelling catheter times and postoperative hospital stays were similar for both the pure laparoscopic and robot-assisted laparoscopic surgeries. According to our latest follow-up, all of the patients were symptomatically recovered. Hydronephrosis in 8 megaureters of 7 patients was relieved as confirmed by postoperative examinations. The results of the follow-up have demonstrated that the salvaged kidneys well drained and resolved of hydronephrosis, and their functions were preserved when compared with the preoperative examinations.

Conclusion

In summary, both pure laparoscopic and robot-assisted laparoscopic surgery for megaureter are technically feasible and safe. However, in our study, the number of cases is insufficient, and the follow-up time is short for some of the cases. More experience in robot-assisted laparoscopic surgery should be accumulated in future work. In the future, more clinical data are required to prove the convenience of robot-assisted laparoscopic surgery in complex genitourinary reconstructive operations.

Acknowledgments

The authors would like to thank Professors Xu Zhang (Department of Urology, PLA General Hospital) for his support, helpful advice and many valuable scientific discussions throughout the project.

Author Contributions

Conceived and designed the experiments: WJF XZ XYZ. Performed the experiments: WJF XZ XYZ PZ JPG JD GFC. Analyzed the data: AXX XM HZL LXS. Contributed reagents/materials/analysis tools: WJF XZ XYZ PZ JPG. Wrote the paper: WJF XZ XYZ PZ.

References

1. Shokeir AA, Nijman RJ (2000) Primary megaureter: current trends in diagnosis and treatment. BJU Int 86: 861–868.
2. Abraham GP, Das K, Ramaswami K, Siddaiah AT, George D, et al. (2012) Laparoscopic reconstruction for obstructive megaureter: single institution experience with short- and intermediate-term outcomes. J Endourol 26: 1187–1191.
3. Hemal AK, Nayyar R, Rao R (2009) Robotic repair of primary symptomatic obstructive megaureter with intracorporeal or extracorporeal ureteric tapering and ureteroneocystostomy. J Endourol 23: 2041–2046.
4. Hemal AK, Ansari MS, Doddamani D, Gupta NP (2003) Symptomatic and complicated adult and adolescent primary obstructive megaureter-indications for surgery: Analysis, outcome, and follow-up. Urology 61: 703–707.
5. Dorairajan LN, Hemal AK, Gupta NP, Wadhwa SN (1999) Primary obstructive megaureter in adults: need for an aggressive management strategy. Int Urol Nephrol 31: 633–641.
6. Bapat S, Bapat M, Kirpekar D (2000) Endoureterotomy for congenital primary obstructive megaureter: preliminary report. J Endourol 14: 263–267.
7. Biyani CS, Powell CS (2001) Congenital megaureter in adults: Endoscopic management with holmium: YAG laser - Preliminary experience. Journal of Endourology 15: 797–799.
8. Mufarrij PW, Woods M, Shah OD, Palese MA, Berger AD, et al. (2008) Robotic dismembered pyeloplasty: a 6-year, multi-institutional experience. J Urol 180: 1391–1396.
9. Patil NN, Mottrie A, Sundaram B, Patel VR (2008) Robotic-assisted laparoscopic ureteral reimplantation with psoas hitch: a multi-institutional, multinational evaluation. Urology 72: 47–50; discussion 50.

10. Thiel DD, Badger WJ, Winfield HN (2008) Robot-Assisted Laparoscopic Excision and Ureteroureterostomy for Congenital Midureteral Stricture. Journal of Endourology 22: 2667–2669.
11. Schimpf MO, Wagner JR (2009) Robot-Assisted Laparoscopic Distal Ureteral Surgery. Jsls-Journal of the Society of Laparoendoscopic Surgeons 13: 44–49.
12. Tatlisen A, Ekmekcioglu O (2005) Direct nipple ureteroneocystostomy in adults with primary obstructed megaureter. J Urol 173: 877–880.
13. Chung H, Jeong BC, Kim HH (2006) Laparoscopic ureteroneocystostomy with vesicopsoas hitch: nonrefluxing ureteral reimplantation using cystoscopy-assisted submucosal tunneling. J Endourol 20: 632–638.
14. Al-Shukri S, Alwan MH (1983) Bilharzial strictures of the lower third of the ureter: a critical review of 560 strictures. Br J Urol 55: 477–482.

Comparative Effects of Snoring Sound between Two Minimally Invasive Surgeries in the Treatment of Snoring

Li-Ang Lee[1,2,3], Jen-Fang Yu[4], Yu-Lun Lo[2,5], Ning-Hung Chen[2,5], Tuan-Jen Fang[1,2], Chung-Guei Huang[6], Wen-Nuan Cheng[7], Hsueh-Yu Li[1,2*]

1 Department of Otorhinolaryngology-Head and Neck Surgery, Chang Gung Memorial Hospital at Linkou, School of Medicine, College of Medicine, Chang Gung University, Taoyuan, Taiwan, R.O.C., **2** Sleep Center, Chang Gung Memorial Hospital at Linkou, Taoyuan, Taiwan, R.O.C., **3** Department of Otolaryngology, Xiamen Chang Gung Hospital, Xiamen, Fujian Province, China, **4** Graduate Institute of Medical Mechatronics, Taiouan Interdisciplinary Otolaryngology Laboratory, Chang Gung University, Taoyuan, Taiwan, R.O.C., **5** Department of Pulmonary and Critical Care Medicine, Chang Gung Memorial Hospital at Linkou, School of Medicine, College of Medicine, Chang Gung University, Taoyuan, Taiwan, R.O.C., **6** Department of Laboratory Medicine, Chang Gung Memorial Hospital at Linkou, College of Medicine, Chang Gung University, Taoyuan, Taiwan, R.O.C., **7** Graduate School of Recreation and Sports Management, Taipei Physical Education College, Taipei, Taiwan, R.O.C.

Abstract

Background: Minimally invasive surgeries of the soft palate have emerged as a less-invasive treatment for habitual snoring. To date, there is only limited information available comparing the effects of snoring sound between different minimally invasive surgeries in the treatment of habitual snoring.

Objective: To compare the efficacy of palatal implant and radiofrequency surgery, in the reduction of snoring through subjective evaluation of snoring and objective snoring sound analysis.

Patients and Method: Thirty patients with habitual snoring due to palatal obstruction (apnea-hypopnea index ≤15, body max index ≤30) were prospectively enrolled and randomized to undergo a single session of palatal implant or temperature-controlled radiofrequency surgery of the soft palate under local anesthesia. Snoring was primarily evaluated by the patient with a 10 cm visual analogue scale (VAS) at baseline and at a 3-month follow-up visit and the change in VAS was the primary outcome. Moreover, life qualities, measured by snore outcomes survey, and full-night snoring sounds, analyzed by a sound analytic program (Snore Map), were also investigated at the same time.

Results: Twenty-eight patients completed the study; 14 received palatal implant surgery and 14 underwent radiofrequency surgery. The VAS and snore outcomes survey scores were significantly improved in both groups. However, the good response (postoperative VAS ≤3 or postoperative VAS ≤5 plus snore outcomes survey score ≥60) rate of the palatal implant group was significantly higher than that of the radiofrequency group (79% *vs.* 29%, P = 0.021). The maximal loudness of low-frequency (40–300 Hz) snores was reduced significantly in the palatal implant group. In addition, the snoring index was significantly reduced in the radiofrequency group.

Conclusions: Both palatal implants and a single-stage radiofrequency surgery improve subjective snoring outcomes, but palatal implants have a greater effect on most measures of subjective and objective snoring. Multi-stage radiofrequency surgery was not tested.

Editor: Oscar Arias-Carrion, Hospital General Dr. Manuel Gea González, Mexico

Funding: This study was financially supported by a grant from the National Science Council, Taiwan (NSC 99-2314-B-182A-099-MY2) and the Chang Gung Memorial Hospital, Taiwan (CMRPG3A1501-2). The funders had no role in study design, data collection and analysis, decision to publish, or preparation of the manuscript.

Competing Interests: The authors have declared that no competing interests exist.

* E-mail: hyli38@ cgmh.org.tw

Introduction

Recent publications have demonstrated reductions in snoring with several minimally invasive surgery (MIS) methods of the soft palate including radiofrequency (RF) surgery and palatal implant (PI) [1,2]. Despite modest effects in the treatment of obstructive sleep apnea [1–4], patients often wish to receive MIS for habitual snoring. However, the efficacy in reducing snoring has mainly been determined by self-reported questionnaires in the past. Further, the definition of surgical success in snoring treatment has not been universally defined. To date, changes in snoring sound characteristics following MIS have not been demonstrated.

Many cohort studies and a few randomized controlled trials or clinical controlled trials have compared MIS with a placebo [5–9], different energy generators [10], different material rigidity [11], or different operative techniques [12,13]. RF of the soft palate produces volumetric tissue reduction [14] and selective scar tissue [5] to reduce obstruction and induce stiffness. However, the RF energy delivered to the soft palate can be inadequate and may result in residual or recurrent snoring [7,15]. PI can decrease palatal flutter by increasing the rigidity of the soft palate through implant identity and tissue fibrosis [16,17]. In addition, PI can be chronically retained in the muscle layer of the soft palate thereby producing a long-term anti-snoring effect [18,19]. Nevertheless, whether PI provides a better efficacy in the treatment of snoring than RF surgery is still unknown.

The primary aim of the current study was to compare the anti-snoring effect between PI and RF by subjective assessments in a randomized controlled parallel trial. The secondary aim was to explore and compare the acoustic changes in snoring sounds after PI and RF.

Materials and Methods

The protocol for this trial and supporting CONSORT checklist are available as supporting information; see Protocol S1 and Checklist S1.

Ethics Statement

This study was approved by the Institutional Review Board of Chang Gung Memorial Hospital and conducted according to the principles expressed in the Declaration of Helsinki. Signed informed consent was obtained from all patients. Full details of the trial protocol can be found in the Supplementary Appendix, available with the full text of this article at www.plosone.org.

Participants and Setting

This study was a prospective, randomized, parallel-controlled, open labeled trial that was conducted from August 1, 2010 to July 30, 2012 in a tertiary medical center (Department of Otorhinolaryngology, Head and Neck Surgery, Chang Gung Memorial Hospital at Linkou, Taoyuan, Taiwan). The flowchart diagram following the CONSORT 2010 guideline demonstrated our study design (Figure 1). No important changes to methods (such as eligibility criteria) have been made after trial commencement. Thirty-four patients with habitual snoring and apnea-hypopnea index (AHI) ≤15 events/h confirmed by standard full-night polysomnography were prospectively recruited from October 1, 2010 to March 30, 2012 for the treatment of snoring by the two MIS methods. Standard level I polysomnography (Nicolet UltraSom System, Madison, WI, USA) was performed in the sleep laboratory to document sleep parameters in each patient. All respiratory events were scored as per standard criteria [20].

The inclusion criteria were: a) age, 18–60 years; b) body mass index, ≤30 kg/m^2; c) length of the soft palate (from the uvula base to the hard palate-soft palate junction) ≥2.5 cm and the width of the base of the uvular ≥1.0 cm (Figure 2). These criteria were basically in accordance with the criteria for a PI procedure as described in the literature [6,9,11,16]. Patients were excluded if they had tonsillar hypertrophy (tonsil size ≥3), high tongue position (Friedman tongue position ≥4), retrognathia, craniofacial abnormalities, trismus, allergy to anesthetic or poorly controlled medical disorders such as hypertension, bleeding tendency, cardiovascular disorder, and stroke. Four patients were excluded due to 'Not meeting inclusion criteria ($n = 3$)' and 'Declined to participate ($n = 1$)'.

Therefore, 30 participants were therefore enrolled in the present study. Subjective assessments of snoring and snoring sound recording were conducted after enrollment. The randomization procedure assured balanced design in subjective snoring severity and we stratified our subjects into two subgroups: 'VAS >7' ($n = 12$) and 'VAS ≤7' subgroups ($n = 18$). Computer-generated lists of random numbers were created using Random Number Generators of SPSS software for allocation of the participants and were stratified by center with a 1:1 allocation using a fixed block size of 6 (Rv. Uniform [0, 1]) in both subgroups. Participants were enrolled by four authors (LAL, YLL, NHC, and HYL). The allocation sequence was concealed from the researcher (CGH) before operation and the MIS procedure was performed by a single surgeon (HYL) who adhered to our computer-generated randomization protocol. Participants were randomly allocated to either PI or RF group (Figure 1). Half of the patients were randomized to the PI group and the remaining patients were randomized to the RF group. Subjective and objective assessments were re-measured 3 months following the MIS.

Snoring Sound Assessment

Subjective snoring questionnaires. The snoring of all subjects was assessed by two subjective surveys: visual analogue scale (VAS) and snore outcomes survey (SOS) questionnaires. The participants, based on descriptions from their spouse or bed partner, were asked to estimate the severity of their snoring using a 10 cm VAS from 0 (no snoring) to 10 (very severe snoring, bed partner leaves the room). The SOS questionnaire was comprised of eight Likert-type items to comprehensively evaluate the duration, loudness, and frequency of snoring. The scale of the SOS was normalized from 0 (worst) to 100 (best) [21]. The Mandarin Chinese version of the SOS has been validated and repeatedly used as an outcome measure in obstructive sleep apnea patients [22].

Objective snoring sound analysis. We collected full-night snoring sounds of each subject in a standard sleep laboratory using a snore detection system as described previously [23]. An external measurement microphone (TEDS type 46AE, G.R.A.S. Corp., Holte, Denmark) was positioned 100 cm above the patient's head to record the snoring sounds in the sleep laboratory [23,24]. Calibration of sound pressure level was performed before each test. The environmental sounds of the study room were recorded for 10 minutes as the background signal and analyzed. The recorded snoring sounds were detected by portable data cards (PXI 4462, National Instruments Corp., Austin, TX, USA) and processed by digital recording software (Sound & Vibration Toolkit for Labview, National Instruments Corp., Austin, TX, USA) at a sample rate of 44,100 Hz. The frequency power spectrum was created by fast Fourier transformation (range, 3.15 Hz–2,000 Hz).

After the patients had fallen asleep naturally and started to snore, we continually recorded the snoring sounds for 6 hours. Snoring sound signals were analyzed by the specially designed computer program Snore Map (Chang Gung Memorial Hospital, Taoyuan, Taiwan, R.O.C.). In accordance with an observer-blind study, the snoring sound recorder and the analyzer (JFY) were blind to the results of the randomization. The details of our snoring sound detection algorithm have been described elsewhere [23]. Using this method, we calculated the snoring index (SI [event/hour]), maximal sound intensity (Imax [dB]), mean sound intensity (Imean [dB]), peak sound frequency (Fpeak [Hz]), and mean sound frequency (Fmean [Hz]) in 4 different frequency domains (40 Hz–2,000 Hz [total-frequency, Total], 40 Hz–

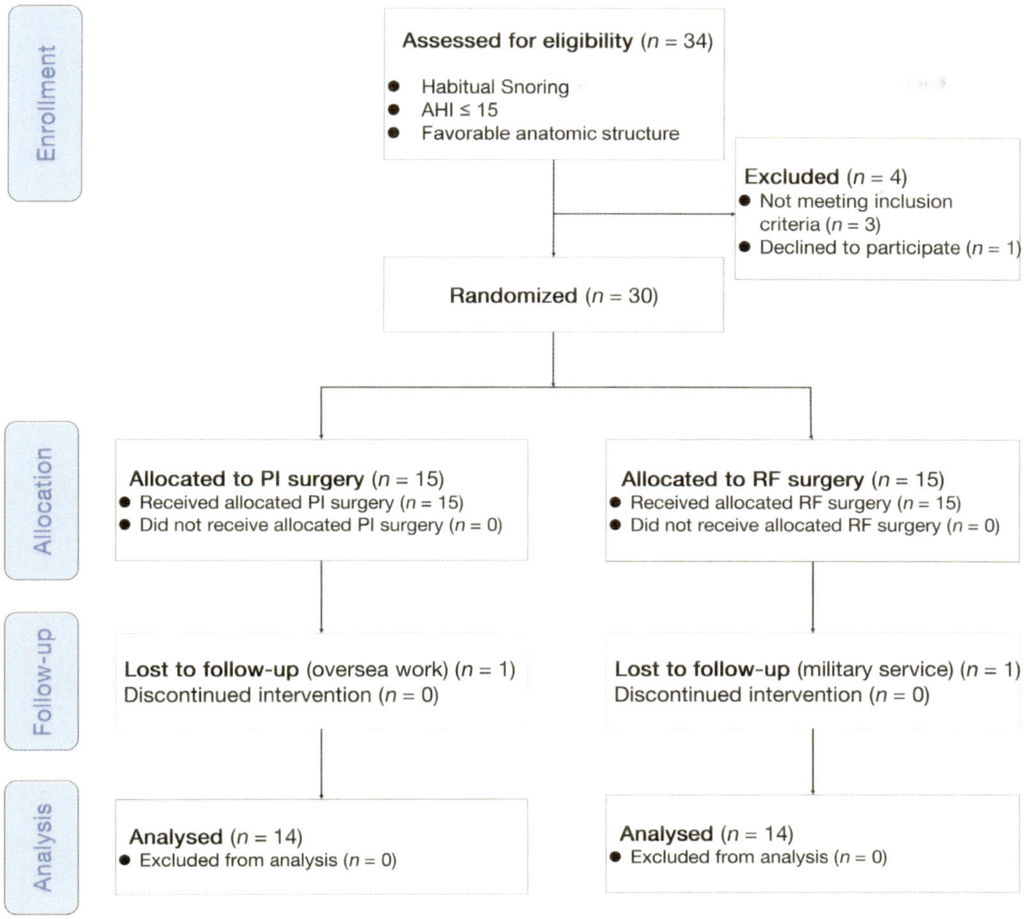

Figure 1. Schematic diagram (CONSORT 2010 flowchart diagram) summarizing the study design. AHI: apnea-hypopnea index. PI: palatal implant; RF, radiofrequency. SOS: snoring outcomes survey. VAS: visual analogue scale.

300 Hz [low-frequency, B1], 301 Hz–850 Hz [mid-frequency, B2], and 851 Hz–2,000 Hz [high-frequency, B3]).

In this study, we focused on the acoustic changes of Total- and B1-frequency domains due to the soft palate producing low frequency snores (<300 Hz) [25] and being operated on by the two different MIS.

MIS

The patients underwent a session of either PI surgery or temperature-controlled RF surgery under local anesthesia on an outpatient basis. Before the MIS procedure, the palate was anesthetized by applying a topical 10% xylocaine spray followed by injection of a local anesthetic mixture of 2% lidocaine with diluted adrenaline (1:100,000). All of the study subjects were given antibiotics (ampicillin 500 mg q6h for 5 days) and analgesics (acetaminophen 500 mg q6h when required).

PI surgery. Using the delivery tool of the PI system (Pillar, Medtronic Inc., Jacksonville, FL, USA), the mucosa of the soft palate close to the hard palate-soft palate junction (approximate 0.5 cm) was punctured in the midline [26]. The needle was inserted to the uvular muscle and moved parallel to the curve of the soft palate towards the tip of the uvula. After reaching the insertion point, the implant was delivered steadily after which the needle was withdrawn. This process was repeated for the second and third implants in the bilateral para-midline with a 0.2 cm horizontal distance from the first implant (Figure 3).

RF surgery. RF energy was delivered via a generator (Somnus Model S2, Gyrus-ACMI Corporation, Maple Grove, MN, USA) with the power set to 10 watts and the maximal target temperature to 85°C. The needle electrode was inserted through the mucosa into the muscle layer at the entry points (approximately 1 cm below the hard palate-soft palate junction). The electrode was kept in place until 600 J had been delivered at the midline and 300 J at both para-midline sites (approximately 1 cm horizontal distance; Figure 4) [13,27].

Outcomes

The mean change in VAS before and after MIS was the primary outcome measurement. The mean changes in SOS and acoustic characteristics of snoring sound were the secondary outcome measurements. Postoperative 'VAS ≤3' was traditionally defined as 'major response' [28]. For a comprehensive profile of the outcomes, we further created another definition of 'fine response': 'postoperative VAS ≤5 plus SOS ≥60' post hoc in the present study. Accordingly, we compare a 'good response' rate, defined herein by a postoperative VAS ≤3 or postoperative VAS ≤5 plus SOS ≥60, between the PI and RF groups.

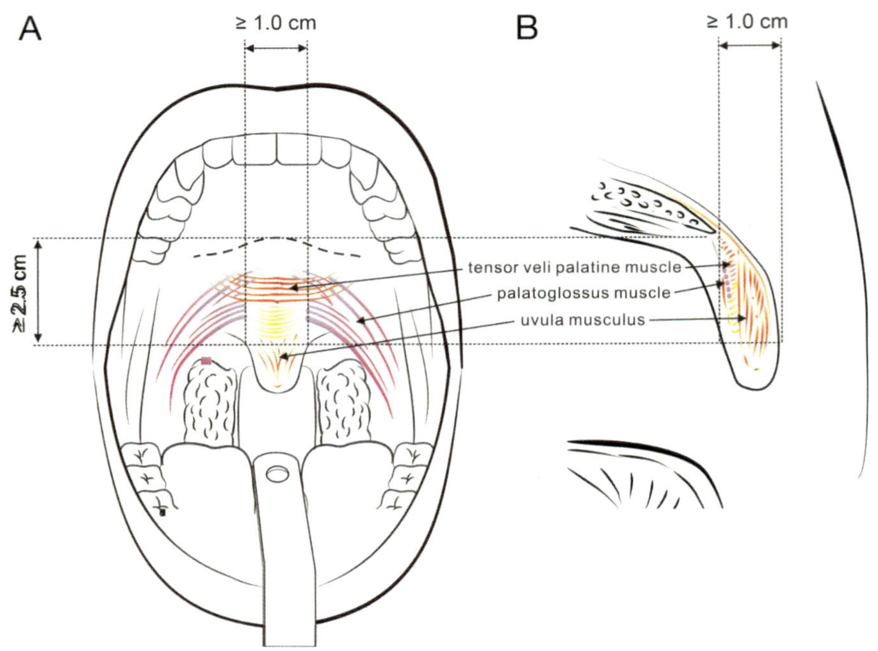

Figure 2. Favorable anatomy for the MIS of the soft palate in anti-snoring treatment. (A) Frontal view showing the longitudinal length from the uvular base to the hard palate-soft palate junction ≥ 2.5 cm and the lateral width of the uvular base ≥ 1.0 cm. (B) Lateral view illustrating the anterior-posterior width of the uvular base ≥ 1.0 cm.

Statistical Analysis

Statistical analyses were performed using SPSS software (version 17.0; SPSS, Inc., Chicago, IL, USA) and G*Power (version 3.1.5; University Kiel, Germany). For the relative small sample size of the present study, we analyzed all variables using non-parametric approaches. The sample size for this study was estimated using the primary outcome effects (VAS) in two previously published studies [6,14]. Using a two-tailed Wilcoxon signed-rank test for calculating the sample size (normal parent distribution; effect size, 1.0; type I error, 0.05; power, 80%), we got a sample size of 11. For considering a 20% drop-out rate to fulfill the criteria of intention-to-treat analysis, we needed at least 14 participants to attend this

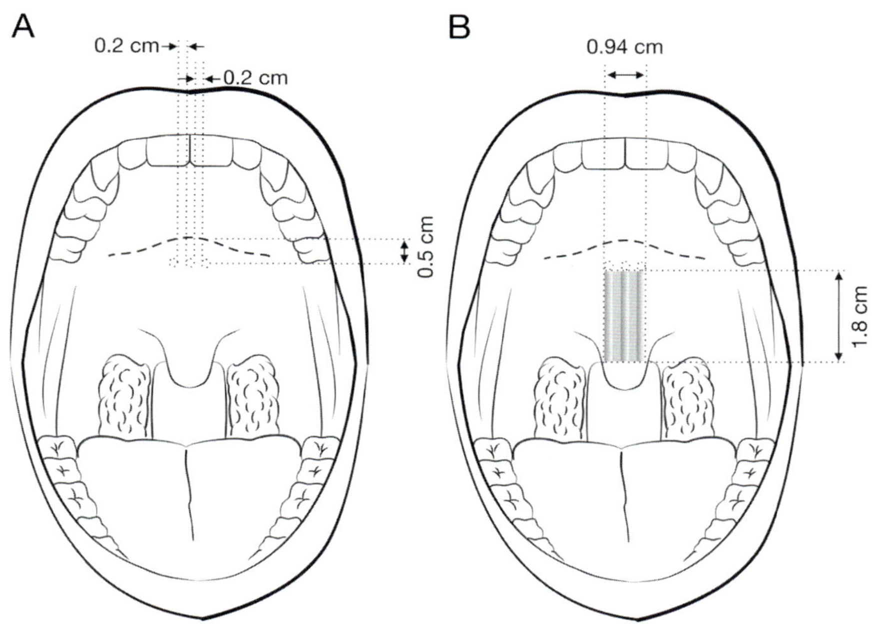

Figure 3. Palatal implant surgery. (A) Preoperative frontal view demonstrating the 3 operative sites of the soft palate (0.5 cm below the hard palate-soft palate junction; 0.2 cm between the midline and para-midline sites). (B) Postoperative frontal view showing the stiffened zone (grey zone) by the implant (1.8 cm×0.94 cm).

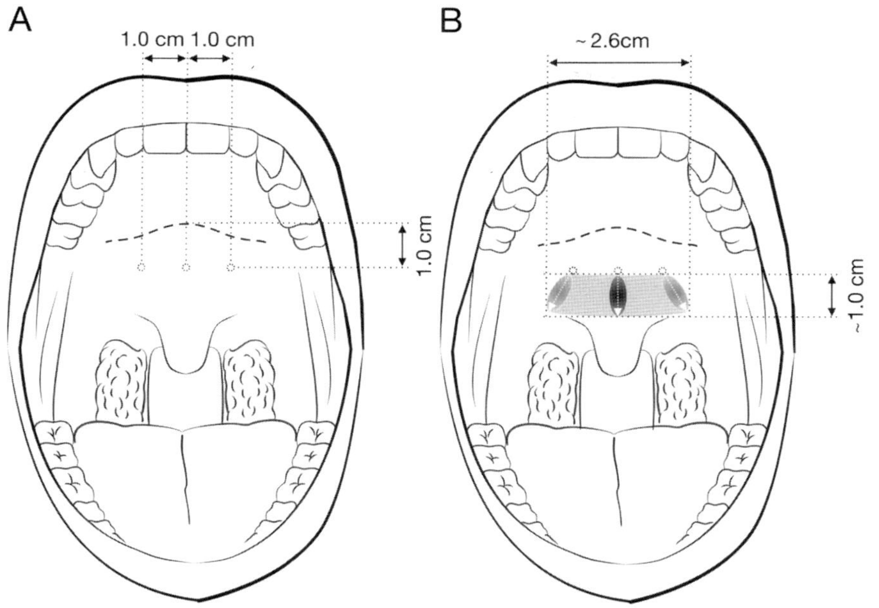

Figure 4. Radiofrequency surgery. (A) Preoperative frontal view illustrating the 3 operative sites of the soft palate (1.0 cm below the hard palate-soft palate junction; 1.0 cm between the midline and para-midline sites). (B) Postoperative frontal view demonstrating the stiffened zone (grey zone) by the RF energy (1.0 cm×2.6 cm).

study. Accordingly, we decided to enroll 30 patients with 15 in each group for showing the difference in mean before and after VAS scores. Two interim analyses were performed at the end of the first year during the trial: 1) the levels of significance maintained an overall P value of 0.05 and were calculated according to the O'Brien-Fleming stopping boundaries, and 2) this final analysis used a Z score of 1.985 with an associated P value of 0.0471 [29]. We planned to stop early if exceptional benefit or harm had been shown.

Further implementing the Kolmogorov-Smirnov test, distributions of patient clinical characteristics, subjective and objective snoring parameters were non-Gaussian and the descriptive statistics of these variables were presented as means (standard errors). Percentage (%) of change ([after value-before value]/[before value] × 100) in subjective snoring as well as in objective acoustic factors and differences between groups were analyzed with the Wilcoxon signed ranks test or the Mann-Whitney U test, as appropriate. Categorical variables were analyzed with the Fisher's exact test or the chi-square test. A P value of less than 0.05 was considered to be statistically significant.

Results

Subjects

Table 1 summarizes baseline anthropological data, polysomnographic parameters, and subjective snoring questionnaire scores for the entire study cohort. There were no significant differences in these parameters between the PI and RF groups. There were no protocol deviation in this study and all participants received the intended intervention after randomization. At the end of study (July 30, 2012), there were 28 patients completed the protocol; two study cases were not available for follow-up (one for oversea work and one for military service; Figure 1). Thus data from 28 patients (PI group, $n = 14$; RF group: $n = 14$) were available for the intention-to-treat analyses. Moreover, no significant complication was noted during the study period.

Comparison of the Effects of PI and RF on Subjective Snoring Questionnaires

Changes in VAS scores after surgery were significant in both groups (PI group: 7.7 [0.4] *vs.* 4.4 [0.6], difference = −3.3, 95% conference interval [CI], −5.0 to −1.6, $P = 0.005$; RF group: 6.6 [0.5] *vs.* 5.2 [0.4], difference = −1.4, 95% CI, −2.7 to −0.1, $P = 0.022$). Significant improvements in SOS scores were also noted in both groups (PI group: 39.4[2.2] *vs.* 62.2 [3.2], difference = 22.8, 95% CI, 15.3 to 30.3, $P = 0.002$; RF group: 41.4 [2.4] *vs.* 54.4 [2.5], difference = 13.0, 95% CI, 7.6 to 18.3, $P = 0.001$). Further, the mean change rate of VAS score in the PI group was significantly different from that in the RF group (−38.8% [9.0%] *vs.* −15.7% [7.2%], difference = 23.1%, 95% CI, −0.6% to 46.8%, $P = 0.029$). The mean change rate of SOS in the PI group was also significantly higher than that in the RF group (61.2% [10.1%] *vs.* 35.4% [7.7%], difference = 25.8%, 95% CI, −0.3% to 51.8%, $P = 0.027$).

Table 2 shows the results comparing the postoperative changes in subjective questionnaire scores after re-categorization between both groups. The rates of ΔVAS ≥1, ΔSOS ≥10, and response (ΔVAS ≥1 or ΔSOS ≥10) in both groups were not different. Twenty-nine percent of the PI group subjects reported mean postoperative VAS ≤3 (major response), and another 50% of the patients (fair response) complained of mild-to-moderate snoring (postoperative VAS ≤5) but had adequate functional outcomes (postoperative SOS ≥60). Only 7% of the RF group had major response after RF surgery, and 21% scored postoperative VAS ≤5 plus SOS ≥60 (fair response). Accordingly, the 'good response' rate was significantly higher in the PI group compared with the RF group (79% *vs.* 29%, difference = 50%, 95% CI, 13% to 72%, $P = 0.021$).

Table 1. Patient characteristics for the entire study cohort ($n=30$).

	Overall ($n=30$)	Palatal implant group ($n=15$)	Radiofrequency group ($n=15$)	Difference* (95% CI)	*P* value
Gender (% male [*n*])	90 (27)	100 (15)	80 (12)	20% (4% to 45%)	0.073
Age (years)	36.7 (1.7)	38.3 (3.1)	35.1 (1.9)	3.3 (−3.2 to 9.7)	0.288
BMI (kg/m^2)	24.2 (0.5)	24.7 (0.8)	23.6 (0.7)	1.1 (−1.0 to 3.2)	0.983
Neck circumference (cm)	37.9 (0.6)	39.0 (0.9)	37.0 (0.9)	2.0 (−0.6 to 4.6)	0.391
Tonsil size	1.0 (0.03)	1.1 (0)	1.0 (0)	0.1 (−0.1 to 0.2)	0.317
Friedman's tongue position	2.4 (0.09)	2.3 (0.1)	2.4 (0.1)	−0.1 (−0.4 to 0.3)	0.710
AHI (events/hour)	7.8 (0.7)	7.9 (0.7)	7.7 (1.1)	0.2 (−2.6 to 3.1)	0.419
PSG-SI (events/hour)	290.2 (38.4)	307.1 (48.0)	273.3 (55.2)	33.8 (−126.0 to 193.6)	0.633
VAS	7.3 (0.4)	7.9 (0.5)	6.8 (0.6)	1.1 (−0.3 to 2.5)	0.384
SOS	40.5 (1.6)	40.4 (2.6)	40.5 (2.5)	−0.1 (−6.9 to 6.7)	0.934

Values were given as mean (standard error). AHI: apnea-hypopnea index. BMI: body mass index. CI: conference interval; PSG-SI: polysomnography-defined snoring index. SOS: snoring outcomes survey. VAS: visual analogue scale.
*Statistical analyses were implemented with the Mann-Whitney *U* test.

Comparison of the Effects of PI and RF on Objective Snoring Sound Analysis

Despite the randomized parallel-controlled trial nature of this study, some conditions were different between the two groups. The patients in the PI group had a significantly higher mean preoperative Total-Imax (70.9 [3.3] *vs.* 57.7 [2.1], difference = 13.2, 95% CI, 4.9 to 21.4, $P=0.004$) and B1-Imax (63.8 [2.5] *vs.* 53.9 [2.0], difference = 9.8, 95% CI, 3.1 to 16.5, $P=0.014$) than those in the RF group (Table 3).

In the PI group, the change of mean B1-Imax (64.5 [1.9] *vs.* 56.7 [1.9], difference = −7.9, 95% CI, −16.4 to 0.7, $P=0.048$) was significant, whereas changes of the other acoustic parameters were insignificant (Table 4). Although the mean B1-SI (121.2 [40.4] *vs.* 54.4 [31.4], difference = −66.9, 95% CI, −145.0 to 11.3, $P=0.041$) was significantly reduced after surgery, the mean postoperative Total-Imax (58.3 [2.2] *vs.* 64.9 [3.3], difference = 6.7, 95% CI, 1.8 to 11.5, $P=0.016$), Total-Imean (48.0 [2.0] *vs.* 56.3 [2.9], difference = 8.3, 95% CI, 2.3 to 14.2, $P=0.009$), and B1-Imean (45.4 [2.0] *vs.* 51.6 [2.6], difference = 6.3, 95% CI, 1.1 to 11.4, $P=0.011$) were significantly increased compared with the preoperative data in the RF group. As expected, the change rates of Total-Imax (−6.8% [5.9%] *vs.* 11.3% [3.8%], difference = −18.1%, 95% CI, −32.5% to − 3.6%, $P=0.022$), Total-Imean (−0.4% [5.6%]. *vs.* 18.2% [6.1%], difference = −17.9%, 95% CI, −34.9% to −0.9%], $P=0.027$), B1-Imax (−9.4% [5.6%] *vs.* 5.6% [3.1%], [difference = −15.1%, 95% CI, −28.3%to −1.9%], $P=0.024$), and B1-Imean (−4.6% [5.3%] *vs.* 14.7% [5.5%], difference = −19.3, 95% CI, −34.9% to −3.3%], $P=0.009$) were significantly different between the PI group and RF group.

Discussion

This is the first study to compare the anti-snoring effects in two MIS of the soft palate, PI and RF, using both objective and subjective evaluations. Clinically, RF surgery is more widely used and investigated, while PI surgery has received increasing attention, although their efficacy in changing the objective characteristics of snoring sounds remains uncertain. Our results suggest that both PI and RF surgeries were safe and improved subjective snoring severity and functional outcomes; however there were differences in their effects on acoustic characteristics. Furthermore, PI surgery had a greater effect on a favorable

Table 2. Comparison of the postoperative changes in subjective questionnaire scores between the palatal implant and radiofrequency surgery groups.

Subgroups, % (*n*)	Palatal implant group ($n=14$)	Radiofrequency group ($n=14$)	Ratio (95% CI)	Difference (95% CI)	*P* value
ΔVAS ≥1	93 (13)	64 (9)	1.44 (0.95–2.19)	29% (−3% to 55%)	0.165
ΔSOS ≥10	93 (13)	57 (8)	1.63 (1.01–2.62)	36% (3% to 61%)	0.077
Postoperative VAS ≤3	29 (4)	7 (1)	4.00 (0.51–31.46)	21% (−8% to 48%)	0.326
Postoperative VAS ≤5 plus SOS ≥60	71 (10)	29 (4)	2.50 (1.02–6.10)	43% (6% to 67%)	0.057
Response (Either ΔVAS ≥1 or ΔSOS ≥10)	93 (13)	71 (10)	1.30 (0.91–1.87)	21% (−8% to 48%)	0.326
Good response (Ether postoperative VAS ≤3 or postoperative VAS ≤5 plus SOS ≥60)	79 (11)	29 (4)	2.75 (1.15–6.58)	50% (13% to 72%)	0.021

CI: conference interval. SOS: snore outcomes survey. VAS: visual analogue scale.

Table 3. Objective snoring sound parameters at baseline for the entire study cohort ($n = 30$).

	Overall ($n = 30$)	Palatal implant group ($n = 15$)	Radiofrequency group ($n = 15$)	Difference* (95% CI)	*P* value
Total domain (40 Hz–2000 Hz)					
SI (events/hour)	116.3 (22.3)	116.3 (23.7)	116.4 (38.4)	−0.1 (−93.2 to 92.9)	0.135
Imax (dB)	64.3 (2.3)	70.9 (3.3)	57.7 (2.1)	13.2 (4.9 to 21.4)	0.004
Imean (dB)	49.1 (1.2)	50.8 (1.3)	47.4 (2.0)	3.4 (−1.4 to 8.3)	0.054
Fpeak (Hz)	580.3 (107.6)	543.3 (150.8)	617.3 (158.6)	−74.0 (−521.6 to 373.6)	0.709
Fmean (Hz)	101.9 (4.8)	101.4 (5.8)	102.3 (7.9)	−0.9 (−21.0 to 19.2)	0.868
B1 domain (40 Hz–300 Hz)					
SI (events/hour)	113.3 (22.3)	113.4 (23.6)	113.3 (38.5)	0.1 (−92.9 to 93.1)	0.135
Imax (dB)	58.9 (1.8)	63.8 (2.5)	53.9 (2.0)	9.8 (3.1 to 16.5)	0.004
Imean (dB)	46.0 (1.1)	47.2 (1.1)	44.8 (1.9)	2.4 (−2.1 to 7.0)	0.093
Fpeak (Hz)	219.0 (8.6)	217.3 (8.9)	220.7 (14.9)	−3.3 (−39.0 to 32.3)	0.934
Fmean (Hz)	100.0 (4.7)	98.0 (6.1)	101.9 (7.4)	−3.9 (−23.7 to 15.8)	0.494

Values were given as mean (standard error). AHI: apnea-hypopnea index. BMI: body mass index. CI: conference interval; PSG-SI: polysomnography-defined snoring index. SOS: snoring outcomes survey. VAS: visual analogue scale.
*Statistical analyses were implemented with the Mann-Whitney *U* test.

surgical response than one-session of RF surgery in this randomized parallel-controlled trial.

Previous functional outcome studies of palatal MIS are limited, and most have used VAS score to measure the differences. The VAS for snoring assessment is a standardized, well-established tool to measure the subjective intensity of snoring. Many reports have shown that the patients who receive MIS for snoring usually have a high (>7) VAS score [1–4]. Nevertheless, only a few studies have demonstrated a MIS reduction in VAS snoring score to ≤3 [14,26–28,30–35]. Although MIS rarely cures snoring in subjective evaluation, it has been shown to effectively alleviate snoring in several randomized placebo-controlled trials [5,6,8,9]. Further, VAS alone cannot reflect the whole profile of snoring and related consequences. Accordingly, full outcome analysis of MIS for snoring should include other snoring-related outcomes such as the Functional Outcomes of Sleep Questionnaire (FOSQ) [36] or SOS [21]. Steward et al. reported that PI surgery could improve FOSQ scores more significantly than placebo [8]. In our previous study, the SOS score significantly increased following one-session of RF surgery [14].

Theoretically, both PI and RF surgery stiffens the muscle layer of the soft palate in order to reduce the palatal flutter [16,37]. Previous studies have indicated that patients with mild obstructive sleep apnea or simple snoring have peak intensities between 100 and 300 Hz (B1-domain) [23,25,38]. As expected, this study found that the two MIS mainly influenced B1-snoring sounds although in different dimensions. That is, the distinct mechanisms of the palatal rigidity can also alter the surrounding airway structures that can then produce different snoring sounds.

To the best of our knowledge, there are currently no reports on changes of the upper airway structure or changes in acoustic characteristics after PI surgery. Clinically, the shape and size of the uvula and soft palate do not change after PI procedure. However, polyethylene teralphate implants can be regarded as an extension of the hard palate to prop up and stiffen the soft palate in a rectangular area by approximately 1.8 cm (length) x 0.94 (0.18 + 0.2 + 0.18 + 0.2 + 0.18) cm (width; Figure 3B). It seems that the PI strengths the uvular muscle (Figure 1A) and consequently confines palatal flutter leading to the reduction in B1-Imax. Of note, VAS and SOS improved significantly in spite of insignificant reductions in other B1-domain parameters in the PI group.

In contrast, RF energy may affect the soft palate in a long oval area by approximately 1.0 cm (length) x 2.6 cm (width) based on our surgical technique (Figure 4B). The location of the RF treatment includes the musculus uvulae (midline position 600 J) and combination of levator veli palatini and palatopharyngeus (para-midline positions 300 J each). Bäck et al. used magnetic resonance imaging to evaluate soft palates that received two sessions of bipolar RF energy, and found that the scar tissue formation resulting in the T1-signal intensity of the soft palate increased significantly three months after treatment [26].

In this study, the subjective improvement rates in the VAS and SOS were significantly lower in the RF group than the PI group despite having the same inclusion criteria with regards to anatomy. Moreover, B1-SI decreased significantly without respect to the increase in B1-Imean. Since the length and width of the soft palate could not be significantly changed by RF surgery despite scaring of the soft palate [26], the non-operated part (at least 0.5 cm; 2.5 – 1.0 – 1.0 = 0.5) and insufficient longitudinal rigidity of the uvular muscle in one single session RF treatment cannot resist a higher inspiratory force resulting in louder B1-snores. In contrast, we presume that RF energy works on the tensor veli palatine and palatopharyngeus muscles in a horizontal direction (Figure 1A) and tenses up the soft palate to resist lower inspiratory force thereby decreasing the occurrence of B1-snores. These findings imply the necessity of more treatment sessions or multiple midline longitudinal injection sites in RF surgery of the soft palate to reduce the intensity of snoring, and the application of additional PI in the tensor veli palatine muscle to decrease SI.

The major limitation to this study is unbalanced randomization in Total-Imax despite insignificant differences in baseline anthropologic, symptomatic, and polysomnographic parameters between the two groups. This may be a methodological flaw in such a prospective randomized controlled trial, although this was not predicted before the study was undertaken. Moreover, the small sample size creates at least a few limitations: unable to do

Table 4. Results of objective snoring sound parameters before and after treatment in the two groups.

	Palatal implant group ($n = 14$)			Radiofrequency group ($n = 14$)			
Parameters	**Before**	**After**	**Mean percentage (%) of change***	**Before**	**After**	**Mean percentage (%) of change***	**Difference of mean percentage (%) of change** (95% CI)**
Total domain (40 Hz–2000 Hz)							
SI (events/hour)	123.8 (24.8)	101.3 (28.8)	−5.9 (25.6)	124.6 (40.3)	73.9 (34.2)	−48.9 (22.1)	43.1 (−11.1 to 97.3)
Imax (dB)	72.1 (3.4)^{A}	65.1 (1.8)	−6.8 (5.9)^{C}	58.3 (2.2)^{A}	64.9 (3.3)^{B}	11.3 (3.8)^{C}	−18.1 (−32.5 to −3.6)
Imean (dB)	50.9 (1.4)	50.6 (2.6)	−0.4 (5.6)^{C}	48.0 (2.0)	56.3 (2.9)^{B}	18.2 (6.1)^{C}	−17.9 (−34.9 to −0.9)
Fpeak (Hz)	570.7 (161.9)	570.0 (146.6)	−6 (24.2)	651.5 (163.4)	477.9 (122.0)	−12.1 (26.2)	6.1 (−33.9 to 69.3)
Fmean (Hz)	100.7 (6.2)	99.6 (8.6)	−0.9 (8.7)	104.6 (8.1)	89.8 (12.7)	−10.9 (11.6)	10.0 (−18.0 to 41.5)
B1 domain (40 Hz–300 Hz)							
SI (events/hour)	120.8 (24.7)	116.2 (30.9)	−1.7 (29.5)	121.2 (40.4)	54.4 (31.4)^{B}	−51.8 (22.5)	50.1 (−3.9 to 110.9)
Imax (dB)	64.5 (2.6)^{A}	56.7 (1.9)^{B}	−9.4 (5.6)^{C}	54.4 (2.1)^{A}	57.4 (2.6)	5.6 (3.1)^{C}	−15.1 (−28.3 to −1.9)
Imean (dB)	47.2 (1.2)	44.7 (2.2)	−4.6 (5.3)^{C}	45.4 (2.0)	51.6 (2.6)^{B}	14.7 (5.5)^{C}	−19.3 (−34.9 to −3.3)
Fpeak (Hz)	222.1 (9.6)	192.9 (15.9)	−10.9 (7.9)	226.4 (13.9)	142.1 (25.6)	−33.5 (11.4)	22.6 (−6.0 to 51.1)
Fmean (Hz)	97.0 (6.6)	95.2 (6.9)	−1.6 (8.4)	103.9 (7.6)	75.0 (9.4)	−24.8 (8.7)	22.2 (−1.5 to 51.3)

CI: conference interval. Fmean: mean sound frequency. Fpeak: peak sound frequency. Imax: maximal sound intensity. Imean: mean sound intensity.

subgroup analyses, risk of unbalanced allocation of patients (i.e., imperfect randomization can be a consequence of the small sample size), and statistical difference between groups is seen only when there are large differences (i.e., smaller differences are not statistically significant, even if clinically important). A future study with a larger sample could overcome these limitations. Although our study indicated PI surgery may be more efficacious in the treatment of snoring for adult patients with simple snoring, it will be important to test the effects of this MIS technique with more anthropologically and ethnically diverse subjects in a larger sample.

Conclusions

Both PI and RF alleviated subjective snoring intensity and improved snoring-related outcomes; however, the changes in magnitude and pattern in the acoustic parameters of snoring differed between these two MIS techniques. Our study indicated PI surgery may be more efficacious than single-stage RF surgery in the treatment of snoring for adult patients with simple snoring, it will be important to test the effects of this MIS technique with more anthropologically and ethnically diverse subjects in a larger sample. Further research evaluating the histoanatomical and acoustic changes within the soft palate to predict treatment outcomes is warranted.

Acknowledgments

The authors would like to thank Mrs. Shin-Jao Lee, Department of Otorhinolaryngology-Head and Neck Surgery, Chang Gung Memorial Hospital at Linkou, Taoyuan, Taiwan, for assisting in data collection, and Mr. Yen-Sheng Chen and Mr. Ding-Li Wang, Graduate Institute of Medical Mechatronics, Taiouan Interdisciplinary Otolaryngology Laboratory, Chang Gung University, Taoyuan, Taiwan, for assisting in snoring sound acquisition.

Author Contributions

Conceived and designed the experiments: LAL, JFY, YLL, NHC, TJF, CGH, WNC, HYL. Performed the experiments: LAL, JFY, YLL, CGH, WNC, HYL. Analyzed the data: LAL, YLL, CGH, WNC, HYL. Contributed reagents/materials/analysis tools: LAL, JFY, YLL, NHC, TJF, CGH, WNC, HYL. Wrote the paper: LAL, JFY, YLL, NHC, TJF, CGH, WNC, HYL. N/A.

References

1. Bäck LJ, Hytönen ML, Roine RP, Malmivaara AO (2009) Radiofrequency ablation treatment of soft palate for patients with snoring: a systematic review of effectiveness and adverse effects. Laryngoscope 119:1241–1250.
2. Choi JH, Kim SN, Cho JH (2013) Efficacy of the Pillar implant in the treatment of snoring and mild-to-moderate obstructive sleep apnea: a meta-analysis. Laryngoscope 123:269–276.
3. Stuck BA, Maurer JT, Hein G, Hörmann K, Verse T (2004) Radiofrequency surgery of the soft palate in the treatment of snoring: a review of the literature. Sleep 27:551–555.
4. Franklin KA, Anttila H, Axelsson S, Gislason T, Maasilta P, et al. (2009) Effects and side-effects of surgery for snoring and obstructive sleep apnea-a systematic review. Sleep 32:27–36.
5. Stuck BA, Sauter A, Hörmann K, Verse T, Maurer JT (2005) Radiofrequency surgery of the soft palate in the treatment of snoring. A placebo-controlled trial. Sleep 28:847–850.
6. Friedman M, Schalch P, Lin HC, Kakodkar KA, Joseph NJ, et al. (2008) Palatal implants for the treatment of snoring and obstructive sleep apnea/hypopnea syndrome. Otolaryngol Head Neck Surg 138:209–216.
7. Bäck LJ, Liukko T, Rantanen I, Peltola JS, Partinen M, et al. (2009) Radiofrequency surgery of the soft palate in the treatment of mild obstructive sleep apnea is not effective as a single-stage procedure: A randomized single-blinded placebo-controlled trial. Laryngoscope 119:1621–1627.
8. Steward DL, Huntley TC, Woodson BT, Surdulescu V (2008) Palate implants for obstructive sleep apnea: multi-institution, randomized, placebo-controlled study. Otolaryngol Head Neck Surg 139:506–510.
9. Maurer JT, Sommer JU, Hein G, Hörmann K, Heiser C, et al. (2012) Palatal implants in the treatment of obstructive sleep apnea: a randomised, placebo-controlled single-centre trial. Eur Arch Otorhinolaryngol 269:1851–1856.
10. Blumen MB, Chalumeau F, Gauthier A, Bobin S, Coste A, et al. (2008) Comparative study of four radiofrequency generators for the treatment of snoring. Otolaryngol Head Neck Surg 138:294–299.
11. Skjøstad KW, Stene BK, Norgård S (2006) Consequences of increased rigidity in palatal implants for snoring: a randomized controlled study. Otolaryngol Head Neck Surg 134:63–66.
12. Bassiouny A, El Salamawy A, Abd El-Tawab M, Atef A (2007) Bipolar radiofrequency treatment for snoring with mild to moderate sleep apnea: a comparative study between the radiofrequency assisted uvulopalatoplasty technique and the channeling technique. Eur Arch Otorhinolaryngol 264:659–667.
13. Balsevičius T, Uloza V, Vaitkus S, Sakalauskas R, Miliauskas S (2013) Controlled trial of combined radiofrequency-assisted uvulopalatoplasty in the treatment of snoring and mild to moderate OSAS (pilot study). Sleep Breath 17:695–703.
14. Fang TJ, Li HY, Shue CW, Lee LA, Wang PC (2003) Efficacy of radiofrequency volumetric tissue reduction of the soft palate in the treatment of snoring. Int J Clin Pract 57:769–772.
15. Blumen MB, Vezina JP, Bequignon E, Chabolle F (2013) Snoring intensity after a first session of soft palate radiofrequency: predictive value of the final result. Laryngoscope 123:1556–1559.
16. Ho WK, Wei WI, Chung KF (2004) Managing disturbing snoring with palatal implants: a pilot study. Arch Otolaryngol Head Neck Surg 130:753–758.
17. Caples SM, Rowley JA, Prinsell JR, Pallanch JF, Elamin MB, et al. (2010) Surgical modifications of the upper airway for obstructive sleep apnea in adults: a systematic review and meta-analysis. Sleep 33:1396–1407.
18. Neruntarat C (2011) Long-term results of palatal implants for obstructive sleep apnea. Eur Arch Otorhinolaryngol 268:1077–1080.
19. Rotenberg BW, Luu K (2012) Four-year outcomes of palatal implants for primary snoring treatment: a prospective longitudinal study. Laryngoscope 122:696–699.
20. Iber C, Ancoli-Israel S, Chesson AL, Quan SF (2007) The AASM manual for the scoring of sleep and associated events: Rules, terminology and technical specifications. 1st ed. Westchester: American Academy of Sleep Medicine.
21. Gliklich RE, Wang PC (2002) Validation of the snore outcomes survey for patients with sleep-disordered breathing. Arch Otolaryngol Head Neck Surg 128:819–824.
22. Chen NH, Li HY, Gliklich RE, Chu CC, Liang SC, et al. (2002) Validation assessment of the Chinese version of the Snore Outcomes Survey. Qual Life Res 11:601–607.
23. Lee LA, Yu JF, Lo YL, Chen YS, Wang DL, et al (2012) Energy types of snoring sounds in patients with obstructive sleep apnea syndrome: a preliminary observation. PLoS One 7:e53481.
24. Ben-Israel N, Tarasiuk A, Zigel Y (2012) Obstructive apnea hypopnea index estimation by analysis of nocturnal snoring signals in adults. Sleep 35:1299–1305.
25. Herzog M, Schmidt A, Bremert T, Herzog B, Hosemann W, et al. (2008) Analysed snoring sounds correlate to obstructive sleep disordered breathing. Eur Arch Otorhinolaryngol 265:105–113.
26. Goessler UR, Hein G, Verse T, Stuck BA, Hormann K, et al. (2007) Soft palate implants as a minimally invasive treatment for mild to moderate obstructive sleep apnea. Acta Otolaryngol 127:527–531.
27. Back LJ, Tervahartiala PO, Piilonen AK, Partinen MM, Ylikoski JS (2002) Bipolar radiofrequency thermal ablation of the soft palate in habitual snorers

without significant desaturations assessed by magnetic resonance imaging. Am J Respir Crit Care Med 166:865–871.
28. Powell NB, Riley RW, Troell RJ, Li K, Blumen MB, et al. (1998) Radiofrequency volumetric tissue reduction of the palate in subjects with sleep-disordered breathing. Chest 113:1163–1174.
29. Galgiani JN, Catanzaro A, Cloud GA, Johnson RH, Williams PL, et al. (2000) Comparison of Oral Fluconazole and Itraconazole for Progressive, Nonmeningeal Coccidioidomycosis. A Randomized, Double-Blind Trial. Ann Intern Med 133:676–686.
30. Coleman SC, Smith TL (2000) Midline radiofrequency tissue reduction of the palate for bothersome snoring and sleep-disordered breathing: a clinical trial. Otolaryngol Head Neck Surg 122:387–394.
31. Amorós-Sebastiá LI (2011) Radiofrequency treatment in simple snoring: tolerance, safety and results. Acta Otorrinolaringol Esp 62:300–305.
32. Blumen MB, Dahan S, Wagner I, De Dieuleveult T, Chabolle F (2002) Radiofrequency versus LAUP for the treatment of snoring. Otolaryngol Head Neck Surg 126:67–73.
33. Iseri M, Balcioglu O (2005) Radiofrequency versus injection snoreplasty in simple snoring. Otolaryngol Head Neck Surg 133:224–228.
34. Sher AE, Flexon PB, Hillman D, Emery B, Swieca J, et al. (2001) Temperature-controlled radiofrequency tissue volume reduction in the human soft palate. Otolaryngol Head Neck Surg 125:312–318.
35. Terris DJ, Coker JF, Thomas AJ, Chavoya M (2002) Preliminary findings from a prospective, randomized trial of two palatal operations for sleep-disordered breathing. Otolaryngol Head Neck Surg 127:315–323.
36. Nordgård S, Stene BK, Skjøstad KW (2006) Soft palate implants for the treatment of mild to moderate obstructive sleep apnea. Otolaryngol Head Neck Surg 134:565–570.
37. Weaver TE, Laizner AM, Evans LK, Maislin G, Chugh DK, et al. (1997) An instrument to measure functional status outcomes for disorders of excessive sleepiness. Sleep. 20:835–843.
38. Courey MS, Fomin D, Smith T, Huang S, Sanders D, et al. (1999) Histologic and physiologic effects of electrocautery, CO2 laser, and radiofrequency injury in the porcine soft palate. Laryngoscope 109:1316–1319.

10

Extending the Body to Virtual Tools Using a Robotic Surgical Interface: Evidence from the Crossmodal Congruency Task

Ali Sengül[1,2,3]*, Michiel van Elk[1,2], Giulio Rognini[1,2,3], Jane Elizabeth Aspell[2], Hannes Bleuler[3], Olaf Blanke[1,2,4]

1 Center for Neuroprosthetics, School of Life Sciences, Ecole Polytechnique Fédérale de Lausanne (EPFL), Lausanne, Switzerland, **2** Laboratory of Cognitive Neuroscience, Brain Mind Institute, Ecole Polytechnique Fédérale de Lausanne (EPFL), Lausanne, Switzerland, **3** Systems Robotic Laboratory, Ecole Polytechnique Fédérale de Lausanne (EPFL), Lausanne, Switzerland, **4** Department of Neurology, University Hospital of Geneva (HUG), Geneva, Switzerland

Abstract

The effects of real-world tool use on body or space representations are relatively well established in cognitive neuroscience. Several studies have shown, for example, that active tool use results in a facilitated integration of multisensory information in peripersonal space, i.e. the space directly surrounding the body. However, it remains unknown to what extent similar mechanisms apply to the use of virtual-robotic tools, such as those used in the field of surgical robotics, in which a surgeon may use bimanual haptic interfaces to control a surgery robot at a remote location. This paper presents two experiments in which participants used a haptic handle, originally designed for a commercial surgery robot, to control a virtual tool. The integration of multisensory information related to the virtual-robotic tool was assessed by means of the crossmodal congruency task, in which subjects responded to tactile vibrations applied to their fingers while ignoring visual distractors superimposed on the tip of the virtual-robotic tool. Our results show that active virtual-robotic tool use changes the spatial modulation of the crossmodal congruency effects, comparable to changes in the representation of peripersonal space observed during real-world tool use. Moreover, when the virtual-robotic tools were held in a crossed position, the visual distractors interfered strongly with tactile stimuli that was connected with the hand via the tool, reflecting a remapping of peripersonal space. Such remapping was not only observed when the virtual-robotic tools were actively used (Experiment 1), but also when passively held the tools (Experiment 2). The present study extends earlier findings on the extension of peripersonal space from physical and pointing tools to virtual-robotic tools using techniques from haptics and virtual reality. We discuss our data with respect to learning and human factors in the field of surgical robotics and discuss the use of new technologies in the field of cognitive neuroscience.

Editor: Nicholas P. Holmes, University of Reading, United Kingdom

Funding: A. Sengül was supported by ARAKNES project, a European Community's Seventh Framework Programme (FP7-ICT-2007-2) and SAFROS project, a European Community's Seventh Framework Programme research project (FP7-ICT-2009.5.2), M. van Elk was supported by a Marie Curie Grant (IEF grant 252713). O. Blanke is supported by the European Science Foundation, the Swiss National Science Foundation, and the Bertarelli Foundation. The funders had no role in study design, data collection and analysis, decision to publish, or preparation of the manuscript.

Competing Interests: The authors have declared that no competing interests exist.

* E-mail: ali.sengul@epfl.ch

Introduction

Complex tool-use is a uniquely human activity and its achievement enabled a remarkable step forward in the evolution of our species. In daily life we use spoons, knives, forks, pencils, rulers and scissors. When enjoying sports we use a variety of equipment such as golf clubs or tennis rackets. In addition, we often interact with tools to control computers, such as a keyboard, computer mouse and joysticks. In a certain sense, even vehicles can be considered as tools that greatly extend the boundaries of our physical body and our bodily capabilities [1,2]. Thus, tools can be used to extend our action space and to perform many tasks of daily life, whether at home, at work, or for recreation [3,4].

To perform common daily tasks easily, we use different tools that can be categorized based on their function and characteristics. Holmes and Spence [5] classified tools into three categories: physical interaction tools, pointing tools and detached tools. Physical interaction tools function as a physical connection between the body and environment (e.g. a brush, a stick, a pen etc.). They are often hand-held objects that are purposefully used to interact with other objects to achieve a goal (e.g. brushing the floor). Many studies have described the changes in the neural representation of multisensory peripersonal space with physical tools in healthy adults [6–8]. The second category consists of pointing tools that are typically used to point at another object (e.g. a laser pointer). There is no direct physical connection between the user and the objects with which they interact. Some studies have investigated the changes in the neural representation of multisensory peripersonal space with pointing tools in healthy participants [9,10]. The last category of tools defined by Holmes and Spence [5] are detached tools. A human operator uses an interface to perform a task at distant locations or even in virtual reality (computer screen). With detached tools there is no direct physical linkage between the user and the target whereas those tools exhibit force and motion coupling between the human and virtual environment. Up to now, the effect of detached tool use on the neural representation of multisensory peripersonal space has not been studied.

Recent advances in robotics have brought attention to a specific class of detached tools: human-robot interfaces. Robotic tools, such as surgery robots and telemanipulators are designed to operate at distant locations or in virtual scenarios under direct human control [11,12]. These unprecedented tools greatly increase the precision, force and accessibility of human manipulation (within the human body or within industrial systems such as piping, turbines etc.). These tools allow increased dexterity by down-scaling position or up-scaling forces. Such devices are also called 'master-slave' systems: they have a master side, which detects the positions and motion of the user and sends this information to a slave robot that is in contact with the remote environment [13]. Surgeons now frequently and efficiently interact with such telemanipulators to perform complex tasks, such as laparoscopic surgery [14–16].

Despite these technical advances in the field of surgical robots and telemanipulators, only little attention has been paid to the psychological and cognitive mechanisms that underlie the interactions with these devices. The aim of these robots is to increase the telepresence and transparency between the surgeon and the environment, as well as the accuracy and intuitiveness of the use of the system. The precise role of the different factors that contribute to the extension of one's body and one's peripersonal space during virtual tool use remains unknown. For instance, it is unclear whether the inclusion of sensory modalities, such as touch or haptic feedback, would result in a more realistic interaction and thereby improve the control over the robot. In order to address these questions we here propose a cognitive neuroscience approach to robotics. More specifically, we measured the multisensory integration of vision and touch when operating a haptic device and evaluated the potential of such newly emerging surgical robotic devices at the level of their perception as a tool by the human brain [17].

The integration of information from different sensory modalities by the human brain is a complex process that has received a lot of attention in cognitive neuroscience. Previous studies have shown for instance, that the space around the body (near extrapersonal space or peripersonal space) is represented in the brain differently than the extrapersonal space that is far from the body [18]. Peripersonal space representation is based on the multisensory integration of visual, tactile, somatosensory, and auditory cues in the frontal and parietal lobes of the human cortex [18]. The brain representation of peripersonal space is highly plastic and has been shown to adapt dramatically to physical tool use, for example by extending or projecting peripersonal space beyond its normal range to also include the end of a handheld tool. Several studies using single unit recordings in macaque monkeys and the spatial modulations of multisensory behavior in healthy participants and brain-damaged patients have supported the idea that tool use extends multisensory peripersonal space [19–21]. One method for studying the integration of multisensory information in relation to tool use is the crossmodal congruency task [21,22]. In this task, participants are required to respond to the elevation of tactile stimuli to the thumb and index finger, while at the same time ignoring visual distractors presented at the end of the tool. Participants are asked to make speeded elevation judgments (up vs down) to the vibrotactile stimulus while ignoring the visual distractors. The crossmodal congruency effect (CCE) is defined as the reaction time difference between incongruent conditions (light and vibration in opposite position, i.e. up vs. down) and congruent conditions (light and vibration both up or both down). The CCE is considered a reliable measure of multisensory integration in peripersonal space, as it has been shown that the CCE is enhanced for objects that can be easily integrated in the body representation, such as rubber hands and virtual bodies [21,22]. CCEs have been shown to reflect changes in hand ownership [23,24] as well as full-body ownership [25]. Recently, CCEs have been used to study the effect of tool-use and in particular whether humans experienced changes in the representation of peripersonal space. It has been found, for instance, that after active tool use, visual distractors presented at the tip of the tool interfered with tactile stimuli presented at the hand of the participant holding the tool, suggesting that the peripersonal space representation was changed with tool use [8,21,22] and that peripersonal space was extended by active tool use [8].

Although several tool-use studies have now established these changes in the representation of peripersonal space by using the CCE, they were all done with simple physical tools such as golf clubs, rakes or sticks. Advanced robotic tools such as haptic devices or master/slave systems have to our knowledge not yet been investigated in this context (but see Moizumi et al., 2007). Compared to physical tools, these advanced tools behave like 'tele-arms' and user movements from the master side are mapped on the remote tools. For instance, in the case of a surgical robotic system, the slave robot performs the movements of the surgeon who can be working at a different physical location. One of the aims in surgical robotics is to increase the immersion and telepresence of the surgeon into the remote site by using appropriate display and telepresence technologies to regain virtually direct access to the operation - comparable to the experience during open surgery. Hence, the study of the neurocognitive aspects of these advance tools is important from an engineering perspective. For instance, studying how the peripersonal space representation changes with virtual robotic tool use would provide an objective evaluation of the telepresence and the usability of the surgical robotic systems. This will give new insights in the design of usable and immersive surgical robotic system that can easily be integrated by the brain and are experienced by the surgeons as a 'tele-arm'. In addition, virtual tools enable to study the different factors involved in the remapping of peripersonal space (e.g. providing haptic feedback, changing the mapping from the arm movements to the tool movements etc.; cf. Sengül et al. in prep.). The present study provides the first step towards investigating virtual tool use using cognitive neuroscience methods.

We tested whether the peripersonal space representation would change 'naturally' even in the case of a telemanipulated tool, i.e. without a mechanical connection between the hand (master side) and the point of physical action (slave side). As a benchmark, the well-known experiment of Maravita et al. [8], performed with physical tools (golf clubs), was reproduced here in a new technological context (multimodal haptic interface operating on a VR physical scene). The participant's task was to cross or uncross the virtual golf clubs in experiment 1 and to just hold the tool interface in experiment 2, in which the crossing and uncrossing was done by the experimenter. Subsequently, participants were required to make speeded elevation discriminations of vibrotactile stimuli delivered to the thumb and index finger – using a foot pedal while ignoring visual distractors presented at the end of the virtual tool. Unlike physical tools, virtual robotic tools behave like 'tele-arms'. User movements from the master side are mapped on the remote tools. In combination with appropriate displays (3D monitors or head mounted displays) and telepresence technologies (realistic 3D graphics), they aim to enable a high level of immersion into the remote site. Because of these different physical and information processing mechanism in virtual-robotic tools compared to physical tools, we hypothesize that the neural representation of the peripersonal space would change quickly due to the immersive nature of these tools. In the first study we tested whether the active use of virtual-robotic tools would alter the spatial dependency of CCEs in a similar way as found in Maravita's (2002) experiment with physical tools [8]. That is, we expected that visual distractors would interfere with tactile stimuli applied to the hand that is holding the tool and this should be the case not only for the uncrossed posture but also for the crossed posture. In the second study we tested whether the spatial modulation of the CCE according to the tool posture (i.e. crossed or uncrossed) is the result of the active use of the tools or not. To this end in the second experiment the tools were not crossed actively, but passively by the experimenter. We expected an interference of visual distractors with the tactile stimuli connected to the hand by the tool for both the uncrossed posture and the crossed posture due to the immersive and 'tele-arm'-like nature of the virtual robotic tools, thereby facilitating a remapping of peripersonal space even when the tool is only used passively.

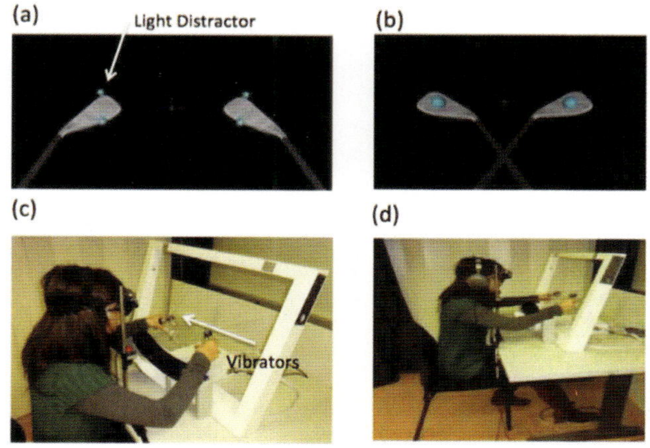

Figure 1. Virtual reality views and experimental setup used in the experiments. (A) Virtual tools in an uncrossed posture: the small balls on the upper and lower part of the tools are the visual distractors. They are presented simultaneously with the vibrotactile stimuli to distract the participants. They can be presented at the same positions as the vibrotactile stimuli (congruent) or at different positions (incongruent). (B) Virtual tools in a crossed posture: The big balls in the middle of the tools have two functions. First they indicate that the CCE phase is finished. Second they indicate the position to locate the tools to keep the distance between each tool constant. The big cross in the middle of the tools is the fixation point. (C, D) A cable driven haptic device (the Da Vinci Simulator) with a large workspace was used. Participants interacted with the virtual object through the handles of the device. Their interactions were shown through a head mounted display. To mask the noise of the vibrators and environmental noise, headphones were used to present white noise. Participants responded to vibrotactile stimuli using the foot pedal. A chin rest system was used to prevent undesired movement of the head. The participant has given written informed consent (according to the PLoS guidelines) for the publication of her picture.

Materials and Methods

Subjects

A total of 19 healthy right-handed participants took part in these experiments: Ten participants (2 female, ages 21–24, mean age (SE): 22.3 (1.2) years) in study 1. Nine participants (3 female, ages 19–28, mean age (SE) 23.2 (2.6) years) in study 2. All participants had normal or corrected to normal vision, no disorder of touch and had no history of neurological or psychiatric conditions. Each experiment took approximately 60 minutes per participant. The participants were informed about the general purpose of the research, were fully debriefed and were given the opportunity to ask questions and to comment on the research after the experiment. All participants gave written informed consent and were compensated for their participation. The experimental procedure was approved by the local research ethics committee – La Commission d'éthique de la recherche Clinique de la Faculté de Biologie et de Médecine – at the University of Lausanne, Switzerland and was performed in accordance with the ethical standards laid down in the Declaration of Helsinki.

Materials and Apparatus

We employed a robotic system consisting of a bimanual haptic interface for the training of operations with the da Vinci surgery system (Mimic's dV-Trainer^{TM}, Mimic Technologies Inc., Seattle USA [26] see Figure 1D). The da Vinci system is a well-known surgical robotic system that is used for minimally invasive surgical procedures. This novel device is the first test-bed for the telerobotic surgical simulator. The tracking of the hand movements and force feedback are provided through a cable-driven system. Since it is a cable driven system, it has a large workspace. It provides 7 Degrees of Freedom (DOF) in motion for each hand and it can render high forces in 3-translation directions (x,y,z) without instability. The system has two lightweight grippers that enable transparent interactions with virtual reality making realistic bimanual manipulations possible. The participants were seated at a table and held two haptic interfaces, one in their left and one in their right hand. The index and thumb of both hands were positioned in the haptic device as shown in Figure 1D and their movements and interactions with virtual objects were presented on a head mounted display (HMD, eMagin Z800 3DVisor, 1.44 megapixel resolution).

An open source platform, CHAI 3D, and a set of C++ libraries were used for the modeling and for simulating the haptics, and for visualization of the virtual world. This platform supports several commercial haptic devices and it is possible to extend it to support new custom force feedback devices. We have extended this platform by adding the drivers and libraries of our custom force feedback device.

Two vibrotactile target stimulators (Precision MicroDrive shaftless vibration motors, model 312-101, 3 V, 80 mA, 9000 rpm (150 Hz) 1.7 g with a diameter of 12 mm and a length of 3.4 mm) were attached to the participants' thumb and index finger. Foam and rubber padding was used to insulate the vibrotactile stimulators from the surrounding material, thus minimizing any conduction of vibrations through the haptic device itself. For each participant, these stimulators were tested to generate easily localizable and clearly perceptible sensations. Vibrotactile stimuli were driven by electrical signals generated by a desktop computer (Intel Core i7 CPU with 2.8 GHz, 3 GB or Ram, with NVIDIA GeForce 9800 GT Graphic Card). Two data acquisition cards (NI PCI-6014 and NI PCI 6052E) were used to detect pedal responses and to drive vibrotactile stimulators. To minimize any unwanted reflections, the participants were seated in a dimly illuminated room enclosed by black curtains.

The participants viewed two virtual-robotic tools through a head mounted display. The distance between the tools subtended approximately 35° of visual angle. Visual distractor stimuli subtended approximately 0.9° of visual angle, positioned at the upper and lower locations of tips of the virtual-robotic tools that had a visual angle of 6.4°. For the modeling, simulating the haptics, and visualization of the virtual world, CHAI 3D and a set of C++ libraries were used. A virtual world with two virtual golf clubs was developed, see Figure 1 A and B.

A fixation cross was positioned at the vertical and horizontal mid-point of the corresponding four LEDs on the two tools. A chin rest system was used to prevent undesired movement of the head. In order to measure the participant's response, two pedals were attached to the floor next to the participant's right foot. The pedal separation was adjusted to fit the participant's foot size. One of the pedals was placed under the heel and the other under the toe of the participant's right foot. The participant raised his toes to indicate that the vibrations were felt at the index finger or raised his heels to indicate that the vibrations were felt at the thumb. White noise was presented over the headphones at an adequate level so that participants could not hear the sound of the vibrotactile stimulators or the operation of the other hardware during the experiments.

Experimental Design and Procedure

The experiments were designed in a 2×2×2 factorial manner. The 3 within-participants factors were congruency of the elevation of the vibrotactile stimuli with respect to the visual distractors (congruent vs. incongruent), the vibrotactile target side relative to the visual distractor side (same vs. different), and the type of posture (uncrossed vs. crossed). There were two blocks of 16 practice trials each, which were not analyzed. Experimental blocks began when the participant achieved an accuracy of more than 85 percent. A total of 480 experimental trials were given, divided into 15 blocks, with 240 trials for the straight tools and 240 trials for the crossed tools. Participants actively crossed or uncrossed the tools between every four trials in study 1 and changed passively (tool crossing made by the experimenter rather than the participants by crossing the tools only visually on the screen) at the end of 240 trials in study 2. Each of the 16 conditions (4 visual distractors×4 vibrotactile target locations) was presented 15 times (crossed or uncrossed), in a pseudo-randomized order determined by the computer.

Participants sat in front of a table and the table height was adjusted for each participant. They held the two haptic interfaces, with their thumbs next to the lower vibrotactile stimulator and their index fingers next to the upper stimulator. They were instructed to make speeded elevation discriminations to the vibrotactile stimuli. They were told that visual distractors would be presented simultaneously with the vibrotactile stimuli but that they should ignore them as much as possible while they were responding. They were instructed not to close their eyes and fixate on the central fixation cross until the end of the trial. The participant's right foot rested on the two pedals. They were instructed to hold both pedals pressed, which was the default condition and to release the toes in response to tactile stimuli applied to the index finger or to depress the heel if the stimuli were applied to the thumb. This toe/heel response mapped to index/thumb to make it compatible with upper/lower elevation of the vibrotactile and visual stimuli. In each trial, the visual distractor stimulus was presented 100 ms before presentation of the vibrotactile stimulus (SOA 100 ms) as previous work showed that this maximizes the CCE [27].

Participants moved two virtual golf clubs via the handle of a bimanual haptic simulator. In the first study, for some trials they held two tools in a straight position and for some trials they actively crossed the tools. Tool posture was changed actively after every four CCE trials. After every four CCE trials, to indicate that the CCE task was finished, two light balls were shown. This instructed the participant to cross or to uncross the tools. These two light balls also functioned to indicate where to position the tools in order to keep the distance between the tools constant for the crossed and uncrossed posture. In the second study the tools were not changed actively after every four CCE trials but only changed at the end of 240 trials. Virtual robotic tools were crossed by the experimenter rather than the participants as in the Maravita et al.'s experiment with physical tools [8] and only visual feedback of the crossed golf clubs was presented.

Analysis

For CCE analysis, trials with an incorrect response were discarded from the RT analysis but they were analyzed in the percentage error analysis. Trials with RTs larger than 1.500 and less than 200 milliseconds were removed. Next, RT outliers were removed using a criterion of 3 standard deviations above or below the subject's mean RT. These led to a rejection of a mean ± SE of 4.9±0.45% of all trials in experiment 1, and 6.7±0.65% of all trials in experiment 2. Data from all trials that resulted in correct responses were analyzed by using a repeated-measures three-way analysis of variance (ANOVAs) on the mean values of RTs. The three factors in the ANOVA design were: Congruency (congruent/incongruent), Side (same/different) and Tool posture (uncrossed/crossed). Paired t-tests were used for post-hoc comparisons on the CCEs. In addition, following previous studies on the CCE, the inverse efficiency (IE) was calculated by dividing the reaction time by the accuracy (proportion correct) for each condition, thereby controlling effectively for any speed-accuracy trade-off in the reaction time data [22].

Results

Study 1: Active tool use

Congruency effects derived from RT data from the first experiment are represented in Figure 2 and Table 1. The ANOVA performed on RTs from Experiment 1 revealed a main effect of congruency ($F(1, 9) = 32.90$, $p<0.001$) and a significant interaction between congruency and side ($F(1, 9) = 9.07$), $p<.05$) confirming that CCEs were significantly larger in the same side conditions compared to the different side conditions ($t(9) = 3.02$; $p<.05$). Crucially, we also found a three-way interaction between Congruency, Side and Tool Posture ($F(1, 9) = 37.88$, $p<0.001$).

To determine the driving factor of this three-way interaction, we performed post-hoc comparisons between the same side CCE versus the different side CCE for the RT measures for each tool posture. This analysis revealed that the CCE differed significantly between same side and different side for the uncrossed ($t(9) = 5.80$; $p<0.001$) and crossed condition ($t(9) = 3.30$; $p<0.01$) (see Figure 2 and Table 1). As inspection of Figure 2 reveals, the direction of these effects differed for uncrossed versus crossed conditions. In line with data obtained with physical tools, for the uncrossed condition the same side CCEs were larger than the different side CCEs, whereas for the crossed condition the different side CCEs were larger than the same side CCEs. These data indicate that active tool use results in a remapping of peripersonal space, depending on the position of the tools.

The ANOVA on the error rates revealed a main effect of congruency ($F(1, 9) = 21.75$, $p<0.01$) and a tendency for a three-way interaction between Congruency, Side and Tool Posture ($F(1, 9) = 3.97$, $p = 0.077$). The ANOVA on the IE data revealed a main effect of congruency ($F(1, 9) = 40.21$, $p<0.001$ and a significant interaction between congruency and side ($F(1, 9) = 5.52$), $p<.05$) and a three-way interaction between Congruency, Side and Tool

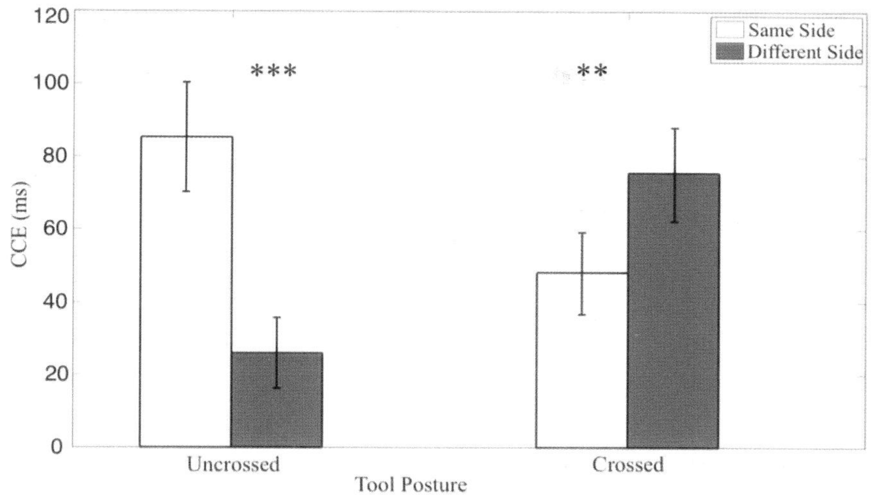

Figure 2. Crossmodal congruency effect (CCE) with standard error in Experiment 1. The CCE was calculated as incongruent reaction times minus congruent reaction times. White bars represent the condition in which visual stimuli were presented to the same visual hemifield with tactile stimuli, black bars represent trials in which the visual stimuli were presented to the different hemifield. The bars on the left side are for the uncrossed posture and bars on the right side are for the crossed posture.

Posture ($F(1, 9) = 14.99$, $p<0.01$) (see Table 1). Thus the analysis of the IE confirms the main findings from the analysis of Reaction Times and Error rates, indicating that the CCE side effect is modulated by the posture of the virtual tools (i.e. crossed or uncrossed). More importantly, this analysis provides further support that this effect cannot be accounted for by a speed-accuracy trade-off between the different experimental conditions.

Study 2: Passive tool use

Reaction time data from the second experiment are represented in Figure 3 and Table 2. The ANOVA performed on RTs from Experiment 2 revealed a main effect of tool posture ($F(1, 8) = 5.37$, $p<0.05$), a main effect of congruency ($F(1, 8) = 142.00$, $p<0.001$) and a significant interaction between side and congruency ($F(1, 8) = 17.63$), $p<0.005$) reflected in a stronger same side CCE than a different side CCE ($t(8) = 4.6$; $p<0.005$). Crucially, we found a

Table 1. Mean reaction times (RT) in milliseconds, percentage of errors (%) and inverse efficiency (IE) for Experiment 1.

Experiment 1				
Same Side				
Tool Posture		**Congruent**	**Incongruent**	**Mean CCE**
	RT	682.4(26.2)	730.8(21.7)	48.3(10.9)
Crossed	%	1.43(0.63)	1.59(0.49)	0.16(0.71)
	IE	691.6(26.3)	741.3(19.2)	49.7(11.8)
	RT	678.8(25.9)	764.1(32.5)	85.4(15.0)
Uncrossed	%	0.94(0.49)	4.57(0.97)	3.63(1.12)
	IE	686.1(27.3)	804.2(41.1)	118.1(20.7)
Different Side				
Tool Posture		**Congruent**	**Incongruent**	**Mean CCE**
	RT	673.5(26.3)	749.2(27.1)	75.6(12.5)
Crossed	%	1.32(0.58)	4.10(1.00)	2.78(0.91)
	IE	682.3(25.7)	786.4(34.0)	104.2(17.3)
	RT	718.7(27.1)	744.7(27.6)	26.0(9.8)
Uncrossed	%	1.41(0.57)	2.91(0.70)	1.50(0.67)
	IE	728.7(28.0)	763.8(28.2)	35.1(12.5)

The left column represents data for congruent conditions, the middle column for incongruent conditions. The right column represents the crossmodal congruency effect (CCE; i.e. difference between incongruent and congruent conditions). The first rows represent data for the crossed tool posture and the second rows represent data for the uncrossed posture. The upper panel represents data for visual stimuli at the same side as the tactile vibrations, the lower panel represents data for visual stimuli at the different side compared to the tactile vibrations. Values in parentheses are standard errors.

three-way interaction between Congruency, Side and Tool Posture ($F (1, 8) = 12.18$, $p<0.01$). We also performed post-hoc comparisons between the same side CCE versus the different side CCE for the RT. This analysis revealed that the CCE difference between same side and different side was significant for the uncrossed ($t(8) = 4.58$; $p<0.01$) but not significant for the crossed case ($t(8) = 0.11$; $p = 0.91$ NS)(see Figure 3 and Table 2). As can be seen in Figure 3, same side CCEs were larger than the different side CCEs only for the uncrossed condition but not for the crossed conditions. This finding indicates that passive tool use did not result in a complete remapping of peripersonal space, according to the position of the tools.

The ANOVA performed on error rates revealed a main effect of congruency ($F (1, 8) = 21.21$, $p<0.01$), a main effect of tool posture ($F (1, 8) = 5.42$, $p<0.05$) and an interaction between tool posture and congruency ($F (1, 8) = 13.36$, $p<0.01$). We also found a three-way interaction between Congruency, Side and Tool Posture for the percentage of errors ($F (1, 8) = 5.78$, $p<0.05$). We performed post-hoc comparisons between same side CCE versus different side CCE for the error rates. This analysis revealed that the difference between same side and different side was significant for the uncrossed posture ($p<0.01$) but not significant for the crossed posture. The ANOVA performed on the IE data revealed a main effect of tool posture ($F (1, 8) = 17.70$, $p<0.01$), a main effect of congruency, ($F (1, 8) = 78.71$, $p<0.001$) and an interaction between side and congruency ($F (1, 8) = 30.28$, $p<0.01$). We also found a three-way interaction between Congruency, Side and Tool Posture ($F (1, 8) = 10.87$, $p<0.05$) (see Table 2). Thus, the ANOVA on the IE data confirms the main findings of the analysis of the RT and error data and provides further support that no speed-accuracy trade-off underlies the present results.

In experiment 1, we found a significant three-way interaction between Congruency, Side, and Tool posture, as expected. In experiment 2, this interaction was also significant. In order to directly investigate the difference between active and passive tool crossing, we performed a between-experiments comparison, using a 4-way ANOVA with Experiment as a between-participants variable. The 4-way ANOVA performed on RTs revealed a main effect of tool posture ($F (1, 17) = 5.01$, $p<0.05$), a main effect of congruency ($F (1, 17) = 97.38$, $p<0.001$), a significant interaction between side and congruency ($F (1, 17) = 27.67$), $p<0.001$) and a three-way interaction between Congruency, Side and Tool Posture ($F (1, 17) = 42.52$, $p<0.001$). The 4-way interaction was not significant ($F (1, 17) = 0.57$, $p = 0.46$ NS) suggesting a remapping according to tool posture for both active and passive tool crossing.

In addition, to explore the pattern of interference reversal statistically, we analyzed the interference effect by pairs of blocks [8]. We could not find any significant correlation of the same side distractors or different side distractors with block number for the straight or crossed tools. Only a tendency for a negative correlation of same side distractors with the block number for the active straight tool was observed ($r = -0.86$ $p = 0.059$). The result of this analysis suggests that there is no learning effect of remapping. This analysis provides further evidence that the remapping of peripersonal space using virtual tools happens instantaneously.

Discussion

In the present study we investigated the integration of visuo-tactile cues in the case of a multimodal robotic interface controlling a virtual-robotic tool. At least three findings support the notion that the use of such 'virtual-robotic' tools facilitates the integration of multisensory information in peripersonal space. First, our results show that there was an interaction of vision and touch as reflected in the crossmodal congruency effect (CCE) for virtual robotic tools. Second, it was found that actively crossing the tool resulted in a remapping of peripersonal space, as reflected in a stronger CCE when visual stimuli appeared at a different side than the tactile vibration, at the tip of the tool that was held in the stimulated hand. Third, it was found that this remapping of peripersonal space did not depend on active tool use, as passive crossing of the tools resulted in a change in the CCE side effect as well. These results therefore extend previous findings on visuo-tactile integration in tool-use [20,22,26] to the domain of virtual tools, haptic interfaces and surgical robotics.

First, the results of both experiments showed an interference effect of visual distractors presented on the virtual-robotic tools on

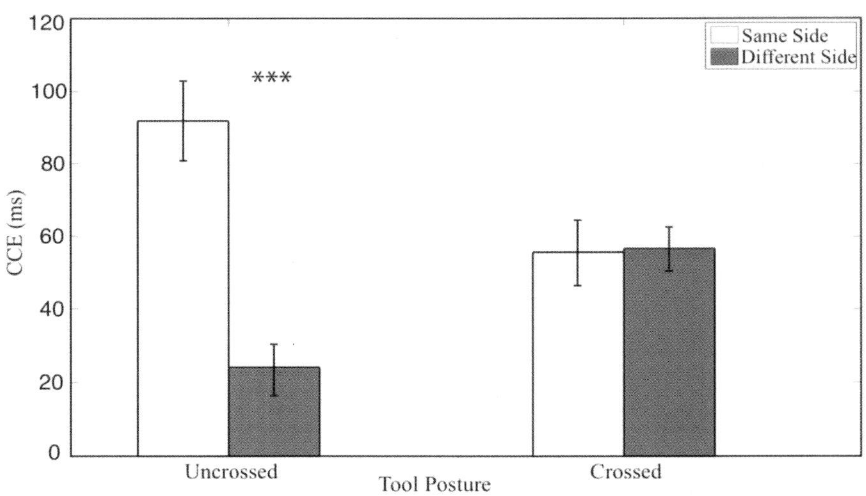

Figure 3. Crossmodal congruency effect (CCE) with standard error in Experiment 2. The CCE was calculated as incongruent reaction times minus congruent reaction times. White bars represent the condition in which visual stimuli were presented to the same visual hemifield with tactile stimuli, black bars represent trials in which the visual stimuli were presented to the different hemifield. The bars on the left side are for the uncrossed posture and on bars on the right side are for the crossed posture.

Table 2. Mean reaction times (RT) in milliseconds, percentage of errors (%) and inverse efficiency (IE) for Experiment 2.

Experiment 2				
Same Side				
Tool Posture		**Congruent**	**Incongruent**	**Mean CCE**
	RT	601.0(19.7)	656.7(22.6)	55.7(8.8)
Crossed	%	1.33 (0.55)	3.79 (1.02)	2.46 (1.22)
	IE	609.2(20.6)	681.8(21.7)	72.7(4.5)
	RT	591.7(18.0)	683.5(24.8)	91.8(11.1)
Uncrossed	%	2.63 (0.92)	9.62 (0.99)	6.99 (1.13)
	IE	607.7(19.2)	754.4(26.4)	146.7(14.6)
Different Side				
Tool Posture		**Congruent**	**Incongruent**	**Mean CCE**
	RT	595.5(22.6)	652.2(23.7)	56.7(5.9)
Crossed	%	2.67 (0.72)	6.24(1.79)	3.57(2.23)
	IE	624.2(28.4)	683.6(25.7)	59.4(22.1)
	RT	643.9(24.1)	668.0(21.6)	24.1(6.3)
Uncrossed	%	4.16(1.12)	3.55(1.28)	−0.61(1.22)
	IE	671.1(24.1)	692.8(22.4)	21.7(10.8)

The left column represents data for congruent conditions, the middle column for incongruent conditions. The right column represents the crossmodal congruency effect (CCE; i.e. difference between incongruent and congruent conditions). The first rows represent data for the crossed tool posture, the second rows represent data for the uncrossed posture. The upper panel represents data for visual stimuli at the same side as the tactile vibrations, the lower panel represents data for visual stimuli at the different side compared to the tactile vibrations. Values in parentheses are standard errors.

tactile discrimination judgments. The interfering effect of the visual stimuli on the virtual-robotic tools was reflected in slower reaction times and increased error rates when participants responded to incongruent compared to congruent vibrotactile stimuli, which is known as the crossmodal congruency effect (CCE). The results of the first experiment showed that visual distractors presented at the end of the left tool interfered more strongly with judging tactile stimuli applied to the left hand compared to the right hand (and vice versa for visual distractors presented at the right tool). Therefore, these findings suggest that both the passive and the active use of a virtual-robotic tool can alter multisensory integration in peripersonal space, reflecting a remapping of peripersonal space similar to the effects found for active physical and pointing tool use [6,8,9,18]. Thus, when the participants used the virtual-robotic tools actively, our data suggest that they functioned as an extension of their arms. This extension produced a stronger association between the vibrotactile stimuli on the hands and the visual stimulation at the end of the tool. The effect of visual distractors on tactile discrimination responses has often been related to findings in monkeys, indicating that the response properties of neurons in parietal areas reflect the functional aspects of tool use (i.e. incorporation of the tool in the body; cf. [10,19]; but for critical discussion, see: [22]). A similar neural mechanism has been proposed to underlie the effects of multisensory integration after tool use, as seen in healthy humans as well as brain damaged patients [21]. For instance, Farne el al. [28] studied the extension of peripersonal space with physical tool-use in visuo-tactile neglect patients and found that visuo-tactile extinction can be modulated by tool use (i.e. stronger left tactile extinction with right lights when a tool is wielded on the right side).

Second, in the first experiment it was found that when the virtual-robotic tools were actively crossed, visual distractors from the opposite visual field interfered more strongly with tactile stimuli applied to the hand that was holding the tool. In the crossed condition the tip of the tool held by the left hand was in the right visual field and visual distractors presented at the tip of this tool interfered more strongly with tactile stimuli applied to the left compared to the right hand. The opposite was true for the tool held by the right hand. Thus, visual stimuli were primarily associated with the hand that was holding the tool rather than the spatial side at which the stimuli appeared. This finding suggests that actively crossing the tool resulted in a remapping of peripersonal space, as reflected in a stronger CCE when visual stimuli appeared at a different side than the tactile vibration, at the tip of the tool that was held in the stimulated hand. The finding that active crossing of the virtual-robotic tool resulted in a remapping of peripersonal space extends previous studies on real-world tools [8,19,20]. These studies showed that crossing the tools actively remapped the visuo-tactile representation of peripersonal space [8].

The results of the second experiment, obtained in a different participant sample, showed that when participants held uncrossed tools, the CCE was larger when the visuotactile stimuli were presented at the same side compared to the different side. In contrast to the results obtained in the first experiment, when the tools were passively crossed, the CCEs for visuotactile stimuli presented at the same and different side were comparable in size. Thus, the passive crossing of the virtual-robotic tools did not completely remap the peripersonal space representation, as it did in the first experiment. It did affect the representation of peripersonal space, as reflected in the fact that the difference between the same and different side CCE differed between crossed and uncrossed postures (i.e. a significant 3-way interaction was found). This result is different to that in previous studies (see [8]), in which passively moving the real-world tool always resulted in a stronger CCE for visuotactile stimuli appearing at the same compared to the different side, irrespective of whether the tools were crossed or not. Our findings suggest that virtual-robotic tools may alter multisensory integration even when the tool is not actively used and thus affect multisensory integration differently than the physical tools. This could also be due to different physical and information processing mechanism of the virtual robotic tools such as the immersive nature and 'tele-arm' like behavior of these tools. In our experiments the real hands were not visible, as the participants were wearing head mounted displays. The absence of visual information about the hands may have facilitated the integration of the virtual tools in the body representation, thereby resulting in a remapping of the visuo-tactile representation of peripersonal space even in the case of passive tool use.

The results of this study are novel and extend previous studies for several reasons. Up to now, studies on the representation of peripersonal space in humans have used mainly tools that physically link peripersonal space and extrapersonal space - such as golf clubs, rakes, long sticks to press a button or to reach a distant object [6,8]. It has been found, for instance, that peripersonal space was extended by active tool use [8]. However, there is an alternative interpretation with respect to the extension of peripersonal space with the tool. Holmes et al. have shown that multisensory spatial interactions were enhanced at the tips of the tools rather than in the middle of tools, suggesting that peripersonal space is not extended but projected towards the part of the tool that is most relevant for the task. According to this interpretation, tools act as spatial attentional cues rather than entities which cause an extension of peripersonal space [29]. In fact, virtual robotic tools can help to shed light on the question of whether peripersonal space is projected or extended, by enabling novel experimental paradigms with virtual robotic tools that would be difficult to perform with physical tools. For instance, in a recent study we inserted a movable joint in the middle of the tool, thereby making the middle part of the tool more relevant to the action at hand (e.g. as if the middle part of the tool represents one's wrist or elbow; cf. Sengül et al. in prep.). It was found that peripersonal space was selectively projected towards the part of the tool that was relevant to the task at hand (i.e. controlling the tool by moving the wrist or the elbow), thereby providing further support for the idea that peripersonal space is indeed projected to distant locations that are task-relevant and attended.

The results of the present study also extend previous studies with pointing tools [9,10]. For instance, Iriki et al (2001; cf. [10]) conducted a study in which monkeys trained to control a tool via a computer screen with the arms out of view. It was found that the visual receptive field size of visuo-tactile neurons in parietal areas was enlarged to include the tool viewed through the video monitor. Interestingly, when only a cursor was presented instead of a tool, much fewer neurons with such properties were found. It could be that for monkeys it is more difficult to integrate abstract visual information into their body representation. In contrast, for humans the interaction with virtual objects is omnipresent in our everyday lives (e.g. the use of computers, video games, PC tablets, etc.) and as a consequence virtual tools may be more easily integrated in the representation of our body. In support of this view, Bassolino et al. showed that the space where a pointing tool (i.e. a computer mouse) was actually held (i.e. close to hand) was extended to the space where it operates (i.e. the computer screen) even though these spaces were not physically connected [9].

Furthermore, the findings of this study are in line with the findings of Moizumi et al. [30], reporting a remapping of touch in VR with humans holding the arms in a crossed or uncrossed position. In this study a temporal order judgment task was used and it was found that when the arms were uncrossed participants' ability to report tactile vibrations applied to the hand was modulated by whether the virtual tools were crossed or uncrossed. In contrast, when the arms were crossed, the direction of the force feedback primarily determined the perceived order of tactile judgments, indicating the importance of haptic force feedback for disambiguating the referral of tactile sensations. The present study extends these findings [30], by showing that virtual tool use changes visuo-tactile instead of only tactile interactions in virtual space. In addition, our findings indicate that both active crossing and passive crossing of the virtual tool results in a remapping of the peripersonal space. Finally, we would like to point out that we investigated peripersonal space representations, using a new class of virtual tools that are increasingly used in surgical robotics. In surgical robotics, an important aim is to increase the telepresence of the surgeon in the remote site. Studying how peripersonal space representation as measured through the CCE changes with virtual robotic tools could be an objective assessment method for the evaluation of the telepresence by analysing whether the remote site was represented as within peripersonal space or not.

We note that the present work on the relation between the CCE and peripersonal space representations, is also consistent with the findings by Rognini et al., who showed that visuo-tactile CCEs can be obtained in a robotically mediated environment using virtual hands [26]. The present study, however, shows that visuo-tactile integration on a robotic platform does not only occur for virtual hands but also for virtual-robotic tools. Moreover, Rognini et al. measured the integration of visuo-tactile cues online: during the holding and moving of virtual objects with virtual hands. In the present study, we measured visuo-tactile CCEs after using a telemanipulation tool. Hence we propose that measuring such CCE post-effects can also be used as an objective assessment of how we learn to use robotic tools.

Together, the results of these studies show that cognitive neuroscience measures can be used to investigate the integration of visual and tactile cues in robotic technologies. This suggests that CCE measurements may be used as an objective assessment of human factors. Up to now, human factors in robotics, especially in surgical robotics was quantified by means of questionnaires or performance based measurements such as task completion time or task accuracy [31–33]. These studies focused on a specific task such as needle insertion during surgical procedures, neglecting more basic and repeated behavioral changes of multisensory integration driven by tool-use [34–36]. Here we propose a new methodology to study 'human factors' in a surgical interface with a more objective assessment technique by quantifying visuo-tactile integration measured by the CCE. This extends and changes the standard analysis of human factors in the field of surgical robotics by injecting insights and methods from cognitive neuroscience into this emerging field between neuroscience, psychology, and engineering. Understanding how the brain codes peripersonal space and which factors contribute to the integration of tools into the brain's body representation may turn out to be of pivotal importance for the design of future robots that can be more easily used and controlled for the benefit of patients nearby and at distance. For instance, an important issue in the field of medical and surgical robotics is the feeling that the surgeon is holding, and operating with a surgical tool – as if he were controlling a real tool to operate his patient. The present study provides a first step to study more objectively the relation between real tools and virtual-robotic tools, by showing that similar neurocognitive mechanisms are involved in using real and virtual-robotic tools.

In summary, the present paper presented two experiments on multisensory integration through the use of a virtual-robotic tool. It was found that virtual-robotic tool use changed the integration of visuo-tactile information in peripersonal space, as reflected in a cross-modal congruency effect (CCE). This result illustrates that, in order to change the representation of peripersonal space, it is not necessary to have a physical connection between the space where the tool is held and the space where the tool operates. The results are consistent with previous studies on the cross-modal congruency effect (CCE). This study establishes that telemanipulators consisting of haptic devices and virtual reality can be used in cognitive neuroscience investigations, thereby opening up exciting new possibilities for neuroscience experimentation and improved incorporation of human factors into the future design of minimally invasive surgical robots.

Acknowledgments

We thank the anonymous reviewers and N. P. Holmes for their helpful and constructive comments.

Author Contributions

Conceived and designed the experiments: AS GR JA OB. Performed the experiments: AS. Analyzed the data: AS. Contributed reagents/materials/analysis tools: AS GR. Wrote the paper: AS MvE GR JA HB OB.

References

1. Iriki ATM (in press) Triadic (ecological, neural, cognitive) niche construction: a scenario of human brain evolution extrapolating tool-use and language from the control of reaching actions. Phil Trans R Soc B.
2. Ishibashi H, Hihara S, Iriki A (2000) Acquisition and development of monkey tool-use: behavioral and kinematic analyses. Canadian Journal of Physiology and Pharmacology 78: 958–966.
3. Goldenberg G, Spatt J (2009) The neural basis of tool use. Brain 132: 1645–1655.
4. Peeters R, Simone L, Nelissen K, Fabbri-Destro M, Vanduffel W, et al. (2009) The Representation of Tool Use in Humans and Monkeys: Common and Uniquely Human Features. J Neurosci 29: 11523–11539.
5. Holmes NP, Calvert GA, Spence C (2006) Beyond the body: visual, prosthetic and technological contributions to bodily perception and awareness; In: Knoblich GT, I.M.; Grosjean, M.; Shiffrar, M., editor. New York: Oxford Univ. Press.
6. Holmes NP, Sanabria D, Calvert GA, Spence C (2007) Tool-use: Capturing multisensory spatial attention or extending multisensory peripersonal space? Cortex 43: 469–489.
7. Maravita A, Iriki A (2004) Tools for the body (schema). Trends Cogn Sci 8: 79–86.
8. Maravita A, Spence C, Kennett S, Driver J (2002) Tool-use changes multimodal spatial interactions between vision and touch in normal humans. Cognition 83: B25–B34.
9. Bassolino M, Serino A, Ubaldi S, Ladavas E (2010) Everyday use of the computer mouse extends peripersonal space representation. Neuropsychologia 48: 803–811.
10. Iriki A, Tanaka M, Obayashi S, Iwamura Y (2001) Self-images in the video monitor coded by monkey intraparietal neurons. Neurosci Res 40: 163–173.
11. Rosen J, Hannaford B, Satava R (2011) Surgical Robotics: Systems Applications and Visions. London: Springer
12. Suematsu Y, del Nido PJ (2004) Robotic pediatric cardiac surgery: present and future perspectives. Am J Surg 188: 98S–103S.
13. Stone R. Haptic feedback: A potted history, from telepresence to virtual reality. 2000; Glasgow, UK, 1–7. Springer-Verlag Lecture Notes in Computer Science.
14. Kenngott HG, Fischer L, Nickel F, Rom J, Rassweiler J, et al. (2012) Status of robotic assistance-a less traumatic and more accurate minimally invasive surgery? Langenbeck Arch Surg 397: 333–341.
15. Rassweiler J, Safi KC, Subotic S, Teber D, Frede T (2005) Robotics and telesurgery–an update on their position in laparoscopic radical prostatectomy. Minim Invasive Ther Allied Technol 14: 109–122.
16. Tavakoli M, Aziminejad A, Patel RV, Moallem M (2007) High-fidelity bilateral teleoperation systems and the effect of multimodal haptics. Ieee Transactions on Systems Man and Cybernetics Part B-Cybernetics 37: 1512–1528.
17. Octavia JR, Raymaekers C, Coninx K (2011) Adaptation in virtual environments: conceptual framework and user models. Multimed Tools Appl 54: 121–142.
18. Ladavas E, Serino A (2008) Action-dependent plasticity in peripersonal space representations. Cogn Neuropsychol 25: 1099–1113.
19. Iriki A, Tanaka M, Iwamura Y (1996) Coding of modified body schema during tool use by macaque postcentral neurones. Neuroreport 7: 2325–2330.
20. Maravita A (2006) From body in the brain, to body in space: sensory and intentional aspects of body representation; Grosjean IGKMSM, editor. Oxford: Oxford University Press.
21. Maravita A, Iriki A (2004) Tools for the body (schema). Trends in Cognitive Sciences 8: 79–86.
22. Holmes NP (2012) Does tool use extend peripersonal space? A review and re-analysis. Experimental Brain Research 218: 273–282.
23. Pavani F, Spence C, Driver J (2000) Visual capture of touch: out-of-the-body experiences with rubber gloves. Psychol Sci 11: 353–359.
24. Zopf R, Savage G, Williams MA (2010) Crossmodal congruency measures of lateral distance effects on the rubber hand illusion. Neuropsychologia 48: 713–725.
25. Aspell JE, Lenggenhager B, Blanke O (2009) Keeping in touch with one's self: multisensory mechanisms of self-consciousness. PLoS One 4: e6488.
26. Rognini G, Sengül A, Aspell JE, Bleuler H, Blanke O (2012) Visuo-tactile integration and body ownership during self-generated action. Eur J Neurosci (in revision).
27. Shore DI, Barnes ME, Spence C (2006) Temporal aspects of the visuotactile congruency effect. Neurosci Lett 392: 96–100.
28. Farne A, Iriki A, Ladavas E (2005) Shaping multisensory action-space with tools: evidence from patients with cross-modal extinction. Neuropsychologia 43: 238–248.
29. Holmes NP, Calvert GA, Spence C (2004) Extending or projecting peripersonal space with tools? Multisensory interactions highlight only the distal and proximal ends of tools. Neuroscience Letters 372: 62–67.
30. Moizumi S, Yamamoto S, Kitazawa S (2007) Referral of tactile stimuli to action points in virtual reality with reaction force. Neuroscience Research 59: 60–67.
31. Lee EC, Rafiq A, Merrell R, Ackerman R, Dennerlein JT (2005) Ergonomics and human factors in endoscopic surgery: a comparison of manual vs telerobotic simulation systems. Surg Endosc 19: 1064–1070.
32. Prasad SM, Maniar HS, Soper NJ, Damiano RJ, Klingensmith ME (2002) The effect of robotic assistance on learning curves for basic laparoscopic skills. Am J Surg 183: 702–707.
33. Santos-Carreras L, Hagen M, Gassert R, Bleuler H (2011) Survey on Surgical Instrument Handle Design: Ergonomics and Acceptance. Surg Innov.
34. Narazaki K, Oleynikov D, Stergiou N (2006) Robotic surgery training and performance: identifying objective variables for quantifying the extent of proficiency. Surg Endosc 20: 96–103.
35. Okamura AM (2009) Haptic feedback in robot-assisted minimally invasive surgery. Curr Opin Urol 19: 102–107.
36. Santos-Carreras LB, Sengül A, Gassert R, Bleuler H (2010) Influence of force and torque feedback on operator performance in a VR-based suturing task. Applied Bionics and Biomechanics 217–230.

11

Minimally Invasive Surgical Versus Catheter Ablation for the Long-Lasting Persistent Atrial Fibrillation

Jiangang Wang[1], Yan Li[1], Jiahai Shi[2], Jie Han[1], Chunlei Xu[1], Changsheng Ma[1], Xu Meng[1]*

1 Department of Atrial Fibrillation Center, Beijing Anzhen Hospital, Capital Medical University, Beijing, China, **2** Department of Cardiothoracic Surgery, Affiliated Hospital of Nantong University, Nantong, China

Abstract

Objective: To assess the efficacy of video-assisted minimally invasive surgical vs. catheter ablation for the long-standing persistent AF.

Methods: We performed a retrospective comparative analysis in a series of 166 long-standing persistent AF patients treated between 2006 and 2009 with either video-assisted minimally invasive ablation (83 patients), or catheter ablations (83 patients). The catheter group was screened using a 'pair-matched case-control' methodology in order to select appropriate statistical comparison candidates out of 169 long-standing persistent AF patients which were potentially suitable for surgery, but have been treated with catheter approaches in order to balance major prognostic factors between the two groups. Follow-up for all patients ranged from 1 to 3.6 years.

Results: No patient died postoperatively. One patient suffered from stroke in the surgical group but recovered before discharge. Freedom from AF was obtained in 59.0% and 74.7% during follow-up in the catheter group and the surgical group respectively ($P = 0.047$). Patients in the catheter group had a significantly higher rate of recurrent arrhythmia ($P = 0.011$, hazard ratio: 0.555, 95% CI: 0.354 to 0.872) compared with the surgically treated group. The freedom from antiarrhythmic drugs was 44.6% in the catheter group and 61.4% in the surgical group ($P = 0.043$).

Conclusions: The video-assisted minimally invasive ablation was safe and effective, and had an optimistic success rate for patients with long-standing persistent AF in our retrospective comparative study. Thus, further randomized studies addressing this issue seem to be justified.

Editor: Shahab A. Akhter, University of Chicago, United States of America

Funding: This work was supported by National Natural Science Foundation of China (Grant No. 30900629), and the Beijing Novo Program, (Grant No. 2010B047). The funders had no role in study design, data collection and analysis, decision to publish, or preparation of the manuscript.

Competing Interests: The authors have declared that no competing interests exist.

* E-mail: mxu@263.net

Introduction

Atrial fibrillation (AF) affects proximately 10 million patients in China, undoubtedly the largest demographic group in the world [1]. Catheter ablation targeting pulmonary vein isolation (PVI) has been evolved over the past decade and has become the common treatment for AF [2], but it often requires repeated procedures, and is associated with serious, although infrequent, complications [3,4]. It has limited success in persistent and permanent AF, although different ablation strategies beyond PVI have been described to improve the outcome in this patient group [5,6]. Wolf and colleagues reported encouraging early experiences with a stand-alone, minimally invasive, video-assisted thoracoscopic surgical technique for the epicardial ablation of AF on a beating heart with the use of dry radiofrequency (RF) bipolar energy [7].

To assess the clinical outcome of surgical ablation we performed a retrospective analysis comparing two pair-matched groups of patients with long-standing persistent AF, one treated with video-assisted minimally invasive ablation, and the other one treated with conventional catheter approach.

Methods

2.1 Objective

In this restrospective study we compared the surgical minimally invasive surgery method versus the internal medicine catheter ablation method in order to evaluate an optimal proceeding for the treatment of long-standing atrial fibrillation and we hypothesised that minimally invasive surgery is the superior approach.

2.2 Patients

Between 2006 and 2009, 91 consecutive patients with long-standing persistent AF were treated with video-assisted thoracoscopic surgical ablation at the Atrial Fibrillation Centre, Beijing Anzhen Hospital. Long-standing persistent AF was defined as continuous AF lasting longer than 1 year, resistant to either electrical or pharmacological cardioversion. Indications for surgical AF ablation were: Drug-refractory; inability to tolerate antiarrhythmic drugs or anticoagulation therapy as well as left ventricular ejection fraction of 30% or greater. The patients should also have been able to provide a written informed consent, their life expectancy should have been at least 2 years and they must have been able to attend scheduled follow-up visits. The exclusion criteria in the surgical group were: left ventricular ejection fraction lower than 30%, sick sinus syndrome, severe pleural adhesions as well as prior attempts with catheter ablation for a treatment of atrial fibrillation, what means that none of the patients in the surgical group, which we have chosen for the comparison, underwent a previous catheter ablation. In order to assess the role of surgery in the treatment of long-standing persistent AF, treatment outcome in this group of patients was compared with that of patients managed with conventional catheter approaches. The inclusion criteria for a treatment with catheter AF ablation were: Symptomatic AF refractory or intolerance to at least one class 1 or 3 antiarrhythmic medication and patients with heart failure and/or reduced ejection fraction. In addition in rare clinical situations, it may be appropriate to perform catheter AF ablation as the first line therapy. The exclusion criteria in the catheter group were: Left ventricular ejection fraction <30 percent, presence of left atrial thrombus on transesophageal echocardiography and prior attempts with catheter or surgical ablation for an atrial fibrillation treatment.

To secure a relatively reliable comparative analysis between patients treated with and without surgery, we performed a matched case-control procedure. From the group of patients treated with catheter approaches we selected cases with similar favorable prognostic factors matching those in the surgical group and from a total of 169 patients treated with catheter approaches, we selected 89 cases which also would have been potentially suitable for surgery. Each patient from the surgical group has then been pair-matched to a patient from the screened catheter group, taking into account the most important prognostic factors, which were duration of AF, left atrial dimension and sex. Patients from both groups for whom no comparable control case could be found were then excluded from further analysis. As a result of this process, 166 patients were selected for a comparative analysis; 83 treated with minimal invasive surgery versus 83 managed with catheter approach (Table 1).

2.3 Catheter ablation

Ablation was guided by an electroanatomical mapping system (CARTO, Biosense Webster) and performed with a temperature-controlled, quadripolar, deflectable catheter with a 3.5-mm irrigated-tip catheter (Navistar, Biosense Webster) to encircle the left and right pulmonary vein (PV) 1 to 2 cm from their ostia, with additional lines in the posterior left atrium or roof and along the mitral isthmus. Two decapolar circular mapping catheters (Lasso, Biosense-Webster Inc) were placed inside the ipsilateral superior and inferior PVs or within the superior and inferior branches of a common PV to verify PVI during radiofrequency current ablation. RF current was delivered at each site until the local electrogram amplitude was reduced by at least 80%. Contiguous lesions were delivered at about 20 mm from the PV ostia. Additional ablation within the circles was performed in most of the patients, outside the PVs, where the local electrogram amplitude exceeded 0.2 mV. Additional lines were created in the posterior wall between the 2 encircling PV lesions and from the lower aspect of the left inferior PV to the mitral annulus. If AF was still present at the end of PVI, transthoracic cardioversion was used to restore sinus rhythm (SR). The end point was defined as the absence of any PV spike recorded on the 2 Lasso catheters placed within the ipsilateral PVs after at least 30 minutes following the PV isolation during SR.

2.4 Surgical Technique

The video-assisted thoracoscopic surgical procedure was developed to perform an electrically PVI bilaterally. In brief a bipolar RF clamp and RF generator system (AtriCure, Inc, Cincinnati, Ohio) is used to achieve linear, transmural ablation lesions. The procedure is conducted after a general anesthesia administered with a double-lumen endotracheal tube and a transesophageal echocardiography used in the operating room is included in order to verify the left atrial appendage (LAA) excisions at the end of the procedures. As shown in Fig. 1 (A–B), each set of PV was encircled and ablated on the left atrium by using an epicardial-placed bipolar RF clamp and no other epicardial lesions were placed. The ligament of Marshall was taken down in all patients and a detailed ganglionic plexus (GP) mapping and ablation was performed. Thoracoscopic LAA exclusion was then performed using a Thoracic Endoscopic Linear Cutter EZ45G (Ethicon Endo-Surgery, Inc, Cincinnati, OH), with non buttressed 4.8-mm staples (Fig.1C). Appropriate stapler angle and adequate appendage coverage was enhanced by direct visualization through the working port.

2.5 Intraoperative Electrophysiologic Testing

Intraoperative electrophysiologic testing was performed, which includes bilateral PV antrum, baseline and post isolation sensing, pacing and GP detection. A baseline positive sensing result (rapid and disorderly atrial potentials) in the PV antrum area could be detected before PVI, and a negative sensing result (no atrial potentials) could be detected in the same area after ablation, which is called entrance block. A positive baseline pacing result is defined as the atrial and ventricular capture, what is the contraction of the atrium and ventricle in response to the electrical stimulus being sent from the temporary pacemaker (Oscor Pace 203H DDD External Dual-Chamber Pacemaker; Oscor Inc, Palm Harbor, Fla). A negative postablation pacing result means that no capture is obtained in the same area after ablation. A combined positive baseline pacing and negative postablation pacing result is called exit block. Achieving both entrance and exit block is regarded as a transmural lesion blocking of the conduction in the PV antrum area. Meanwhile, GP activity detection is included in the electrophysiologic testing procedure, as described by Mehall et al, which consist of a basically mapping by using a high-frequency stimulus (10 V, 800 times per second) for 5 seconds or more [8]. A positive response was defined as sinus bradycardia (<40 beats/min) or asystole, atrioventricular block, or hypotension occurring ventricular asystole of the onset of high-frequency stimulus.

2.6 Postablative Medical Management

Postablative anticoagulation treatment was done according to the American College of Cardiology/American Heart Association/European Society of Cardiology guidelines [9]. The decision whether to apply warfarin or aspirin has been done on the base of the patients Cardiac Failure, Hypertension, Age, Diabetes, Stroke (CHADS) score. Patients received 200 mg of amiodarone orally per day for three months. In the 4th month anticoagulant drug administration was discontinued when SR was present, what was examined by a 24–48 hour Holter monitoring. An AF or atrial flutter (AFL) episode was defined after documentation by means of ECG or Holter monitoring as at least 30 seconds lasting. During the follow-up period, if ECG analysis showed recurrence of AF or AFL which sustained for more than 8 hours and the anticoagulation value was adequately (International normalized ratio >2.0), a direct-current cardioversion was recommended, and a circumferential PV catheter ablation was performed.

2.7 Follow-up procedure

Follow-up controls were obtained from office visits at an outpatient building, mailed medical records received from local

Table 1. Patient characteristics.

	Catheter Group N = 83	Surgical Group N = 83	*P* Value
Age (yrs)	55±12	57±11	0.29
Sex (male/female)	52/31	58/25	0.41
Duration of AF (months)	70±74	71±65	0.16
History of smoking	29	25	0.62
History of alcohol	15	21	0.35
Hypertension	40	37	0.76
Diabetes	11	10	NS
Hyperthyroidism	5	1	0.21
Stroke	7	13	0.23
Permanent pacemaker implantation	5	6	NS
Number of anticoagulant therapy			
Warfarin	28	34	0.42
Aspirin	38	34	0.64
Number of digitalis	28	27	NS
Number of AAD			
Beta receptor blocker	39	43	0.64
Amiodarone	35	37	0.88
LAD (mm)	53±11	51±12	0.25
LVED (mm)	48±5	48±6	0.92
LVEF (%)	61±7	62±9	0.25

AAD = antiarrhythmic drugs; AF = atrial fibrillation; LAD = left atrial dimension; LVED = left ventricular end diastolic dimension; LVEF = left ventricular ejection fraction.

hospitals, and questionnaires. As a standard method for monitoring patient' heart rhythm we used a 24 to 48 hour Holter monitoring and additional twelve-lead ECG analysis for AF or AFL recurrence. Transthoracic UCG were evaluated at discharge and 1, 3, 6 and 12 months postoperatively. After one year, patients were seen every 6 months by their referring cardiologist. Free ECG examinations as well as free 24 to 48 hour Holter monitoring (Del Mar Reynolds Medical, Inc, Irvine, Calif) were offered at the Atrial Fibrillation Centre, Beijing Anzhen Hospital.

2.8 Ethical approval and consent

The protocol was approved by (Institutional Review Board or Ethics Committee of Beijing Anzhen Hospital, Capital Medical University). All participants in this study gave a written informed consent.

2.9 Statistical analysis

Continuous data were presented as the mean ± standard deviation and categorical variables were expressed as the number of cases and percentage. The significance of the differences between the groups was assessed by the Student *t* test or Mann-Whitney *U* test for continuous variables and chi-square test for categorical variables. Cumulative event rates were calculated according to the Kaplan-Meier method. All tests were 2-tailed, and $p<0.05$ was considered significant. The data were analyzed with the SPSS for Windows version 12.0 (SPSS Inc., Chicago, IL, USA).

Results

3.1 Immediate results during hospital observation

All patients successfully underwent the ablation procedure and there was no PV injury, in-hospital mortality, or necessity of reoperation because of bleeding. Circumferential PV catheter ablations were performed within a mean of 39±14 minutes of RF energy. The catheter group had a statistically longer procedure time for the entire ablation (231±27 minutes) than the surgical group for the entire operation (143.4±26.2 minutes) ($P=0.016$). One patient with AF rhythm suffered from stroke in the surgical group, due to poor anticoagulation status (international normalized ratio<2.0), but recovered without any sequelae before discharge.

The changes in the cardiac rhythms during stay in hospital are described in Table 2. During ablation, AF termination (conversion in SR) was seen in 34.9% of the catheter group and in 45.7% of the surgical group of patients, respectively ($P=0.15$). AF organization into AFL occurred more often in the catheter group, 24 patients (28.9%), 13 right sided and 11 left sided, than in the surgical group, 5 patients (6.0%), 2 right sided and 3 left sided

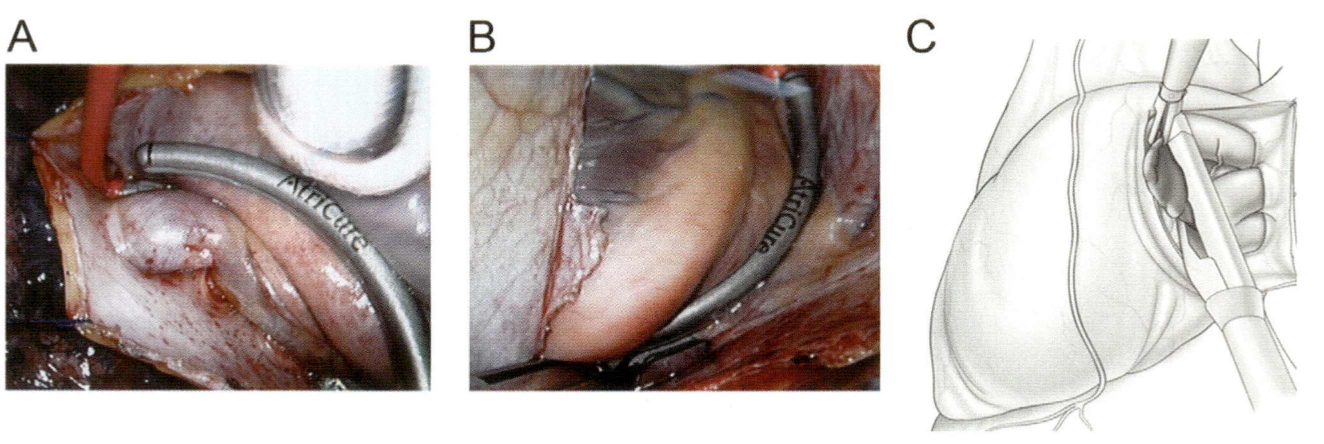

Figure 1. Video-assisted thoracoscopic surgical ablation. (A) Right thoracoscopic view of the bipolar clamp in place on the left atrial antrum, medial to the right PV. (B) Left thoracoscopic view of the bipolar clamp in place on the left atrial antrum, medial to the left PV. (C) The left atrial appendage is excised by stapling it with a stapler.

($P<0.001$). AF was documented to be 39.8% in total of the two groups. Temporary pacemakers were used in 4 patients from the surgical group because of bradycardia.

During hospitalization, AF and AFL recurred in 16 (19.3%) and 22 (26.5%) of the patients in the catheter group after a mean time of 2.0±1.5 days, and 12 (14.5%) and 2 (2.4%) patients in the surgical group after a mean time of 6.0±1.4 days, respectively ($P=0.70$ and $P<0.001$). At discharge from the hospital, SR and AF was maintained in 86.8% and 4.8% of the patients in the catheter group and 63.9% and 28.9% in the surgical group respectively ($P<0.001$).

The average length of stay in hospital was 6.1±2.6 and 4.8±2.5 days in the surgical group and catheter group, respectively ($P=0.56$).

3.2 Follow-up Results

Average followed-up was 2.2years (range 1.0 to 3.6 years) after the procedures. During the follow-up period, two patients (2.4%) died in the catheter group, one for unknown reason and the other one with encephalorraghia. One patient (1.2%) died in the surgical group for unknown reason.

Taking a blanking period of 3 months after surgery into account, 49 (59.0%) and 62 patients (74.7%) did not have a 'single' registration of AF during follow-up in the catheter group and surgical group respectively ($P=0.047$). Additionally, patients in the catheter group had a significantly higher rate of recurrent arrhythmia ($P=0.011$, hazard ratio: 0.555, 95% CI: 0.354 to 0.872). (Fig.2)

In the catheter group, a second ablation procedure was performed in 23 patients with arrhythmia recurrence. Following the 2nd redo procedure, a third redo ablation was performed in 6 patients. Two patients who had failed the third redo ablation were treated then with the surgical procedure and were free from AF after follow-up.

Five patients with recurrent AF, within the surgical group, who agreed to a second treatment, underwent a catheter ablation successfully. Two of these patients were proven to have a bidirectional block based on tests performed during the surgery suffered recurrent AF. Subsequent CARTO electrophysiologic mapping showed complex fractionated atrial electrograms (CFAEs) in both atriums. The CFAEs ablation converted AF into atrial tachycardia, with the average AF cycle length of the 2 patients increasing from 140±12 ms to 214±23 ms after CFAEs ablation. Three-dimensional activation time-sequence mapping of the left atrium, combined with entrainment mapping, was then performed to clarify the underlying focal or macroreentry mechanism. The resulted "Entrainment" refers to higher tachycardia that occurs consistently during high frequency pacing; when the pacing frequency stops or is reduced below the original tachycardia, the tachycardia will drop back to a baseline level. The two patients were found to have several focal gaps originating from the roof and bottom of PVI lines. One of them a gap originating from the roof of the left superior PV down to the left inferior PV. In the third patient with atrial tachycardia a microreentrant cycle around the base of occlusive left appendage was found. An entrainment was performed to verify the reentrant mechanism. Interruption of the circuit as well as ablation of CFAEs mainly located at the posterior of the left atrial terminated the arrhythmia in this patient. The forth patient suffering AFL was identified anticlockwise (anterior of left atrial bottom area to posterior left atrial roof), with the average AF cycle length 302 ms. Ablation at the atrial roof between the two superior PVs, and ablation of CFAEs terminated the AFL. The fifth patients had mitral valve annulus-related atrial flutter. The creation of lesions from the left inferior PV to the mitral valve annulus was required to terminate the AFL in this patient. At the latest follow-up, all five patients were free of arrhythmias and independent of antiarrhythmic drug (AAD).

Frequently, the decision to terminate AAD was made after 3-month monitoring. For patient who had a successful procedure, the freedom from AAD was 44.6% and 61.4% in catheter group and surgical group respectively ($P=0.043$).

During the follow-up, cerebrovascular accidents occurred in two patients (2.4%) of the surgical group, and in one patient (1.2%) of the catheter group. The 1- and 3- year actuarial survival free from stroke rates were both 99.0%±1.0% in the catheter group, and both 96.0%±1.5% in the surgical group, respectively ($P=0.27$).

Eleven (6.6%) patients had to undergo preoperative permanent pacemaker implantation because of sick SR. During the follow-up, in three patients (3.6%) permanent pacemakers were implanted in

Table 2. Cardiac Rhythm in Hospital.

	Catheter Group N = 83	Surgical Group N = 83	p Value
Postoperative period			
SR	29(34.9)	38(45.7)	0.15
AF	30(36.2)	36(43.4)	0.39
AFL	24(28.9)	5(6.0)	<0.001
Pacemaker	0(0)	4(4.9)	0.12
Recurrence of AF/AFL			
AF	16 (19.3%)	12 (14.5%)	0.70
AFL	22 (26.5%)	2 (2.4%)	<0.001
At discharge			
SR	72(86.8)	53(63.9)	<0.001
AF	4(4.8)	24(28.9)	<0.001
AFL	6(7.2)	5(6.0)	NS
Pacemaker	1(1.2)	1(1.2)	NS

Data are presented as the number (%) of patients or mean ± SD. AF, atrial fibrillation; AFL, atrial flutter; SR, sinus rhythm.

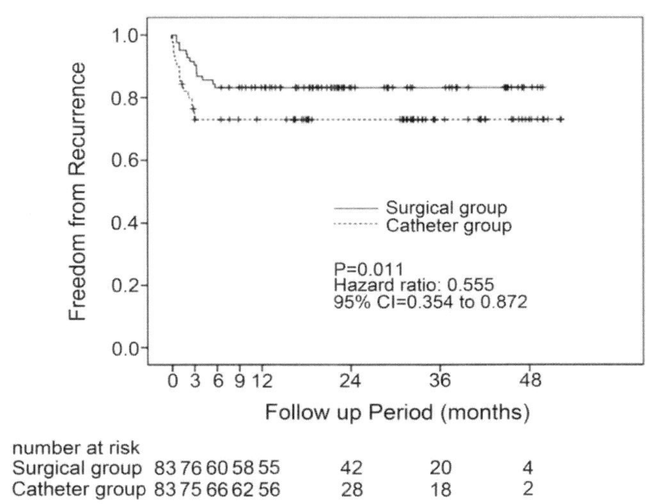

Figure 2. Freedom from recurrence after AF ablation. CI = confidence interval.

the catheter group and in one patient (1.2%) of the surgical group. The 1- and 3- year actuarial survival free from implanting permanent pacemaker were both 97.0%±2.0% in the catheter group, and 100% and 97.0±3.0% in surgical group, respectively ($P = 0.20$).

Discussion

4.1 Main findings

This is the first case-matched retrospective study comparing catheter and video-assisted minimally invasive ablation techniques in patients with long-standing persistent AF. Although at discharge from the hospital, the maintenance of SR was higher in the catheter group, we found that minimally invasive ablation resulted in long-term maintenance of SR in 74.7 percent of the patients (vs. 59.0% in the catheter group, $P = 0.047$). Additionally, a Kaplan-Meier analysis showed that patients in the catheter group had a significantly higher rate of recurrent arrhythmia.

4.2 Catheter ablation

Catheter-based PVI is relatively effective in maintaining SR for paroxysmal AF (65% to 70% success rate); for non paroxysmal AF, however, the PVI success rate is dramatically lower (20% to 30%) [10–12]. Therefore, different strategies adjunctive to PVI or using other concepts have been developed. These strategies include: creation of various ablation lines (mitral isthmus, roof line, posterior lines to isolate the posterior wall); ablation based on the CFAEs as well as cardiac autonomic denervation [13–16]. Oral et al evaluated catheter ablation with chronic AF. After a follow-up period of 7–14 months, only a mean of 33% of patients were in SR [17]. Tilz et al reported on 205 consecutive patients with long-standing persistent AF who underwent PVI, left linear and CFAEs catheter ablation. After a mean of 1.7±0.8 procedures, 135 of 199 patients (67.8%) remained in SR. Eighty-six patients (43.2%) remained in SR following PVI performed as the sole ablative strategy [16] and our results are in accordance with these previous reports who also adopted this technique. The PVI procedure appears to have a low success rate; however, the comparative advantages of a minimally invasive procedure have not been systematically evaluated yet.

4.3 Minimally invasive ablation

The success rate achieved in the most challenging surgical groups of patients, those with long-standing persistent AF, was not clear. Earlier in our series, the long-standing persistent AF group shows 44.4% and 71.4% SR restoration rates at 3 and 6 months postoperatively, respectively [18]. Similar research also reports 67% and 72% success rates, respectively [19,20].

Meanwhile our results show an optimistic therapeutic effect for long-standing persistent AF. This could be either due to a successful addition of bipolar ablation or due to the additional GP-ablation. During the minimally invasive operation, the energy is delivered between the jaws together with a transmurality feedback algorithm, and the transmurality of the isolation lesion is theoretically ensured. Besides the transmurality algorithm and facilitated multiple isolation lesions, the epicardial electrophysiologic testing further helps to evaluate the quality of the atrial lesion. What needs to be specially mentioned is that there are possible (24 patients in the surgical group (28.9%)) persistent regular and small potentials sensed even if ablations were done on a certain side. Often, these diminutive potentials recorded after ablation can represent "far-field" left atrial potentials. The effect of this "positive" postablation sensing and GP detection results on short-term and midterm therapeutic outcomes is under observation in a concurrent study. In this study pacing results show that all patients who were in SR after bilateral ablations did not show "atrial and ventricular capture" and accordingly achieved "exit block".

Investigators have showed that conversion of a premature depolarisation to AF depends on GP stimulation [21]. They could even initiate ectopic foci from the PV by GP stimulation alone. It is clear that the autonomic nervous system plays a key role in the initiation and maintenance of AF. Pappone first showed that patients with a vagal response during ablation had a higher success rate in comparison to patients without a vagal response [22]. Scherlag were the first to compare PVI with and without GP-ablation in a prospective study [23]. The follow-up data suggest better outcome with additional GP-ablation. The reported success rates vary between 29% and 84% [24]. Earlier in our series, ectopic foci outside the PV played an important role in persistent AF [19]. GP-ablation is, therefore, expected to contribute to the success of procedures for long-standing persistent AF.This study supports the feasibility of amputation of the LAA through the minimally invasive technique. In addition after amputation of the LAA, postoperative thromboembolic events were substantially reduced. During the follow-up, only two patients had cerebrovascular events.

4.4 Study limitations

The main limitation of this study is the retrospectivity. A larger, randomized and prospective trial with catheter based and minimally invasive ablation for lone AF is underway and will better define the efficacy of these two procedures in accordance with published guidelines.

A second limitation is that PVI with GP-ablation is not adequate to treat long-standing persistent AF. Patients with long-standing persistent AF pose a challenge because various pathophysiologic changes that occur in the atria of such patients may adversely affect the success of various treatment strategies. We reported electrophysiologic findings in patients presenting with recurrent atrial arrhythmia after minimally invasive procedures. Gaps at the roof and bottom of the PVI ring may contribute to the underlying mechanism of recurrent arrhythmias [18]. The connecting lesions between the left superior PV and left appendage and right inferior PV to the mitral valve annulus, as well as the roof line of the LA are all important; however, it is difficult to ablate these sites when the heart is beating using the present device during minimally invasive procedures. With the recently available Coolrail (AtriCure, Inc, West Chester, Ohio, USA), totally left-sided maze III lesion sets can be achieved relatively easy. In long-standing persistent AF, the efficacy of this procedure could benefit from its more extensive lesion set.

Our results suggest that in patients with long-standing persistent AF, the minimally invasive PVI with GP-ablation had the better ability to maintain SR. A further randomized study assessing the role of minimally invasive surgery in AF patients seems to be justified.

Author Contributions

Conceived and designed the experiments: XM. Performed the experiments: JGW CSM. Analyzed the data: JGW CSM. Contributed reagents/materials/analysis tools: JGW CSM. Wrote the paper: JGW. Read and approved the manuscript: JGW JHS JH CLX CSM YL.

References

1. Zhou Z, Hu D, Chen J, Zhang R, Li K, et al. (2004) An epidemiological survey of atrial fibrillation in China. Chin J Intern Med 43: 491–494.
2. Haissaguerre M, Jais P, Shah DC, Takahashi A, Hocini M, et al. (1998) Spontaneous initiation of atrial fibrillation by ectopic beats originating in the pulmonary veins. N Engl J Med 339: 659–666.
3. Cappato R, Calkins H, Chen SA, Davies W, Iesaka Y, et al. (2010) Updated worldwide survey on the methods, efficacy, and safety of catheter ablation for human atrial fibrillation. Circ Arrhythm Electrophysiol 3: 32–38.
4. Scanavacca MI, D'vila A, Parga J, Sosa E (2004) Left atrial-esophageal fistula following radiofrequency catheter ablation of atrial fibrillation. J Cardiovasc Electrophysiol 15: 960–962.
5. Willems S, Klemm H, Rostock T, Brandstrup B, Ventura R, et al. (2006) Substrate modification combined with pulmonary vein isolation improves outcome of catheter ablation in patients with persistent atrial fibrillation: a prospective randomized comparison. Eur Heart J 27: 2871–2878.
6. Oral H, Knight BP, Tada H, Ozaydin M, Chugh A, et al. (2002) Pulmonary vein isolation for paroxysmal and persistent atrial fibrillation. Circulation 105: 1077–1081.
7. Wolf RK, Schneeberger EW, Osterday R, Miller D, Merrill W, et al. (2005) Video-assisted bilateral pulmonary vein isolation and left atrial appendage exclusion for atrial fibrillation. J Thorac Cardiovasc Surg 130: 797–802.
8. Mehall JR, Kohut RM, Jr., Schneeberger EW, Taketani T, Merrill WH, et al. (2007) Intraoperative epicardial electrophysiologic mapping and isolation of autonomic ganglionic plexi. Ann Thorac Surg 83: 538–541.
9. Fuster V, Ryden LE, Cannom DS, Crijns HJ, Curtis AB, et al. (2006) ACC/AHA/ESC 2006 Guidelines for the Management of Patients with Atrial Fibrillation: a report of the American College of Cardiology/American Heart Association Task Force on Practice Guidelines and the European Society of Cardiology Committee for Practice Guidelines (Writing Committee to Revise the 2001 Guidelines for the Management of Patients With Atrial Fibrillation): developed in collaboration with the European Heart Rhythm Association and the Heart Rhythm Society. Circulation 114: e257–354.
10. Wokhlu A, Hodge DO, Monahan KH, Asirvatham SJ, Friedman PA, et al. (2010) Long-term outcome of atrial fibrillation ablation: impact and predictors of very late recurrence. J Cardiovasc Electrophysiol 21: 1071–1078.
11. Hunter RJ, Berriman TJ, Diab I, Baker V, Finlay M, et al. (2010) Long-term efficacy of catheter ablation for atrial fibrillation: impact of additional targeting of fractionated electrograms. Heart 96: 1372–1378.
12. Tzou WS, Marchlinski FE, Zado ES, Lin D, Dixit S, et al. (2010) Long-term outcome after successful catheter ablation of atrial fibrillation. Circ Arrhythm Electrophysiol 3: 237–242.
13. Elayi CS, Verma A, Di Biase L, Ching CK, Patel D, et al. (2008) Ablation for longstanding permanent atrial fibrillation: results from a randomized study comparing three different strategies. Heart Rhythm 5: 1658–1664.
14. Scharf C, Boersma L, Davies W, Kanagaratnam P, Peters NS, et al. (2009) Ablation of persistent atrial fibrillation using multielectrode catheters and duty-cycled radiofrequency energy. J Am Coll Cardiol 54: 1450–1456.
15. Mikhaylov E, Gureev S, Szili-Torok T, Lebedev D (2010) Additional left atrial septal line does not improve outcome of patients undergoing ablation for long-standing persistent atrial fibrillation. Acta Cardiol 65: 153–160.
16. Tilz RR, Chun KR, Schmidt B, Fuernkranz A, Wissner E, et al. (2010) Catheter ablation of long-standing persistent atrial fibrillation: a lesson from circumferential pulmonary vein isolation. J Cardiovasc Electrophysiol 21: 1085–1093.
17. Oral H, Chugh A, Good E, Wimmer A, Dey S, et al. (2007) Radiofrequency catheter ablation of chronic atrial fibrillation guided by complex electrograms. Circulation 115: 2606–2612.
18. Zeng Y, Cui Y, Li Y, Liu X, Xu C, et al. (2010) Recurrent atrial arrhythmia after minimally invasive pulmonary vein isolation for atrial fibrillation. Ann Thorac Surg 90: 510–515.
19. Li H, Li Y, Sun L, Liu X, Xu C, et al. (2008) Minimally invasive surgical pulmonary vein isolation alone for persistent atrial fibrillation: preliminary results of epicardial atrial electrogram analysis. Ann Thorac Surg 86: 1219–1225.
20. Yilmaz A, Geuzebroek GS, Van Putte BP, Boersma LV, Sonker U, et al. (2010) Completely thoracoscopic pulmonary vein isolation with ganglionic plexus ablation and left atrial appendage amputation for treatment of atrial fibrillation. Eur J Cardiothorac Surg 38: 356–360.
21. Scherlag BJ, Yamanashi W, Patel U, Lazzara R, Jackman WM (2005) Autonomically induced conversion of pulmonary vein focal firing into atrial fibrillation. J Am Coll Cardiol 45: 1878–1886.
22. Pappone C, Santinelli V, Manguso F, Vicedomini G, Gugliotta F, et al. (2004) Pulmonary vein denervation enhances long-term benefit after circumferential ablation for paroxysmal atrial fibrillation. Circulation 109: 327–334.
23. Scherlag BJ, Nakagawa H, Jackman WM, Yamanashi WS, Patterson E, et al. (2005) Electrical stimulation to identify neural elements on the heart: their role in atrial fibrillation. J Interv Card Electrophysiol 13 Suppl 1: 37–42.
24. Pokushalov E, Romanov A, Artyomenko S, Turov A, Shugayev P, et al. (2010) Ganglionated plexi ablation for longstanding persistent atrial fibrillation. Europace 12: 342–346.

12

Comparison of ESWL and Ureteroscopic Holmium Laser lithotripsy in Management of Ureteral Stones

Yon Cui[1]¶, Wenzhou Cao[1]¶, Hua Shen[1], Jianjun Xie[1], Tamara S. Adams[2], Yuanyuan Zhang[3], Qiang Shao[1]*

1 Department of Urology, Suzhou Municipal Hospital, Suzhou, China, **2** Center for Cancer Genomics, Wake Forest University School of Medicine, Winston-Salem, North Carolina, United States of America, **3** Wake Forest Institute for Regenerative Medicine, Wake Forest University Health Sciences, Winston-Salem, North Carolina, United States of America

Abstract

Background: There are many options for urologists to treat ureteral stones that range from 8 mm to 15 mm, including ESWL and ureteroscopic holmium laser lithotripsy. While both ESWL and ureteroscopy are effective and minimally invasive procedures, there is still controversy over which one is more suitable for ureteral stones.

Objective: To perform a retrospective study to compare the efficiency, safety and complications using ESWL *vs.* ureteroscopic holmium laser lithotripsy in management of ureteral stones.

Methods: Between October 2010 and October 2012, 160 patients who underwent ESWL or ureteroscopic holmium laser lithotripsy at Suzhou municipal hospital for a single radiopaque ureteral stone (the size 8–15 mm) were evaluated. All patients were followed up with ultrasonography for six months. Stone clearance rate, costs and complications were compared.

Results: Similarity in stone clearance rate and treatment time between the two procedures; overall procedural time, analgesia requirement and total cost were significantly different. Renal colic and gross hematuria were more frequent with ESWL while voiding symptoms were more frequent with ureteroscopy. Both procedures used for ureteral stones ranging from 8 to 15 mm were safe and minimally invasive.

Conclusion: ESWL remains first line therapy for proximal ureteral stones while ureteroscopic holmium laser lithotripsy costs more. To determining which one is preferable depends on not only stone characteristics but also patient acceptance and cost-effectiveness ratio.

Editor: Jonathan A. Coles, Glasgow University, United Kingdom

Funding: Suzhou Science and Technology Foundation Grant –Leading Project for Medical Science (No. SYSD2010149). The funders had no role in study design, data collection and analysis, decision to publish, or preparation of the manuscript.

Competing Interests: The authors have declared that no competing interests exist.

* E-mail: sq7166822@163.com

¶ These authors contributed equally to this work.

Introduction

Urolithiasis has plagued human beings for thousands of years. Advances in medicine have enabled us to better treat urolithiasis with few complications. Most urinary stones that pass through the renal calyces to the renal pelvis and subsequently to the ureter cause serious symptoms. The most common symptoms of ureteral stones are pain, hydronephrosis and hematuria. There are many options for urologists to treat ureteral stones that range from 8 mm to 15 mm (Table1), including ESWL and ureteroscopic holmium laser lithotripsy [1,2,3]. While ESWL and ureteroscopy are effective and minimally invasive procedures, there is still controversy over which one is more suitable for ureteral stones. Different studies have reported variable outcomes of ESWL and ureteroscopy, despite the fact that both treatments use advanced instruments, offer few complications and high satisfaction among urologists [4–8]. We conducted the current study to compare objective outcomes of patients with ureteral stones treated with ESWL or ureteroscopy.

Materials and Methods

Study Population

Patients that underwent ESWL ($n = 80$) and ureteroscopy ($n = 80$) between October 2010 and October 2012 at Suzhou Municipal Hospital for a single radiopaque ureteral stone ranging from 8 mm to 15 mm were included in the study (Table 2). Patients with bilateral or multiple stones, radiolucent stones, ureteral stricture, acute urinary tract infection, repeated treatment and distal ureteral stones were excluded. Patients were provided with an explanation of the advantages, drawbacks, and complications associated with each procedure prior to voluntarily selecting a treatment option. The study protocol was approved by the Institutional Review Board of Suzhou Municipal Hospital and written informed consent was obtained before treatment.

Table 1. Management of Ureteral Calculi: Guidelines on Urolithiasis of EAU, AUA and CUA.

	Proximal ureter	Mid-ureter	Distal ureter	
	(All size)	(All size)	(All size)	
EAU options	ESWL, URS, PNL, Lapa and open surgery	ESWL, URS, PNL	URS, ESWL	
	Proximal ureter		Distal ureter	
	<1 cm	>1 cm	<1 cm	>1 m
AUA options	Observation,ESWL	ESWL,URS,PNL,Laparoscopic and open surgery	Observation, URS, ESWL	URS, ESWL
	Proximal ureter		Distal ureter	
	<0.8 cm	>0.8 cm	<0.8 cm	>0.8 cm
CUA options	Observation, ESWL	ESWL, URS, PNL, Laparoscopic and open surgery	Observation, URS	URS

Note: EAU- European Association of Urology; AUA-American Urological Association; CUA-Chinese Urological Association; URS-Ureteroscopy; PNL- Percutaneous nephrolithotomy; Lapa-laparoscopy.

Study Design

Ureteral stones were diagnosed by Kidney-Ureter-Bladder (KUB) X-Ray film (Figure 1) and ultrasonography then the longest diameter of each stone was calculated before treatment. Patients that underwent ESWL were evaluated by urine analysis, serum creatinine level and coagulation profile. In addition, ESWL was performed using the third-generation Dornier lithotripter (Dornier, Germany) as an outpatient procedure. Voltage was set at 10–12 Kv and shockwave was set at 3,000–3,500 shocks for the first treatment. Patients were discharged after 2 hours surveillance with routine antibiotics and evaluated one week later by KUB to assess stone passage (Figure 2). ESWL was repeated if residual stones were observed at follow-up. Following the guidelines of the Chinese Urology Association (CUA), if a stone remained after three sessions of ESWL, we performed ureteroscopy in order to avoid ureterostenosis [3].

Patients that underwent ureteroscopy were evaluated by urine analysis, serum creatinine level, coagulation profile, EEG, chest radiograph and KUB X-Ray film (Figure 3). Ureteroscopy was performed using 8/9.8-Fr, 12° rigid ureteroscope (Richard Wolf, Germany) under general anesthesia. For ureteroscopic lithotripsy, a holmium laser (Dahua Systems, Wuxi, China) was used at a setting of 1.2–1.5 J and 10–15 Hz. After stones were broken into

Table 2. Characteristics of the patients on both groups.

	ESWL	Ureteroscopy	*P* value
Age(year),	40.6±9.8	41.5±10.5	0.69
Sex, male/female	49/31	56/24	0.478
Stone site			0.302
Right	38(47.5%)	34(42.5%)	
Left	42(52.5%)	46(57.5%)	
Stone location			0.446
Upper ureter	56(70.0%)	62(77.5%)	
Mid-ureter	24(30.0%)	18(22.5%)	
Stone diameter(mm)	9.8±3.5	10.2±4.3	0.65

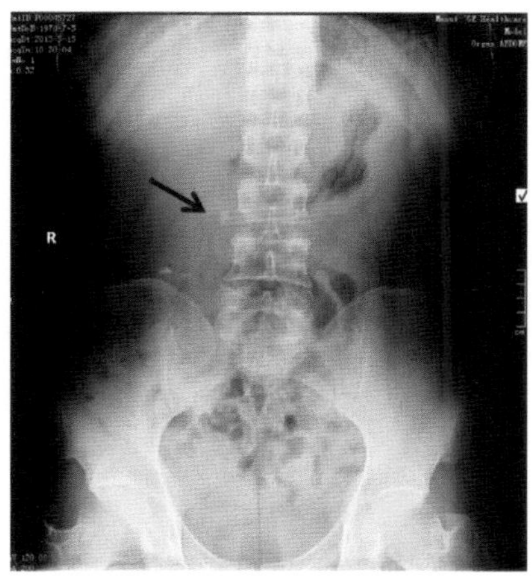

Figure 1. Rightureteral calculus (arrow) before ESWL.

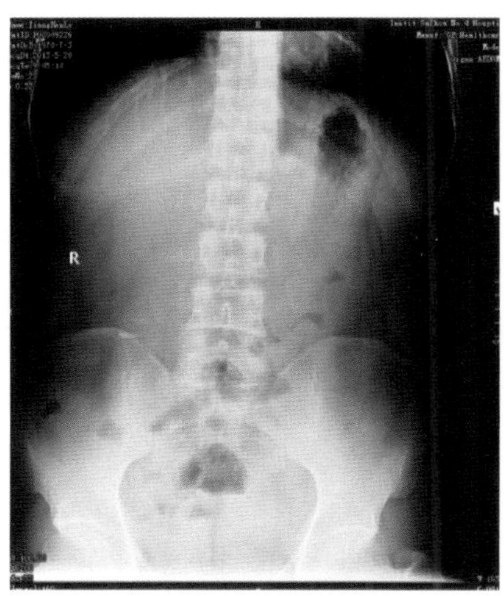

Figure 2. Calculusafter ESWL.

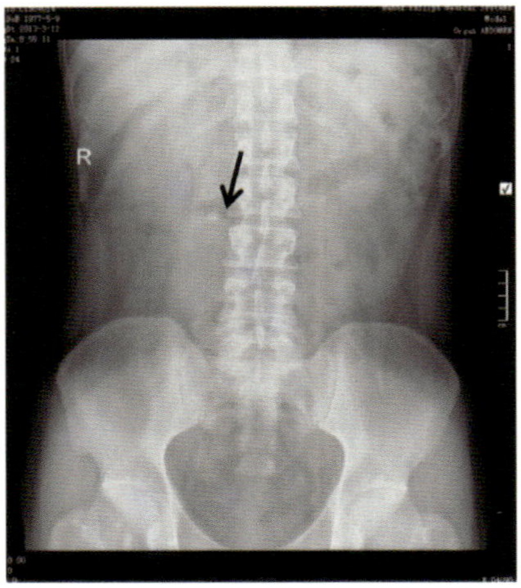

Figure 3. Right ureteral calculus (arrow) before ureteroscopy.

pieces <2 mm one 6.0F double-J was indwelled (Figure 4). Both antibiotics and analgesia were routinely used. All patients were discharged postoperative 1–2 days after catheter removal. Patients were evaluated by KUB one week postoperative (Figure 5) and the stent were removed postoperative 2 weeks.

Statistical Analysis

Fisher's exact or chi-square test was used to compare categorical variables between the groups. The Student's t test was used to compare continuous variables. All statistical analyses were two-sided with $p<0.05$ defined as statistically significant. We used SAS software, version 9.2 (SAS, Cary, NC), for statistical analyses.

Results

Both procedures were successfully achieved at the same time no severe complications during treatment occurred (renal haematoma for ESWL and ureteral perforation or ureteral avulsion for ureteroscopy). The detailed procedural indexes of patients are listed in Table 3. Between the two procedures, overall procedural time, analgesia requirement, total cost, gross hematuria and voiding symptom were significantly different while the stone clearance rate and treatment time were similar. In ureteroscopy group there were two cases which stones shifted to the pelvis and couldn't be reached by rigid ureteroscope; one week later residual stones were removed by ESWL. In ESWL group there were six cases which stones couldn't be removed completely finally were managed by ureteroscopy. All patients were followed up for 3–6

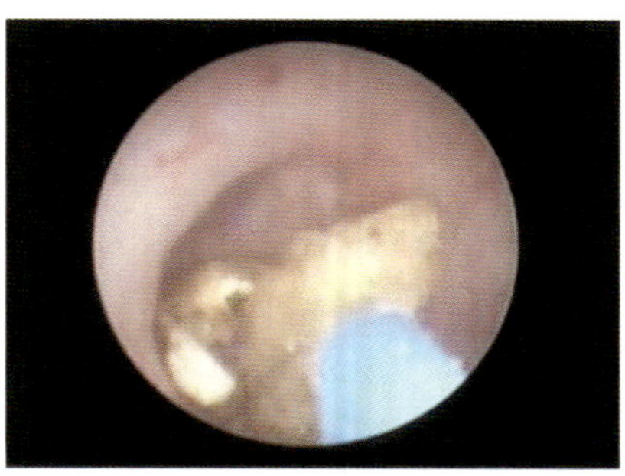

Figure 4. Ureteroscopic holmium laser lithotripsy.

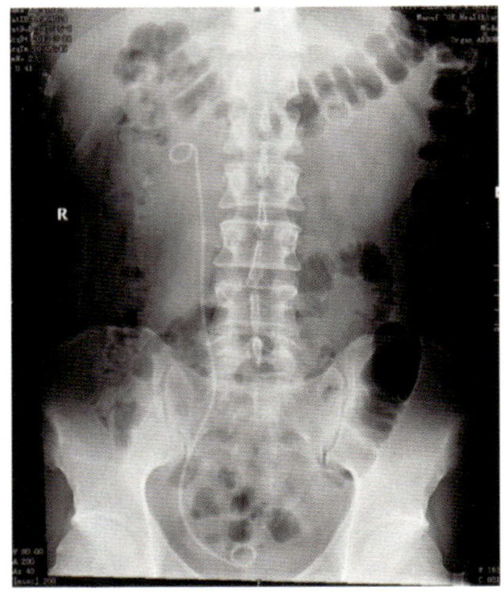

Figure 5. Calculus-freeafter ureteroscopy.

months and there were no obvious residual stones or ureterostenosis at the end of follow-up.

Discussion

Both ESWL and ureteroscopy are minimally invasive treatment options for patients with proximal ureteral stones. The use of ESWL began in the1980s, has stone clearance rate of nearly 90% and has resulted in the fading of open surgical procedures for ureteral stones [9–11]. With subsequent development of ESWL instrument it eliminated the limitations and promoted the efficiencies. Ureteroscopy was first described in 1912 [12], but its use was not widely accepted until the late 1970's, at which time it became a standardized procedure [13]. Along with laser lithotripsy, an impressive 95% or more of the patients treated with were stone free after a single procedure [14,15]. Most of the comparative studies between ESWL and ureteroscopy are not conclusive and sometimes ambiguous. While some studies are in favor of ESWL [7], others concluded that ureteroscopy is the preferable approach [16–18]. We compared several objective outcomes of each procedure method, including stone clearance rate, treatment time, procedural time, complications and costs.

Stone clearance rates in our study were 92.5% for ESWL versus 97.5% for ureteroscopy and not significantly different. These rates were similar to those in previous studies [15,16]. In ureteroscopy group we broke stones into pieces<2 mm during surgery, moreover evaluation of stone clearance based on KUB imaging one week later it might improve the stone passage; in ESWL group stone clearance rate evaluated according to final outcomes which patients maybe experience more than one session of ESWL. As Table 4 showed that the stone clearance rate of uerteroscopy was significantly different with one session of ESWL. Multiple sessions of ESWL resulted in a similar outcome to ureteroscopy. This could explain why the stone clearance rate of ESWL varied from 80%–100% [4,7]. Furthermore, the stone clearance rate of ESWL was determined by stone composition and stone hardness. Holmium laser lithotripsy is a reliable method of stone disintegration irrespective of the stone composition and hardness, it is carried out through all types of ureteroscope [19], but stone migration will make operation failure [20,21]. With the instrument development and operation skill promotion we still cannot avoid ureteroscopic lithotripsy failure. Ureteroscopy with laser lithotripsy has an

Table 3. Detailed procedural indexes of patients.

	ESWL	ureteroscopy	*P* value
Stone clearane rate	74(92.5%)	78(97.5%)	0.61
Treatment time(min)	40.0±10.0	42.5±11.3	0.29
overall procedural time(h)	3.0±1.0	48.0±8.5	<0.05
Analgesia(tramadol mg)	0	80.5±31.6	<0.05
Cost(US $)	120±25	1180±258	<0.05
Introprocedural Complications			
renal haematoma	0	0	
ureteral perforation (avulsion)	0	0	
Early complications			
renal colic	9(11.25%)	2(2.5%)	<0.05
Gross hematuria	16(20%)	2(2.5%)	<0.05
Voiding symptom	5(6.25%)	27(33.75%)	<0.05
Late complications			
residual calculus	0	0	
Ureterostenosis	0	0	
post-procedure satisfaction	72(90%)	67(83.75)	>0.05

Note: "overall procedural time" for ESWL include the repeated procedures in some cases; "overall procedural time" for ureteroscopy included anesthesia time, operation time and hospitalization time.

Table 4. Stone clearance rate according to ESWL sessions.

	ESWL1	ESWL2	ESWL3	Ureteroscopy
Stone clearance rate (%)	77.5	87.5	92.5	97.5
P value (*vs.*ureteroscopy)	0.018	0.20	0.61	

ESWL1:1st session ESWL and so far.

advantage over one session of ESWL with regard to stone clearance rate and efficiency [22–24], but ESWL still is the first line option for proximal ureteral calculi because of fewer cost and easy performance. Moreover, ESWL will be preferred option when ureteroscopy fails.

We did not observe a difference in treatment times between the two groups (Table 3). However, there was a significant difference in total procedural time between both groups. For ESWL group it took the shockwave lithotripsy time and two hours' surveillance then patients went back home until follow up a week later as well as for ureteroscopy group it included operation and hospitalization time which is much more (3.0±1.0 *vs.* 48.0±8.5 hours). Patients underwent ESWL experienced a fast recovery and returned to daily activity within two days while some patients underwent ureteroscopy suffered from voiding symptoms until the ureteral stent was removed postoperative two weeks [25,26]. The procedural time difference resulted the cost difference (120±25*vs.*1180±258US $). Even if patients underwent three sessions of ESWL, the cost between the two options was still significantly different. Moreover, as a surgical procedure, ureteroscopy require general anesthesia and post-operation analgesia while as an outpatient procedure, ESWL doesn't require the both. Conclusively, patients underwent ESWL had a higher cost-effectiveness ratio than patients underwent ureteroscopy.

We compared complications between the two procedures. We didn't found any severe complications such as renal haematoma for ESWL and ureteral perforation or ureteral avulsion for ureteroscopy during both procedures; secondly we found patients underwent ESWL experienced a high percentage of hematuria and renal colic than patients underwent ureteroscopy. Macroscopic bleeding and renal colic for ESWL were caused by stone fragment movements and ureteral mucosa damage [27,28], as most stone fragments were cleared during operation fewer hematuria and renal colic were observed after ureteroscopy. Most hematuria and renal colic will vanish after stone passage without special management. Finally we found more patients underwent ureteroscopy suffered voiding symptoms than patients underwent ESWL (67.5% *vs.* 7.5%). In our procedure of ureteroscopy each patient indwelled ureteral stent and moved out two weeks later it should be the reason patients underwent ureteroscopy suffered more voiding symptom. According to Joshi et al and Lamb et al [29,30] reporter, voiding symptoms and other discomforts after receiving a ureteral stents was unavoidable for ureteroscopy procedure. There is evidence that α-blockers alleviate ureteral stent discomfort, but they don't work completely [31]. Voiding symptoms might be the reason why many patients stated on a questionnaire that they feared of ureteroscopy. At the end of six months follow up there were no residual stones or ureterostenosis in both groups.

A post-procedure questionnaire revealed a similar satisfaction rate that 90% of patients who underwent ESWL were satisfied with the procedure *vs.* 83.75% of patients who underwent ureteroscopy. Most patients who underwent ureteroscopy felt dissatisfied because of voiding symptoms and higher costs of the procedure. To our knowledge, there are no other reports with similar data in a Chinese cohort. This study was performed in one hospital and only included 160 cases so that all conclusions need further multi-center prospective study to validate.

In conclusion, ESWL as an outpatient procedure does not require analgesia or anesthesia; it remains the first line therapy for proximal ureteral stones while ureteroscopic laser lithotripsy as a surgical procedure requires general anesthesia, hospitalization and much more costs. Determining which procedure is preferable depends on stone characteristics, patient acceptance and cost-effectiveness ratio.

Author Contributions

Conceived and designed the experiments: QS. Performed the experiments: YC WY. Analyzed the data: YC. Contributed reagents/materials/analysis tools: HS JX TA YZ. Wrote the paper: QS YC.

References

1. Preminger GM, Tiselius HG, Assimos DG, Alken P, Buck C, et al. (2007) 2007 guideline for the management of ureteral calculi. J Urol 178: 2418–2434.
2. Turk C, Knoll T, Petrik A, Sarica K, Skolarikos A, et al. (2013) Guidelines on Urolithiasis,European Association of Urology (UPDATE MARCH 2013).
3. Na YQ, Sun G, Ye ZQ, Sun YH, Sun ZY, et al. (2011) Guideline of Chinese urological disease diagnosis and treatment- Urolithiasis, People's Health Publishing House, Beijing. p. 241–264.
4. El-Faqih SR, Husain I, Ekman PE, Sharma ND, Chakrabarty A, et al. (1988) Primary choice of intervention for distal ureteric stone: ureteroscopy or ESWL? Br J Urol 62: 13–18.
5. Chang SC, Ho CM, Kuo HC.(1993) Ureteroscopic treatment of lower ureteral calculi in the era of extracorporeal shock wave lithotripsy: from a developing country point of view. J Urol 150: 1395–1398.

6. Biri H, Kupeli B, Isen K, Sinik Z, Karaoglan U, et al. (1999) Treatment of lower ureteral stones: extracorporeal shockwave lithotripsy or intracorporeal lithotripsy? J Endourol 13: 77–81.
7. Pearle MS, Nadler R, Bercowsky E, Chen C, Dunn M, et al. (2001) Prospective randomized trial comparing shock wave lithotripsy and ureteroscopy for management of distal ureteral calculi. J Urol166: 1255–1260.
8. Marchant F, Storme O, Osorio F, Benavides J, Palma C, et al. (2009) Prospective trial comparing shock wave lithotripsy and ureteroscopy for management of distal ureteral calculi. Actas Urol Esp 33: 869–872.
9. Chaussy C, Brendel W, Schmiedt E.(1980) Extracorporeally induced destruction of kidney stones by shock waves. Lancet 13: 1265–1268.
10. Chaussy C, Schmiedt E, Jocham D, Brendel W, Forssmann B, et al. (1982) First clinical experience with extracorporeally induced destruction of stones by shockwaves. J Urol 127: 417–420.
11. Chaussy C, Eisenberger F, Forssmann B.(2007) Extracorporeal shock wave lithotripsy (ESWL®): a chronology. J Endourol 21: 1249–1253.
12. Young HH, McKay RW.(1929) Congenital valvular obstruction of the prostatic urethra. SurgGynecolObstr 48: 509.
13. Lyon ES, Kyker JS, Schoenberg HW. (1978) Transurethral ureteroscopy in women: a ready addition to the urological armamentarium. J Urol 119: 35–36.
14. Teichman JM, Rao RD, Rogenes VJ, Harris JM.(1997) Ureteroscopic management of ureteral calculi: electrohydraulic versus holmium:YAG laser lithotripsy. J Urol 158: 1358–1361.
15. Liu DY, He HC, Wang J, Tang Q, Zhou YF, et al. (2012) Ureteroscopic lithotripsy using holmium laser for 187 patients with proximal ureteral stones. Chin Med J 125: 1542–1546.
16. Peschel R, Janetschek G, Bartsch G. (1999) Extracorporeal shockwave lithotripsy versus ureteroscopy for distal ureteral calculi: A Prospective randomized study. J Urol 162: 1909–1912.
17. Turk T, Jenkins A. (1999) A comparison of ureteoscopy to in situ extracorporeal schockwave lithotripsy for the treatment of distal ureteral calculi. J Urol 161: 45–47.
18. Lotan Y, Gettman MT, Roehrborn CG, Cadeddu JA, Pearle MS. (2002) Management of ureteral calculi: A cost comparison decision making analysis. J Urol 167: 1621–1629.
19. Tawfiek ER, Bagley DH. (1999) Management of upper urinary tract calculi with ureteroscopic techniques. Urology 53: 25–32.
20. Kurahashi T, Miyake H, Oka N, Shinozaki M, Takenaka A, et al. (2007) Clinical outcome of ureteroscopic lithotripsy for 2,129 patients with ureteral stones. Urol Res 35: 149–153.
21. Yencilek F, Sarica K, Erturhan S, Yagci F, Erbagci A. (2010) Treatment of ureteral calculi with semi-rigid ureteroscopy: where should we stop? Urol Int 84: 260–264.
22. Aboumarzouk OM, Kata SG, Keeley FX, McClinton S, Nabi G.(2012)Extra-)Extracorporeal shock wave lithotripsy (ESWL) versus ureteroscopic management for ureteric calculi. Cochrane Database Syst Rev. 2012 May 16.
23. Lindqvist K, Holmberg G, Peeker R, Grenabo L. (2006) Extracorporeal shockwave lithotripsy or ureteroscopy as primary treatment for ureteric stones: a retrospective study comparing two different treatment strategies. Scand J Urol Nephrol 40: 113–118.
24. Lam JS, Greene TD, Gupta M. (2002) Treatment of proximal ureteral calculi: holmium:YAG laser ureterolithotripsy versus extracorporeal shock wave lithotripsy. J Urol 167: 1972–1976.
25. Park J, Shin DW, Chung JH, Lee SW. (2012) Shock wave lithotripsy versus ureteroscopy for ureteral calculi: a prospective assessment of patient-reported outcomes. World J Urol 18. [Epub ahead of print].
26. Chaussy C, Bergsdorf T. (2009) The Preferred Treatment for Upper Tract Stones Is Extracorporeal Shock Wave Lithotripsy (ESWL) or Ureteroscopic: Pro ESWL. Urology 74: 259–262.
27. Wilson WT, Preminger GM. (1990) Extracorporeal shock wave lithotripsy: Anupdate. Urol Clin N Am 17: 231–242.
28. Vural A, Oguz V, Oktenl C, Yenicesu M, Caglar K et al. (1998) Detection of Source of Haematuria after Extracorporeal Shock Wave Lithotripsy (ESWL) by Automated Measurement of Urinary Red Cell Volume. Int Urol Nephrol. 30: 31–37.
29. Joshi HB, Newns N, Stainthorpe A,MacDonagh RP, Keeley FX Jr, et al. (2003) Ureteral stent symptom questionnaire: development and validation of a multidimensional quality of life measure. J Urol 169: 1060–1064.
30. Lamb AD, Vowler SL, Johnston R, Dunn N, Wiseman OJ. (2011) Meta-analysis showing the beneficial effect of α-blockers on ureteric stent discomfort. BJU Int 108: 1894–1902.
31. Wang CJ, Huang SW, Chang CH. (2009) Effects of tamsulosin on lower urinary tract symptoms due to double-J stent: a prospective study. Urol Int 83: 66–69.

Cryosurgery with Pulsed Electric Fields

Charlotte S. Daniels*, Boris Rubinsky

Department of Mechanical Engineering, University of California, Berkeley, Berkeley, California, United States of America

Abstract

This study explores the hypothesis that combining the minimally invasive surgical techniques of cryosurgery and pulsed electric fields will eliminate some of the major disadvantages of these techniques while retaining their advantages. Cryosurgery, tissue ablation by freezing, is a well-established minimally invasive surgical technique. One disadvantage of cryosurgery concerns the mechanism of cell death; cells at high subzero temperature on the outer rim of the frozen lesion can survive. Pulsed electric fields (PEF) are another minimally invasive surgical technique in which high strength and very rapid electric pulses are delivered across cells to permeabilize the cell membrane for applications such as gene delivery, electrochemotherapy and irreversible electroporation. The very short time scale of the electric pulses is disadvantageous because it does not facilitate real time control over the procedure. We hypothesize that applying the electric pulses during the cryosurgical procedure in such a way that the electric field vector is parallel to the heat flux vector will have the effect of confining the electric fields to the frozen/cold region of tissue, thereby ablating the cells that survive freezing while facilitating controlled use of the PEF in the cold confined region. A finite element analysis of the electric field and heat conduction equations during simultaneous tissue treatment with cryosurgery and PEF (cryosurgery/PEF) was used to study the effect of tissue freezing on electric fields. The study yielded motivating results. Because of decreased electrical conductivity in the frozen/cooled tissue, it experienced temperature induced magnified electric fields in comparison to PEF delivered to the unfrozen tissue control. This suggests that freezing/cooling confines and magnifies the electric fields to those regions; a targeting capability unattainable in traditional PEF. This analysis shows how temperature induced magnified and focused PEFs could be used to ablate cells in the high subzero freezing region of a cryosurgical lesion.

Editor: Vladimir N. Uversky, University of South Florida College of Medicine, United States of America

Funding: CD was supported by National Science Foundation. The funders had no role in study design, data collection and analysis, decision to publish, or preparation of the manuscript.

Competing Interests: The authors have declared that no competing interests exist.

* E-mail: daniels.charlotte@gmail.com

Introduction

Minimally and non-invasive surgeries are positioned to transform the field of medicine with shorter hospital stays, reduced surgical trauma, improved immune response and greater precision [1]. These benefits are primarily due to less intrusive procedures and more targeted tissue ablation. Various minimally invasive surgical procedures exist, each with their advantages and disadvantages and particular use. This study explores the feasibility and the advantages of the combined use of two minimally invasive surgical techniques: cryosurgery and pulsed electric fields (PEF).

Cryosurgery is a minimally invasive surgical technique that uses freezing to ablate undesirable tissue [2,3]. Freezing is induced with cryosurgical probes, cooled by an internally circulated cryogen, inserted into or placed in close vicinity to the undesirable tissue. During cryosurgery the frozen lesion propagates as a function of time outward from the cryoprobe, into the tissue, until the undesirable tissue is completely frozen. The time scale of typical cryosurgical procedures is on the order of magnitude of single to tens of minutes. The temperature distribution in the frozen lesion ranges from the cryosurgical probe temperature at the interface between the cryoprobe and the tissue, to the change of phase temperature for physiological solutions, -0.56°C, on the outer edge of the frozen lesion [4]. Cryosurgery has many advantages. One is that freezing has a profound effect on the physical properties of tissue and therefore cryosurgery can be monitored with virtually every medical imaging modality [2,5,6]. Because of cryosurgery's time scale, imaging allows the physician real time control over the extent of freezing with excellent clinical results [7].

Cryosurgery, however, also has limitations. These limitations are related to the mechanism of cell death by freezing and the incomplete cell death in certain ranges of subfreezing temperatures [2,3,8,9,10]. A recent review [3] points out that: "The tissue temperature is a key factor in causing injury… As a guide for the treatment of neoplasms, the many experiments suggesting that about -20°C is adequate for tissue destruction should be viewed with caution. Certainly extensive tissue damage occurs in the -20 to -30°C range, but tumor cell destruction at the temperature range is uncertain and incomplete." This means that on the outer rim of the frozen lesion, cells in the temperature range from at least -30°C to -0.56°C can survive the procedure. Medical imaging can only discriminate between frozen and unfrozen tissue. This is problematic because the region seen as frozen via imaging contains a substantial number of surviving cells, especially on the outer rim. Therefore, the accuracy of targeting pathogenic tissue and the reliability of ablation are compromised. Indeed the same review [3] suggests that: "The greatest opportunity for improved efficacy (of cryosurgery) is in the management of the periphery of the cryogenic lesion where cell destruction is partial. Therapy adjunctive to cryosurgery, such as chemical agents, cytotoxic drugs, or irradiation should prove helpful in completing destruction of cells in the periphery of the frozen volume." Cryoadjunctive strategies to enhance cancer cell sensitivity to freezing is the subject of several investigations [3,8,9,11,12,13]. The goal of this study is to explore, with a mathematical model, the feasibility of using pulsed electric fields delivered through the cryosurgical probe during cryosurgery as a cryoadjunctive modality to ablate cells in the temperature range in which they survive freezing.

The PEF modality, also known as electroporation or electropermeabilization, utilizes pulsed electric fields that target the cellular membrane, increasing membrane permeability through the formation of nanoscale defects [14,15]. The electric field is delivered between two electrodes placed into or in the vicinity of the targeted tissue. Typical PEF parameters currently utilized in medicine and biotechnology employ 0.1 to 10^7 V/m electric fields, nanosecond to millisecond pulse lengths, and one to several hundred pulses. PEFs can have two different effects on the cell membrane as a function of the electric parameters: reversible and irreversible electroporation. In reversible electroporation the permeabilization of the cell membrane is transient. In tissue, reversible electroporation is used for insertion of DNA molecules into cells for gene therapy [16,17,18]. Reversible electroporation is also used with toxic chemicals for tissue ablation in a procedure known as electrochemotherapy [19,20,21]. In irreversible electroporation (IRE), the effect of membrane permeabilization is permanent and leads to cell death. Recently, IRE has emerged as an important minimally invasive technique for tissue ablation [22,23,24,25]. An important attribute of the PEF modalities is that their time scale is extremely rapid (nanoseconds to milliseconds). While this is advantageous because it significantly reduces the time of the surgical procedure, it is so rapid that it essentially precludes real time control, which is a major disadvantage. Our hypothesis is that combining PEF with cryosurgery will facilitate real time control over the delivery of the electric fields, for reasons that will be discussed next.

There are several earlier studies that are relevant to the work presented in this paper. We have shown in a previous paper that lowering the temperature of the PEF electrode, and the consequent local cooling of the tissue, has the effect of confining the electric fields to the cooled region [26]. Furthermore, it was found that the cooling magnifies the electric fields in the cooled region relative to electric fields produced by the same pulses in physiological temperature tissue [26]. That paper [26], dealt with temperatures above freezing. To the best of our knowledge, there are currently no studies on the application of pulsed electric fields on frozen biological tissues. However, there are studies on the effects of temperature on electroporation and on the effects of hyperosmolality on electroporation. We believe that these studies should provide us with some guidelines on what to expect during the electroporation of frozen tissue at the outer rim of the frozen lesion during cryosurgery. The biophysical phenomena on which we focus in this paper are related to the process of freezing at the outer edge of the frozen lesion during cryosurgery. It has been established that the process of freezing at the outer edge of the frozen lesion, where cooling rates are low, is characterized by extracellular freezing and shrinking of the cell to accommodate for the difference in osmotic pressure between the interior of the unfrozen cell and the increased osmolality of the exterior frozen milieu [2,3,27,28,29]. Therefore, during typical cryosurgical protocols, the cells on the outer rim of the frozen region, where cells survive freezing, are: a) unfrozen, b) below freezing temperatures and c) in a hyperosmotic solution.

Several studies have investigated the effects of temperature on PEF. For instance, Diaz investigated the effect of low temperatures on electroporation efficacy. He accomplished electroporation on kidney epithelial cells at temperatures as low as $-2°C$ [30]. Additionally, Gallo demonstrated the trend between temperature and electroporation; as temperature decreases, initial permeabilizing voltage increases [31]. Gallo's study operated on the stratum corneum in the range 0 to 80°C. The same relationship between temperature and electroporation was found in *alga Valonia*, rye leaf protoplast, and mammalian cell lines [32]. From the studies discussed here, we anticipate that: a) electroporation will occur at temperatures that are lower than the lipid phase transition temperature of cells, and b) the strength of the electric field required for electroporation will increase with a decrease in temperature of the electroporated cells. The effect of hyperosmolarity on electroporation was also studied. It was found that when electroporation is carried out in a hypertonic media, cells are permeabilized at a lower voltage than cells maintained in isotonic media and exposed to the same electric pulse parameters [33].

The studies discussed above motivated the foundation of this paper: investigation of a method that combines cryosurgery with PEF to ablate the entire frozen region during cryosurgery, including the tissue in the temperature range of $-30°C$ to $-0.56°C$, located at the frozen lesion outer rim. Electrical conductivity in ionic solutions is a function of temperature, exhibiting a positive correlation. Consequently, the electrical conductivity of frozen and cooled tissue is substantially lower than those at physiological temperatures. As a result of the temperature dependency of tissue electrical properties we hypothesized that applying PEFs through a cryoprobe during freezing and thawing will concentrate the entire electric field to the low temperature region. Additionally, we hypothesize that cells on the margin of the frozen lesion will experience electroporation. Consequently, the entire frozen lesion will contain cells ablated by the combined mechanisms of cryosurgery and PEF, improving the accuracy of cryosurgical procedures. Since the extent of the frozen region can be monitored in real time by medical imaging and because cryosurgery dominates the time scale of the combination cryosurgery/PEF, the combined treatment, including the effect of the PEF, can be controlled by physicians in real time, through imaging of the frozen lesion.

The goal of this paper is to investigate the combination of cryosurgery and PEF through a mathematical analysis of temperature and electric fields produced by the application of PEFs during cryosurgery. The focus of this study is to examine the effect of changes in temperature and freezing on electric fields and the subsequent implications for affecting cryosurgery treated tissue with PEF.

Methods

Theoretical Model

Mathematical Formulation. The analysis of the application of PEF during cryosurgery requires the simultaneous solution of the Laplace equation and the Pennes Bioheat equation. The Laplace equation solves for the electrical potential distribution associated with an electric pulse, and the Pennes Bioheat equation solves for the temperature distribution. The form of the Laplace equation utilized in this study is shown below:

$$\nabla \cdot (\sigma \nabla \phi) = 0, \tag{1}$$

where σ is electrical conductivity, and ϕ is the electrical potential. The electrical potential is subject to voltage boundary conditions applied at the outer edges of the analyzed domain, and the temperature distribution achieved from the solution of the Bioheat equation.

The temperature distribution was obtained from the solution of a modified Pennes Bioheat equation, which was solved simultaneously as the electrical potential equation. The general bioheat equation has the following form:

$$\nabla\cdot(k\nabla T)+\rho_b w_b c_b(T_a-T)+q'''=\rho c_p\frac{\partial T}{\partial t}, \tag{2}$$

where k is thermal conductivity, T is temperature, w_b is blood perfusion, c_b is the heat capacity of blood, T_a is arterial temperature, ρ is the tissue density, c_p is the tissue heat capacity and $q'''=Q_{met}+Q_{ext}$. Where Q_{met} is the metabolic heat generation and $Q_{ext}=\sigma|\nabla\phi|^2$is a term that accounts for Joule heating, where ϕ is electrical potential calculated from Equation 1 and σ is the electrical conductivity of the tissue. In this study, it was assumed that there is blood flow and metabolism in the unfrozen tissue while the blood flow and metabolism in the frozen region was set to zero. The effect of Joule heating on the temperature distribution was considered in both the frozen and unfrozen tissues. The equations were solved subject to temperature boundary conditions on the outer surface of the analyzed domain and to the energy balance at the change of phase interface. The initial temperature was assumed to be physiological body temperature.

The mathematical analysis of both the Laplace equation for electrical potential distribution and the various versions of the Pennes Bioheat equation for temperature distribution was performed using a finite element based numerical analysis executed by Comsol Multiphysics (version 4.1). For heat transfer with phase transformation, the enthalpy method was employed to account for the effects of freezing and thawing during cryosurgery. The enthalpy method is a well-established technique for numerical analysis of the phase transition phenomenon in biological media [34]. To validate the use of the commercial software in this work, we tested the convergence of the numerical parameters employed in the analysis against known solutions of the corresponding heat transfer problem. Specifically, a heat transfer with phase change model without electrical parameters was compared to benchmark problems of this kind and validated the approach and results of this paper.

Electrical and Thermal Properties. Physiological saline was used as a first order simulation of biological tissue. The electrical conductivity for saline was derived analytically for subzero temperatures using composite theory and the thermodynamic phase diagram for saline. The equation for freezing point depression was used to calculate the volume of solution as a function of temperature. Data from J.J. Arps [33] was curve fitted to calculate the electrical conductivity of the composite medium. The derived electrical conductivity for subzero temperatures was combined with experimental data for higher temperatures [35], resulting in the following piecewise function:

$$\sigma(T)=\begin{cases}\dfrac{4.556}{T-273.15}\times\exp\left(\dfrac{T-273.15}{4.99962}\right)-\dfrac{4.5559}{T-273.15}+2.365e-8, T\leq 272.59\\ 0.03(T-273.15)+0.7, T>272.59\end{cases} \tag{3}$$

Equation 3 describes the behavior of electrical conductivity in [S/m] as a function of temperature [K], both above and below freezing. The correlation coefficient of this equation relative to experimental data was tabulated to be *r = 0.99989*.

In addition to electrical conductivity, electrical permittivity is also a function of temperature. The following equation [36] was utilized to take into account the temperature dependence of electrical permittivity:

$$\varepsilon(T)=10^{\left(1.94404-1.99\times10^{-3}(T-273.15)\right)}, \tag{4}$$

where ε is electrical permittivity and T is temperature. This equation is valid for low frequency permittivity, experienced by typical PEF pulse parameters, which are in the range of 0.1-20E-3 seconds.

The values for biological tissue utilized in the Pennes Bioheat equation are listed in Table 1 [22] and the thermal properties used are listed in Table 2.

For consistency with the electric field analysis, properties for physiological saline solution were also used to model the thermal behavior of biological tissue. All three values for frozen media in Table 2 were defined at temperatures below freezing, when $T<272.59$. The models defined values for unfrozen media in Table 2 at temperatures above freezing, when $T>273.59$. The transition region between the frozen and unfrozen media was defined using a smoothed Heaviside function. Therefore, the Heaviside function represented a volume fraction of liquid in the frozen media. The term for specific heat was modified to account for latent heat of fusion in order to model the phase transition:

$$C_{\text{mod}}=\sum\nolimits_i C_p+D\lambda, \tag{5}$$

where λ is the latent heat of fusion (333E3 J/kg [40]) and $D=\dfrac{dH}{dT_{trans}}$. Where H is the Heaviside function and T_{trans} represents the phase transition temperature.

Studies on the effect of temperature on electroporation protocols have revealed a negative correlation between temperature and fields. The electric fields required for producing electroporation increase as temperature decreases. The goal of this study is to investigate the ultimate effects of temperature modulation on cryosugery/PEF protocols, such as the fields necessary to induce reversible and irreversible electroporation. To accomplish this, data has been extracted from existing literature to produce a correlation between temperature and the fields at transition values between reversible and irreversible electroporation [37,38]. The equation used in this study was derived from the experimental data acquired in [39] and is given by:

Table 1. Temperature dependent properties used in the Pennes bioheat equation for the purpose of solving the temperature distribution due to the application of the cooling probe.

Thermal Conductivity	Blood Perfusion	Blood Heat Capacity	Metabolic Heat	Tissue Density	Tissue Heat Capacity
0.5 [W/mK]	0.5[kg/m^{3}s]	3640 [J/kgK]	33800[W/m^3]	1000 [kg/m^3]	3750 [J/kgK]

Table 2. Temperature dependent properties used in the heat conduction equation for the purpose of solving the temperature distribution due to the application of the cryosurgical probe.

	Density (ρ) [kg/m^3]	Specific Heat (C_p) [J/kg K]	Thermal Conductivity (k) [W/m K]	Reference
Frozen	918	2052	2.31	[37]
Unfrozen	997	4179	0.613	[37]

$$E(T) = \frac{-39}{3200}T + 63700.45, \quad (6)$$

where T is temperature [°C] and E is electric field [V/m]. This equation was used as an approximate correlation for this study. It was used primarily to demonstrate an accurate methodology, but a substantial amount of additional research is needed to generate precise correlations, which currently have not yet been developed. It should be emphasized that we expect that the hyperosmolarity of the extracellular solution in the high subzero temperature range should reduce the field required for electroporation [32]. Therefore we anticipate that Equation 6 is an upper limit of the electric field required for electroporation at the conditions on the outer rim of the frozen lesion during cryosurgery.

Models. To extract the most salient biophysical aspects of the analysis, we investigated a simple one-dimensional configuration in Cartesian (Figure 1a) and cylindrical coordinates (Figure 1b). Figure 1a shows a slab like structure of tissue, while Figure 1b shows a cylinder of tissue with a concentric cylindrical cryosurgical probe in the center. The analysis was performed to obtain the temperature distribution and the electric field during freezing and thawing of tissue. The results were compared to a control case in which the electric field was calculated for a constant physiological temperature, 310.15 K. The initial temperature was assumed to be the physiological temperature, 310.15 K. At the onset of freezing, a temperature of 268.15 K was imposed on one surface (the left hand side outer surface in the slab like configuration, Figure 1a, and the central cryoprobe in the cylindrical configuration, Figure 1b). The right hand side of the slab and the outer edge of the cylinder were kept at physiological body temperature, 310.15 K. A temperature of 268.15 K (−5°C) was implemented because in very conservative estimates cell survival occurs at temperatures above 258.15 K in cryosurgery [2,3,9,10]. Therefore, this thermal condition represents the outer margin of a frozen cryosurgical lesion where cells survive freezing [2,3]; which is a range of temperatures where phenomena related to the Cryo/PEF concept occur. This range enables a test of the conditions in which PEF can ablate cells on the margin of the frozen lesion where frozen cells survive. Furthermore, this is a subzero temperature at which electroporation was observed to occur [30,39]. The duration of freezing was 90 seconds, after which the cold surface is thermally insulated and natural thawing was induced by constant deep body physiological temperature. The duration of the analyzed thawing period was also 90 seconds. While these periods of time for freezing and thawing are short relative to conventional cryosurgery, they are relevant to the relatively high subfreezing range of temperatures, which is the focus of this analysis. A voltage difference of 1 V between the two outer surfaces of the slab (Figure 1a); and between the cryoprobe surface and the outer surface of the cylindrical tissue (Figure 1b), was used in the calculation of electrical potential to facilitate a general normalized analysis of the electric fields.

An evenly distributed finite element mesh was incorporated into the 6 cm wide slab model. The mesh size was varied in order to validate the accuracy of the solution. The mesh size was refined until the solution was no longer affected by the quality of the mesh. The mesh used in the analysis presented here consisted of roughly 1500 elements.

The second geometry included a typical cryoprobe 3.4 mm in diameter [40], inserted into the center of an infinitely long cylinder of tissue, 6 cm in radius. The finite element mesh utilized for this case incorporated triangular elements, as shown in Figure 1. The element size was smallest adjacent to the cryoprobe, and increased in size as it radiated towards the outer boundary. This was done in order to accurately capture the steep temperature gradient adjacent to the cryoprobe. The mesh was refined until the solution was no longer affected by mesh size. Approximately 3000 elements were utilized to cover a 113 mm^2 surface area.

Results and Discussion

Cartesian Coordinates

The Cartesian coordinate model was chosen for analysis because it provides a simple model which provides fundamental insight into the biophysical processes that occur during the combined application of cryosurgery and PEF. The Cartesian model utilized the boundary conditions specified in Figure 2.

The temperature distribution during freezing is shown in Figure 3a, and the electric field distribution is shown in Figure 3b. The temperature distribution is as expected, increasing from the low temperature at the cryoprobe surface to body temperature. As time progresses, the low temperatures penetrate further into the tissue due to thermal diffusion. Note that at 272.59 K, the nonlinear behavior indicates the region of phase change. Figures 3a and 3b demonstrate the inversely proportional relationship between temperature and electrical conductivity, as described by Equation 3. Lower temperatures yield a lower ionic conductivity and subfreezing temperatures yield a dramatic decrease in electrical conductivity. Figure 3b illustrates the most important feature of the cryosurgery/PEF combination; because of the increased electrical resistance in the frozen and cooled regions of tissue, the highest electric fields are confined to those regions. Figure 4b also shows that the fields beyond the frozen and cooled regions in the normal tissue are substantially lower than those in the frozen/cooled regions. This suggests that the freezing/cooling has the effect of confining the high electric fields to those regions, as originally predicted.

Figures 2c and 2d illustrate the temperature distribution and the electric field during thawing. Figure 3c shows that adjacent to the cryoprobe, the temperature inches upwards because of the insulating boundary conditions applied by the probe during thawing. If thawing were extended beyond 90 seconds, the temperature graph would continue to equilibrate toward the phase transition temperature. The temperature distribution has a point of inversion, which appears to be stationary in time at about

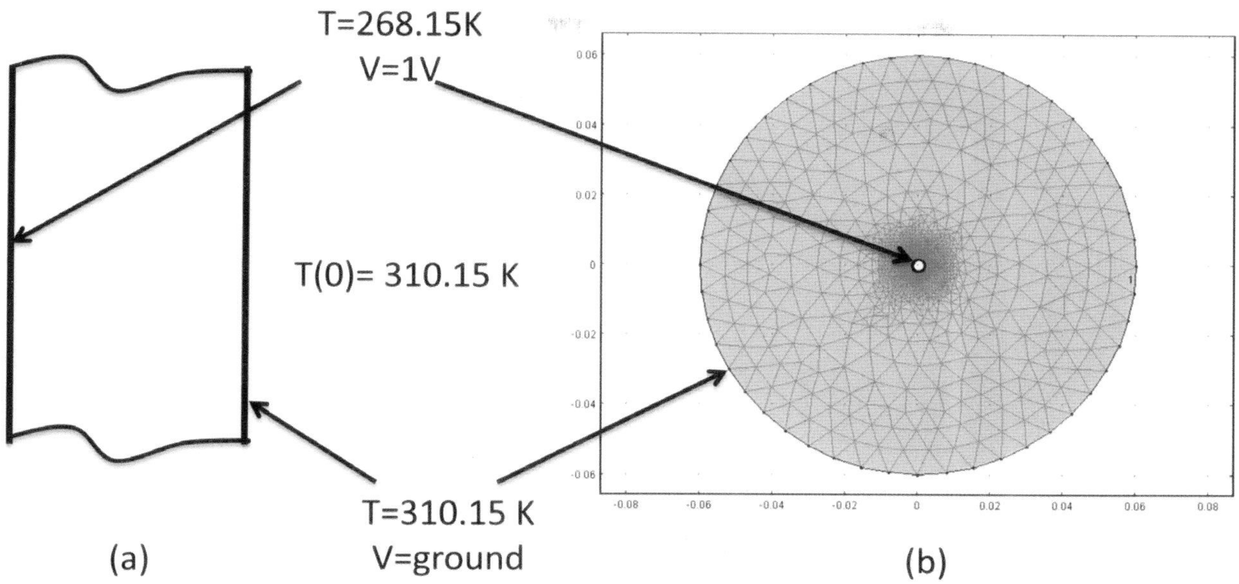

Figure 1. Boundary conditions for the one dimensional Case 1 in a slab-like geometry. Variable resistances *R1* and *R2* represent electric and thermal resistance (in the thermal and electrical equivalent circuits). Boundary conditions utilized in the model are specified at the nodes. The initial temperature was set to physiological temperature, 310.15 K. Figure 1a: geometry of Case 1. Figure 1b: Mesh for Case 2 with one cryoprobe in the center of tissue cylinder. Note that the mesh is extra fine in the vicinity of the probes in order to capture the changes in electric field and temperature that occur due to the effect of the probes.

0.2 cm from the outer surface. This point of inversion corresponds to the position of the change of phase interface.

The temperature history during thawing of frozen media has a peculiarity caused by the effects of the phase transition, which has been studied extensively in the past [41]. This effect appears in Figure 4c. Previous studies have also shown that during thawing of frozen lesions, the temperature of the frozen region increases first to the phase transition temperature, before the frozen tissue begins to thaw, and then remains at this value throughout the thawing process [41]. The explanation for this phenomenon is complex, has been previously discussed in heat transfer papers on cryosurgery, and is not directly relevant to this work. However, the phenomenon is important in the use of cryosurgery with PEF.

Figure 3d shows that the relationship between temperature and electrical conductivity produces an electric field that also has a point of inversion around 0.2 cm, which is the outer edge of the frozen lesion. Figure 3d shows that the electric field in the frozen region drops precipitously during thawing to a constant value of 32 V/m (for the 1 V potential on the cryoprobe). It is apparent that if the temperature in the frozen region during thawing stays at the phase transition temperature, the electrical conductivity in the frozen region will remain constant throughout thawing and (in Cartesian coordinates) the electric field in the frozen region will remain constant as well. This suggests that if PEFs are applied during thawing they will be confined and delivered in the frozen region across cells that are all at the highest possible subfreezing temperature. This could allow for precise design of PEF by utilizing electrical parameters that only affect thawing cells in the frozen tissue at the phase transition temperature.

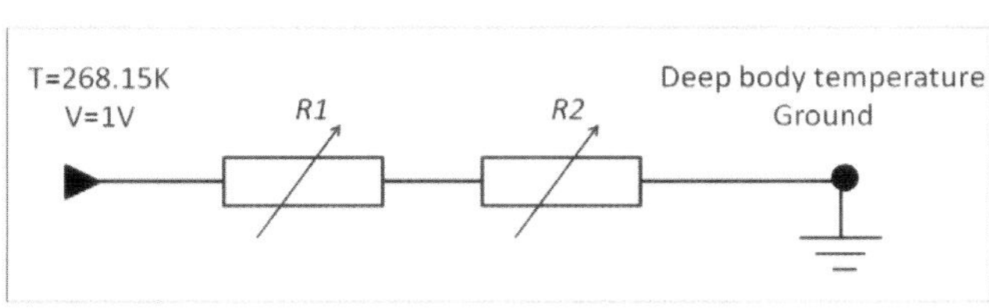

Figure 2. Electric current schematic for the one dimensional 1D Cartesian study in a slab-like geometry. Variable resistances R_1 and R_2 represent electric and thermal resistance (in the thermal and electrical equivalent circuits). Boundary conditions utilized in the model are specified at the nodes.

It is pertinent that the electric field produced during freezing and thawing is compared to a control study. The control study applied the same electrical boundary conditions to tissue held at body temperature. This control study is represented by the dotted horizontal line in Figures 2b (freezing study) and 2d (thawing study). It is evident that the electric field in the frozen/cooled regions is substantially higher than the field produced in the control study in the same region in both freezing and thawing. However, at a distance from the frozen region, in the location of normal body temperatures, the fields are lower than those in the control. This suggests that it should be possible to design cryosurgery/PEF protocols in which the PEF induced cell damage is confined to the frozen/cooled regions and the damage does not extend beyond the cooled regions.

In summary, Figure 3 shows that during both freezing and thawing the electric fields are substantially increased in the frozen/cooled region during cryosurgery with PEF relative to the electric fields in a similar region when PEFs are used with tissue at a constant temperature. The reason for this is illustrated by Figure 2. Figure 2 is an analog representation of the electrical and thermal resistance in the frozen and unfrozen region during cryosurgery. The electrical current flows from one wall of the slab to the other through two resistors in series. The frozen/cooled tissue and the unfrozen tissue equivalent resistances are separated by the phase transition interface. Since the current through the electrodes is constant, it is evident that the resistor of higher magnitude, which in the case in the frozen/cooled region, will experience a higher

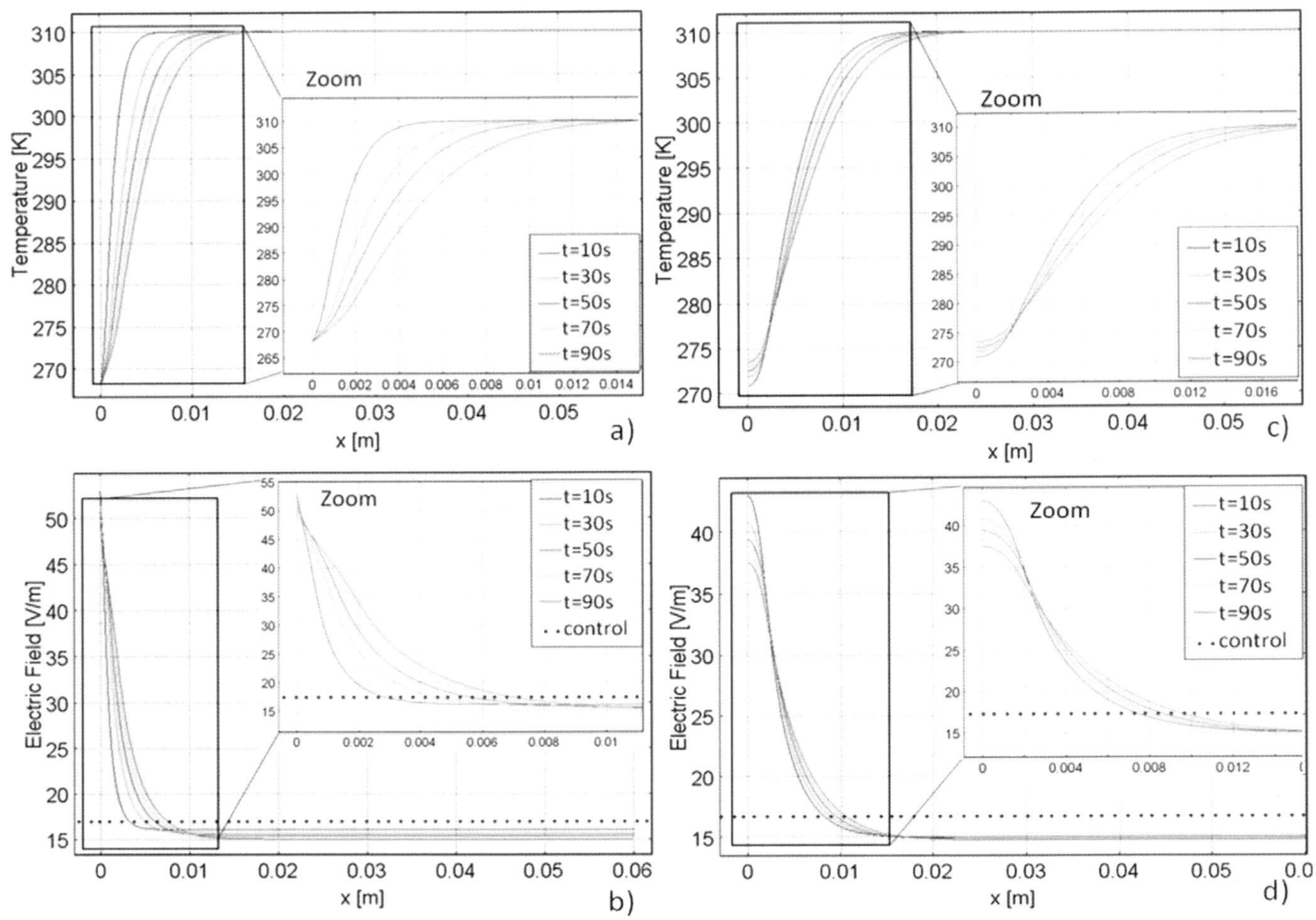

Figure 3. Graphs for the Cartesian coordinate study. Left column: temperature and electric field distribution during 90 seconds of freezing. Right column: temperature and electric field distribution during 90 seconds of thawing. Each line represents a 20 second time increment. The dotted line shows the electric field in tissue held constant at body temperature for the same voltage boundary conditions.

electric field. The large disparity in electrical conductivity between the frozen/cooled region and the unfrozen tissue confines and magnifies the electric field to the frozen/cooled region. The potential-divider circuit in Figure 2 demonstrates the field enhancement in regions of lower conductivity.

It should be emphasized, that this phenomenon occurs because the electric field vector is normal to the boundary of the two regions of different conductivity. If the electric field were parallel to this boundary, then the equivalent circuit would be two resistors in parallel, rather than in series, and there would be negligible field enhancement or possible field decrease, depending on the relative electrical conductivity of the tissues. The particular configuration developed in this study is a direct consequence of the fact that the cryoprobe serves both as the heat sink and as the electric source. The configurations used in this study were chosen particularly to accomplish this effect.

The plots in Figure 3 were obtained for a normalized voltage of 1 V. Combining Figures 2b and Equation 6 suggests that a voltage of about 2000 V applied to the cryoprobe would be sufficient to ablate the analyzed frozen tissue by PEF. This voltage is typical for what is necessary for tissue ablation with irreversible electroporation. The result of applying 2000 V after 90 seconds of freezing to the model in Figure 3 can be seen in Figure 4a and 4b. As can be seen by this graph, the temperature distribution in the tissue is similar to that in Figure 3, where 1 V was applied. However, one difference is evident; the temperature rises to a higher value over a shorter distance adjacent to the leftmost plate. This is because Joule heating occurs when higher voltages are applied.

The electric field distribution for the application of 2000 V is similar to that of the 1 V case. However, the maximum electric field reached with 2000 V is 100,000 V/m. This results in an electric field distribution in the frozen region above 67,000 V/m, the threshold for irreversible electroporation. Figure 3d and Equation 6 suggest that applying an electric potential above 2000 V is sufficient to cause irreversible electroporation in the thawing region in this model.

Figure 4c and 4d illustrate the temperature and electric field distributions when 2000 V is applied after 90 seconds of thawing. The temperature distribution is similar to that seen in Figure 3c (when 1 V is applied). However, the temperature rises to a higher value over a shorter distance when 2000 V is applied due to Joule heating. The lowest temperature is 275 K in the 2000 V case, rather than 274 K as in the 1 V case. The electric field in the 2000 V case has a similar distribution to the 1 V case, except the highest electric field reached in this case is 75,000 V/m. It is important to note that changing the voltage magnitude has a very small effect on the temperature distribution. This is because the

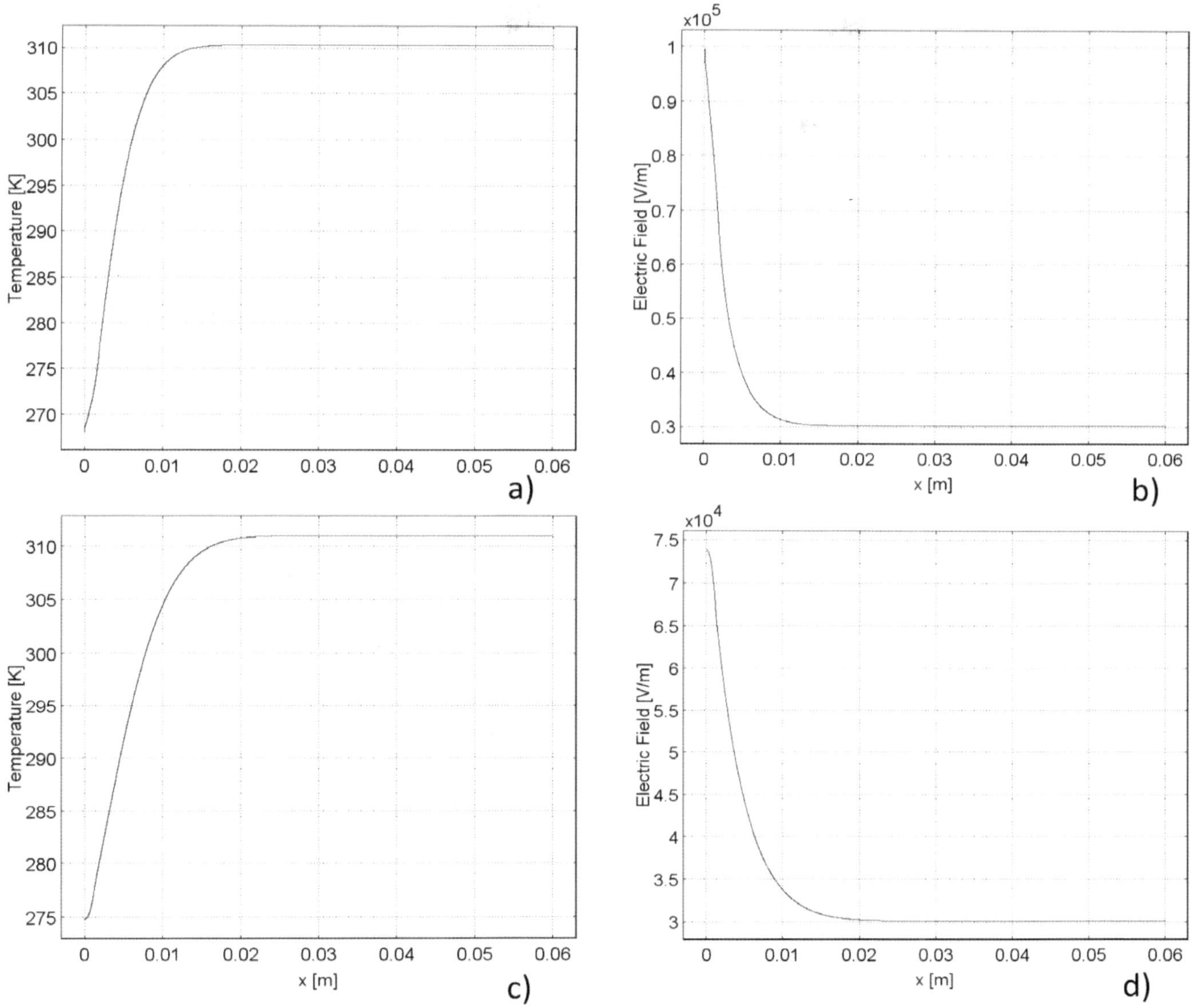

Figure 4. Temperature and electric field plots during freezing and thawing. Left column demonstrates the temperature distribution and right column demonstrates the electric field distribution, both after 90 seconds of freezing with an applied voltage of 2000 V for 90 pulses. The first row illustrates the results due to 90 seconds of freezing and the second row illustrates the results due to 90 seconds of thawing. The trends are similar to those seen in the 1 V cases. However, in the freezing case, the electric field reaches a maximum of 100,000 V/m. In the thawing case the electric field reaches a maximum of 75000 V/m. The temperature rises more quickly at the leftmost plate in both the freezing and thawing cases due to Joule heating.

energy content in an electroporation pulse is very small relative to the enthalpy of phase transition.

It should be emphasized that in this study the range of subfreezing temperatures used are relatively high, above −5°C. In this temperature range cells survive freezing [2,3]. Adding PEF during freezing will ablate the cells in the frozen region that survive freezing and thereby making the cryosurgery/PEF treatment produce tissue ablation to the edge of the frozen lesion. This also suggests that the cryosurgery/PEF technique may not require the cryogenic temperatures used in conventional cryosurgery and cryosurgical systems. Therefore, cooling systems using Joule Thomson, solid state thermoelectric systems or conventional refrigeration cycles may be sufficient for tissue ablation with this method. Figure 3 and this analysis corroborate the initial hypothesis of this study: the effect of freezing and low temperatures on electrical conductivity can actually concentrate the electric field to the cooled/frozen region as well as amplify the electric field in that region, which would require substantial lower voltages on the cryosurgery/PEF probes than on conventional PEF probes.

Cryosurgery/PEF protocols can also be designed to induce cell permeabilization via reversible electroporation for the purpose of gene therapy and drug delivery. For example, Figure 3b shows that the field produced by a 1 V potential difference at the cryosurgical probe ranges from about 50 V/m to about 40 V/m between the −5°C and +5°C isotherms. If an attempt were made to combine cryosurgery with electrochemotherapy PEFs, the fields required for reversible electroporation in the liver are about 36,000 V/m. Therefore a pulse of about 700 V will produce reversible electroporation in the region from −5°C to +5°C. However, Figure 3b shows that the same pulse will produce a field of approximately 10,000 V/m in the body temperature region, which should have no effect on the tissue in that location. In contrast, in the control case (at constant body temperature), Figure 3b shows that a pulse of about 1800 V would be needed to produce the fields required for electrochemotherapy and the fields would affect the entire region between the electrodes.

Cylindrical Coordinates

The purpose of this second study was to examine a more realistic cryosurgical configuration. In Case 2 the geometry consists of a single cryoprobe in a cylindrical section of tissue 6 cm in radius. Geometric details and boundary conditions were previously mentioned in the Models section.

Figure 5a illustrates the temperature distribution at a transection along the diameter. Note that in Figure 5a the gap in the plot is the location of the cryoprobe. As in the 1D Cartesian case, due to thermal diffusion, freezing temperatures penetrate further into the tissue with time. And again, nonlinear behavior at 272.59 K indicates the region of phase change.

The relationship between temperature and electric field is discernable from Figures 4a and 4b. As in the 1D Cartesian study, temperature and electric field are inversely proportional due to the dependence of electrical conductivity on temperature. For this reason, the electric field is highest in the frozen and cooled regions. This result corroborates both the hypothesis of this paper and the results in the 1D Cartesian study. Because of decreased electrical conductivity in the frozen and cooled tissue, the highest electric fields are confined to those regions. Figure 5b shows that the fields beyond the frozen and cooled regions are orders of magnitude lower than those in the frozen/cooled regions. This suggests that freezing/cooling temperatures have the effect of magnifying the high electric fields in those regions. The effect of low temperature on confining the electric field is effectively demonstrated in Figures 6c and 6d. The zoom panel demonstrates that the electric field is confined within the cooled region, which again validates the original hypothesis of this study.

Figures 5a and 5b illustrate the temperature distribution and the electric field during thawing. The temperature distribution during thawing with 1D cylindrical symmetry behaves very similarly to the previously discussed temperature distribution in the 1D

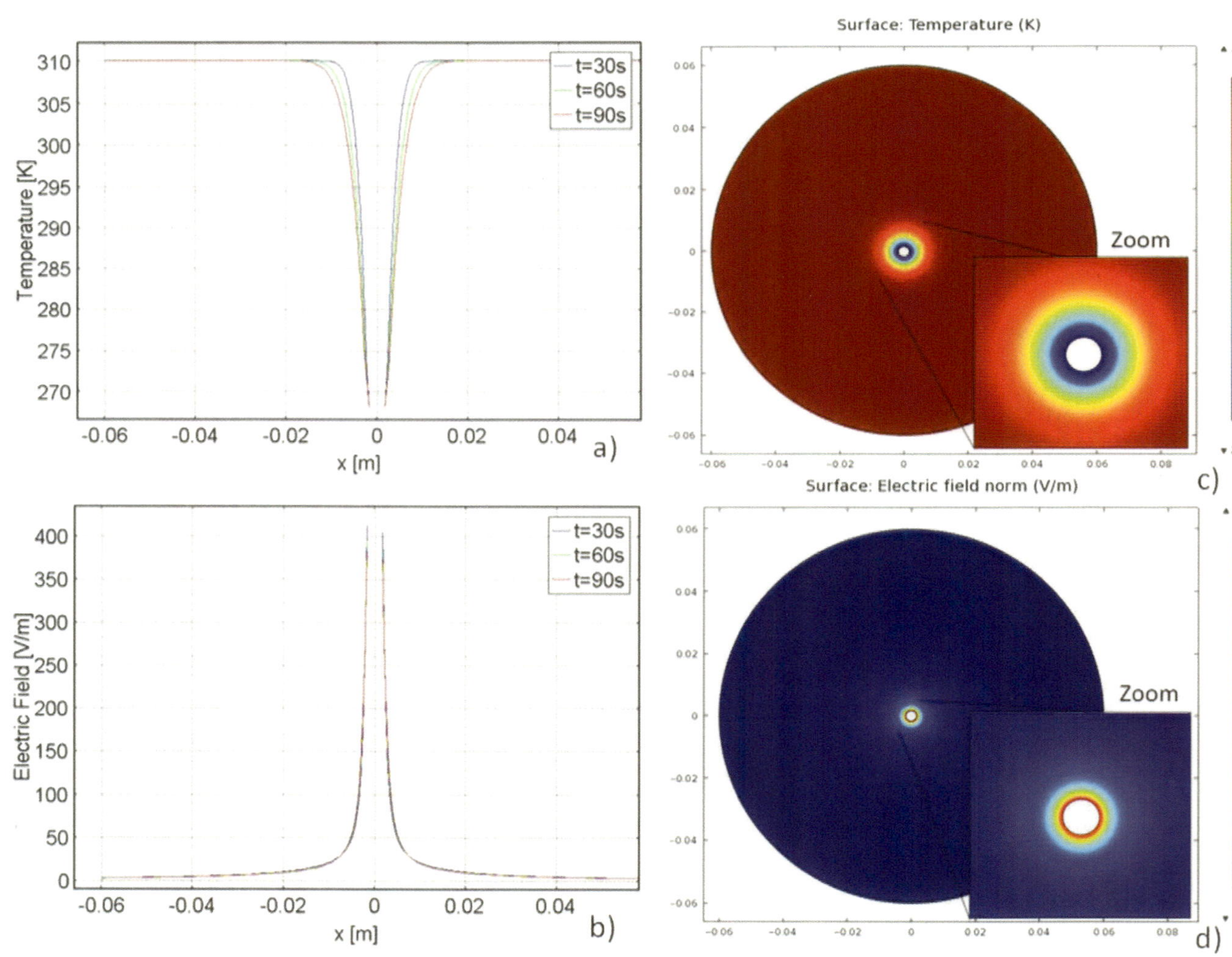

Figure 5. Data for the cylindrical coordinate study. The temperature and electric field distribution are illustrated during 90 seconds of freezing. Left column: graph, right column: surface plot.

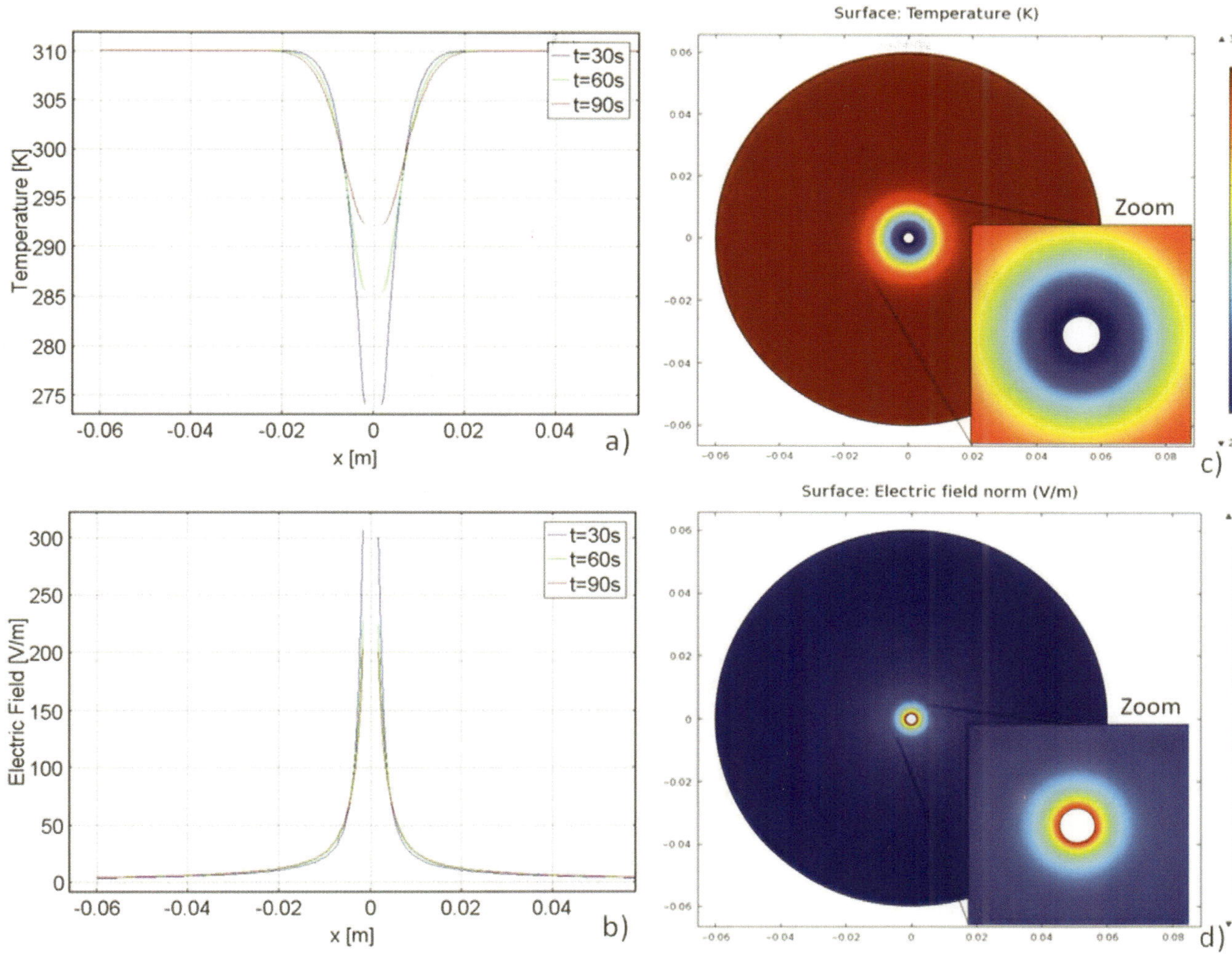

Figure 6. Data for the cylindrical coordinate study. The temperature and electric field distribution are illustrated during 90 seconds of thawing. Left column: graph, right column: surface plot.

Cartesian case. Figure 7c shows that temperatures adjacent to the cryoprobe inch upwards as a result of its insulated boundary conditions. The temperature distribution has a stationary point of inversion at 0.6 cm. Figure 6b shows that the electric field also has a point of inversion around 0.6 cm. Figure 6b also demonstrates that the electric field in the frozen/cooled region during thawing drops dramatically, effectively confining the field. Because of the transient nature of the temperature distribution, the electric field also changes with time. For instance, 30 seconds into thawing the highest electric field near the cryoprobe has dropped from 400 V/m at the end of freezing to 300 V/m.

The location of the highest electric field is the same point in space and time as the lowest temperature, which is consistent with Equation 2. Additionally, the electric field decreases in time as thawing progresses and temperatures rise throughout the domain. The slope of the electric field also follows that of the temperature. The slope of the electric field is steepest at the onset of thawing, when temperatures are lowest. But as thawing progresses, and temperatures begin to rise, the slope of the electric field lessens. This indicates the strong relationship between electric field and temperature in the cryosurgery/PEF procedure and the ability of freezing/cold temperatures to confine the electric field. This observation is most evident from Figures 5c and 5d, which depict surface plots of the temperature and electric field distribution, respectively, during the thawing stage of the cryosurgery/PEF procedure. The zoom panels clearly illustrate that the electric field is confined inside the lower temperature regions during thawing.

Figure 5 shows that the electric field in the frozen region is higher than about 150 V/m for a voltage of 1 V on the cryoprobe. Equation 6 suggests that a voltage of about 400 V imposed on the cryosurgical probe is sufficient to ablate the cells with PEF in the analyzed frozen region. A graph of the electric field and temperature distributions with 400 V applied after 90 seconds of freezing can be seen in Figure 7. When 400 V are applied, the temperature rises to a higher value over a shorter distance than when 1 V was applied (Figure 7a) due to the effect of Joule heating. The electric field with 400 V applied demonstrates the same trend as the case with 1 V applied, but reaches a maximum of 160,000 V/m rather than the peak of 400 V/m seen in the 1 V case.

Figure 6 suggests that here also, similar to the Cartesian one dimensional case, the field produced by 1 V potential at the cryosurgery/PEF probe in the thawing frozen lesion will be higher than about 75 V/m. Therefore, Equation 6 suggests that a voltage

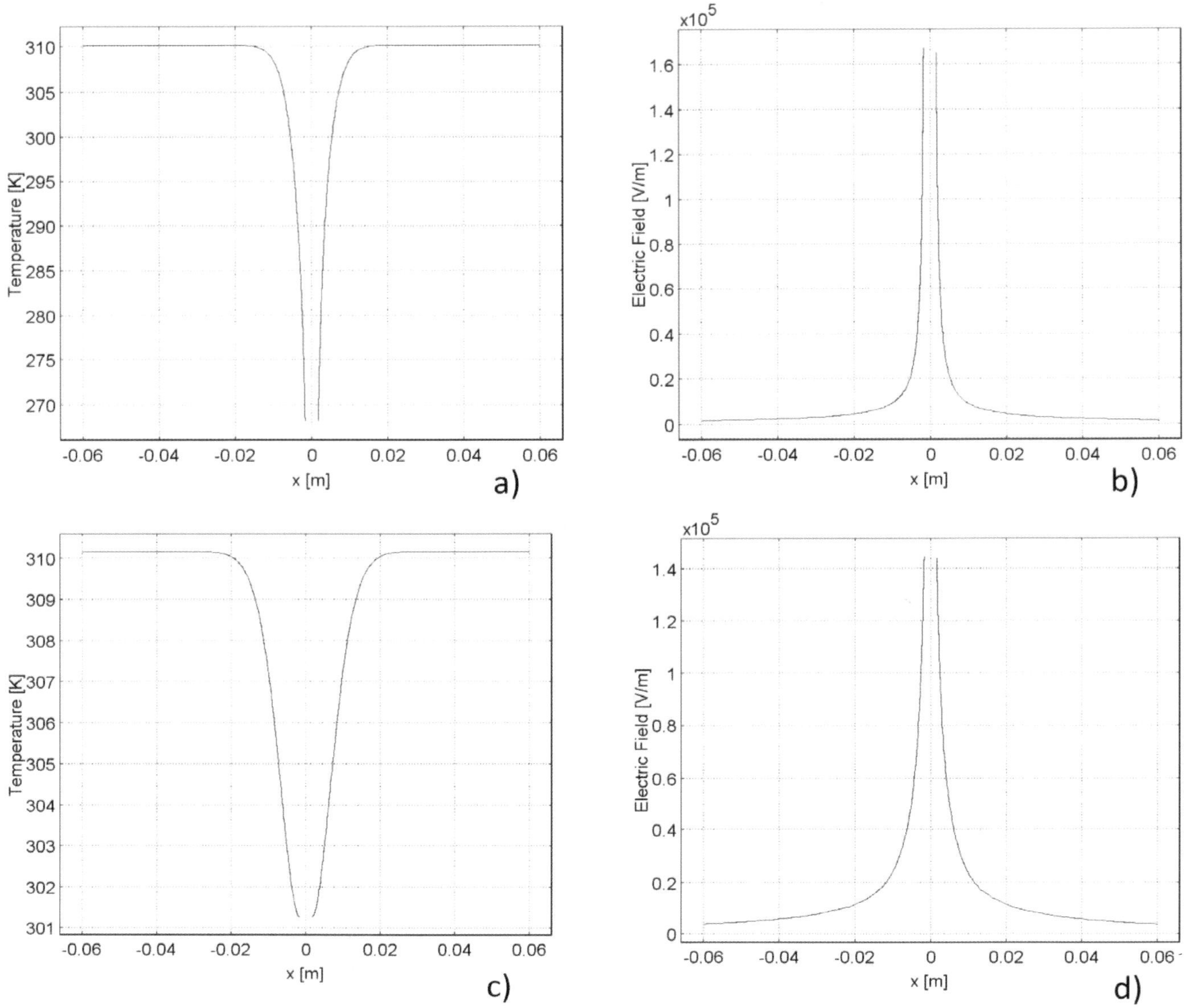

Figure 7. Temperature and electric field distribution during freezing and thawing for the cylindrical coordinate study. Left plot demonstrates the temperature distribution and right plot demonstrates the electric field distribution. The first row illustrates the results after freezing, and the second row illustrates the results after thawing. In each case, a voltage of 400 V is applied for 90 pulses. The trends are similar to those seen in the 1 V cases. However, in the freezing case, the electric field reaches a maximum of 160,000 V/m. In the thawing case, the electric field reaches a maximum of 140,000 V/m. In both instances, the temperature rises higher on the probe due to Joule heating.

of about 850 V on the cryosurgery/PEF probe will be sufficient to ablate the frozen cells during thawing with PEF. Figure 7 illustrates the electric field and temperature distributions after 90 seconds of thawing with an applied voltage of 850 V. Due to the higher voltage, Joule heating affects the temperature distribution. In the case of 850 V, the lowest temperature in the domain is 301 K, whereas with an applied voltage of 1 V the lowest temperature is 293 K. The electric field achieved due to 850 V is also much higher, it reaches a peak of 140,000 V/m, whereas the peak in the 1 V case is only 300 V/m.

The significance of the findings in Figures 4 and 5 is emphasized by a comparison to the control study. The control study applies the same electrical conditions on the cryoprobe as freezing and thawing, but holds the probe and tissue at constant body temperature. The control case represents conventional PEFs delivered by a monopolar probe, which in this case is the cryoprobe. The comparison of the resulting electric fields can be seen in Figure 8. It is clear that the electric field in the frozen/cooled regions during freezing (Figure 8b) and thawing (Figure 8c) are substantially higher than the field produced in the control study in the same region (Figure 8a). The magnitudes of the peak electric field in the freezing and thawing cases are more than double the magnitude of the peak electric field in the control case. However, at a distance from the frozen/cooled tissue, in the region of normal body temperatures, the fields during freezing and thawing are lower than those in the control. This indicates that not only do freezing/cold temperatures amplify the electric field; they also exhibit an effect of targeting the electric field to the cold

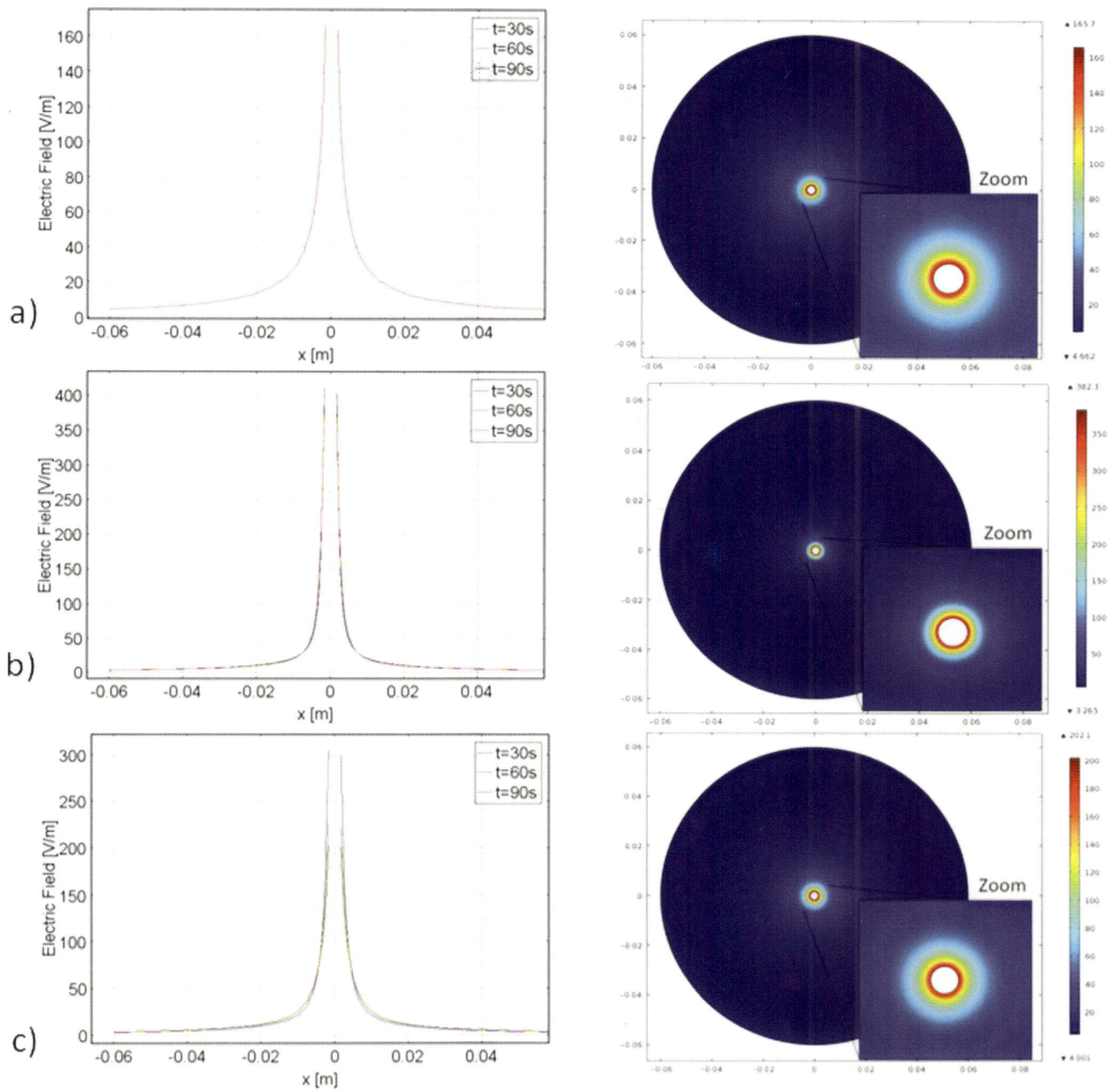

Figure 8. Electric field distribution for the cylindrical coordinate study. From top to bottom row: control, freezing and thawing. Aligned for the purpose of comparison. Right column: surface plot.

region. In fact, once the electric field has decayed and reached a constant value, it is zero in the cryosurgery/PEF case, and above zero in the control PEF case.

Figures 7a, 7b and 7c show that the highest electric field occurs, in descending order: freezing, thawing and control. Figures 7a, 7b and 7c also illustrate the ability of cold/freezing temperatures to concentrate the electric field because the most narrowly spread electric field occurs in the freezing case, followed by thawing and then control. This Figure most clearly demonstrates the ability of freezing/cold temperatures to both amplify and direct the electric fields of PEF.

These results suggest that it will be possible to design a cryosurgery/PEF treatment in which the PEF induced cell damage is confined to the frozen/cooled regions and the damage does not extend beyond these regions. The possibility of designing electrical parameters which concentrate the electric field in the frozen/cooled region suggests that utilizing cryosurgical imaging techniques could possibly image cells ablated due to PEFs. For instance, ultrasound is capable of differentiating between frozen and unfrozen media during cryosurgical procedures [2]. Therefore, by concentrating the electric field to the frozen tissue, imaging frozen tissue with ultrasound will also show cells ablated by PEFs in real time during the procedure. This first order theoretical result indicates the potential feasibility of this technology.

Several additional advantages of the cryosurgery/PEF procedure can be theorized as a result of these two studies. Because cells survive these high subzero freezing temperatures, cryosurgery/PEF would retain PEFs' ability to selectively ablate only cellular membranes without affecting the extracellular matrix, when cryosurgery/PEF is used at high subzero temperatures. Another advantage of this combination may be related to elimination of certain side effects and limitations of PEF [41,42]. The most severe side effects are arrhythmias and involuntary muscle contractions [41,42] caused by low strength electric fields that expand beyond the PEF treatment zone. The solution to arrhythmias through a synchronizer device is described in [42]. Although strong paralytics such as *cisatracurium* or *rocuronium* [41,42] and deep anesthesia are used in clinical NTIRE treatments, muscle contractions are still observed in the proximity to the electrodes. Moreover, diaphragm contractions still take place [42]. Our studies show that the combination of cryosurgery with PEF magnify the electric field in the frozen/cooled region and reduces the electric field beyond the frozen/cooled treatment region. Therefore, it could be anticipated that the detrimental effects of PEFs related to weak electric fields that occur beyond the treatment region will be reduced, or perhaps even eliminated.

During the last three decades, cryosurgery has become widely accepted as a minimally invasive surgical technique and is currently used to ablate undesirable tissues in a large number of clinical applications, such as treatment of cancer and arrhythmias. This suggests that the new concept of cryosurgery enhanced by PEF could be more readily accepted among practitioners of cryosurgery. Cryosurgical probes and apparatuses can easily be modified for a cryosurgery/PEF application. The shaft of any cryoprobe is metal and electrically conductive, and therefore could also be used as an electrode. In fact, many cryosurgical probes also have an electrical conduit through the shaft, housing a thermocouple for the purpose of measuring temperatures at the tip of the cryoprobe. This could be one possible path for the electric pulses. Another possible path could be through direct connection to the metal shaft. To deliver the electric pulse only at the thermally active tip of the cryoprobe, it would be sufficient to apply a thin layer of electric insulation along the cryoprobe shaft, as in typical electroporation needles. The pulsed electric field power supply can either be stand alone, or incorporated in the cryosurgery console and connected to the electrically conductive cryoprobe shaft.

There are several ways in which the PEFs could be delivered during cryosurgery. Currently, typical PEF devices operate only between two electrodes at a time, even when multiple electrodes are inserted in the tissue. Therefore, in a first application modality, one thermally active cryoprobe would be connected to one pole of the power supply. The second pole (or ground) could be connected either to a second cryoprobe inserted into the tissue or to a remote ground pad; for instance on the leg, like during radio frequency ablation. The combined Cryosurgery/PEF effect takes place primarily in regions of tissue in which there is freezing and thawing. Therefore, we anticipate that in typical procedures, the PEF will be delivered at the onset of freezing and through freezing and thawing. To take advantage of the ability of medical imaging to detect the extent of freezing, we anticipate that real time imaging with ultrasound or CT will be employed during the Cryosurgery/PEF procedure and in this way ensure that the PEFs are delivered only in the desired cooled area, with real time control over delivery. In this study we have shown only a few of the possible combinations in which this procedure could be used. It is quite obvious that multiple combinations of cryoprobes or different combinations of cold and heat are possible as a way to increase or reduce the magnitude of the PEFs in desired regions of tissue.

Conclusion

The goal of this study was to evaluate the feasibility and the characteristics of a minimally invasive surgical procedure in which cryosurgery was modulated with PEFs, in the hope that this will improve the effectiveness of cryosurgery and eliminate the problems related to cell survival on the outer rim of frozen tissue as well as produce controlled use of PEF. One dimensional models demonstrated that low and freezing temperatures have a substantial effect on PEF produced electric fields. Furthermore, unanticipated information about the effects of subzero temperature on PEFs was also discovered. This investigation has made clear that both low and subzero temperatures are capable of concentrating the electric field because of the temperature dependence of electrical conductivity. Additionally, this study has demonstrated the ability of low temperatures to increase the magnitude of the electric field.

These results have far reaching implications in terms of imaging strategy and procedural methodology regarding accuracy of treating tissue with cryosurgery. Utilizing cryosurgery/PEF may potentially allow medical imaging of PEF. A further inadvertent consequence of targeted electric fields may be the elimination of muscle contractions during surgery due to the substantial reduction in electric field outside the cryosurgery/PEF treated zone.

Although this is a first order theoretical analysis and additional theoretical and experimental research is needed to further develop this new concept, these primary results act as a promising foundation for future work. For these reasons, this numerical study has indicated the undeveloped potential and the motivation for pursuing cryosurgery/PEF.

Acknowledgments

The authors would like to thank Greg Troszak and Yair Granot for their technical contributions, as well as Peter Minor, and Danielle Levinson for their support.

Author Contributions

Conceived and designed the experiments: CD BR. Performed the experiments: CD. Analyzed the data: CD. Contributed reagents/materials/analysis tools: CD BR. Wrote the paper: CD BR.

References

1. Fuch KH (2002) Minimally invasive surgery. Endoscopy 34: 154–159.
2. Rubinsky B (2000) Cryosurgery. Annual Review of Biomedical Engineering 2: 157–187.
3. Gage AA, Baust JM, Baust JG (2009) Experimental cryosurgery investigations in vivo. Cryobiology 59: 229–243.
4. Rubinsky B, Shitzer A (1976) Analysis of a stefan-like problem in biological tissue around a cryosurgical probe. Journal of Heat Transfer 98.
5. Gilbert J, Onik G, Haddick W, Rubinsky B (1984) The use of ultrasonic imaging for monitoring cryosurgery. IEEE Transactions of Biomedical Engineering 563.
6. Onik G, Cooper C, Goldbery GI, Moss AA, Rubinsky B, et al. (1984) Ultrasonic characteristics of frozen liver. Cryobiology 21: 321–328.
7. Onik G, Rubinsky B, Weaver L, Diamond D, Cobb C, et al. (1991) Ultrasound-guided hepatic cryosurgery in the treatment of metastatic colon carcinoma. Preliminary results Cancer 67: 901–907.

8. Baust JG, Gage AA (2005) The Molecular Basis of Cryosurgery. BJU Int 95: 1187–1191.
9. Baust JG, Gage AA, Klossner D (2007) Issues critical to the successful application of cryosurgical ablation of the prostate. Technology in Cancer Research & Treatment 6: 97–109.
10. Tatsutani K, Rubinsky B, Onik G, Dahiya R (1996) Effect of thermal variables on frozen human primary prostatic adenocarinoma cells. Urology 48: 441–447.
11. Koushafar H, Rubinsky B (1997) Effect of antifreeze proteins on frozen primary prostatic adenocarcinoma cells. Urology 49: 421–425.
12. Mir LM, Rubinsky B (2002) Treatment of cancer with cryochemotherapy. British Journal of Cancer 86: 1658–1660.
13. Jiang J, Goel R, Schmechel S, Vercellotti G, Forster C, et al. (2010) Pre-conditioning cryosurgery: cellular and molecular mechanisms and dynamics of TNF-alpha enhanced cryotherapy in an in vivo prostate cancer model system. Cryobiology 61: 280–288.
14. Weaver JC, Chizmadzhev YA (1996) Theory of electroporation: a review. Bioelectrochemistry and Bioenergetics 41: 135–160.
15. Pakhomov AG, Miklavcic D, Marko S, Eds M (2010) Advanced Electroporation Techniques in Biology and Medicine CRC Press.
16. Neumann E, Schaefer-Ridder M, Wang Y, Hofschneider PH (1982) Gene transfer into mouse lyoma cells by electroporation in high electric fields. EMBO 7: 841–845.
17. Jaroszeski M, Gilbert R, Nicolau C, Heller R (1999) In vivo gene delivery by electroporation. Advanced Drug Delivery Reviews 35: 131–137.
18. Somiari S, Glasspool-Malone J, Drabick JJ, Gilbert RA, Heller R, et al. (2000) Theory and in vivo application of electroporative gene delivery. Molecular Therapy 3: 178–87.
19. Okino M, Mohri H (1987) Effects of a high-voltage electrical impulse and an anticancer drug on in vivo growing tumors. Jpn J Cancer Re 78: 1319–21.
20. Mir LM, Orlowski DS, Belehradek R, Paoletti C (1991) Electrochemotherapy potentiation of antitumour effect of bleomycin by local electric pulses. European Jounal of Cancer 27: 68–72.
21. Mir LM, Glass LF, Sersa G, Teissie T, Domenge D, et al. (1998) Effective treatment of cutaneous and subcutaneous malignant tumours by electrochemotherapy. British Journal of Cancer 77: 2336–42.
22. Davalos R, Mir LM, Rubinsky B (2004) Tissue Ablation with Irreversible Electroporation. Annals of Biomedical Engineering 33: 223–231.
23. Edd JF, Horowitz L, Davalos R, Mir L, Rubinsky B (2006) In vivo results of a new focal tissue ablation technique: irreversible electroporation. IEEE Transactions of Biomedical Engineering 53: 1409–1415.
24. Rubinsky B, Onik G, Mikus P (2007) Irreversible electroporation: a new ablation modality - clinical implications. Technology in Cancer Research and Treatment 6: 37–46.
25. Onik G, Mikus P, Rubinsky B (2007) Irreversible electroporation: implications for prostate ablation. Technology in Cancer Research and Treatment 6.
26. Daniels CS, Rubinsky B (2011) Temperature modulation of electric fields in biological matter. PLoS ONE 6.
27. Rubinsky B, Pegg DE (1988) A mathematical model for the freezing process in biological tissue. Proceedings of the Royal Society of London 234.
28. Rubinsky B, Lee CY, Bastacky J, Onik G (1990) The process of freezing and the mechanism of damage during hepatic cryosurgery. Cryobiology 27: 85–97.
29. Bischof J, Christov K, Rubinsky B (1993) A morphological study of cooling rate response in normal and neoplastic human liver tissue: cryosurgical implications. Cryobiology 30: 482–492.
30. Diaz-Rivera RE, Rubinsky B (2006) Electrical and thermal characterization of nanochannels between a cell and a silicon based micro-pore. Biomedical Microdevices 8: 25–34.
31. Gallo SA, Sen A, Hensen ML, Hui SW (2002) Temperature-dependent electrical and ultrastructural characterizations of porcine skin upon electroporation. Biophysics Journal 82: 109–119.
32. Kanduser M, Miklavcic D (2009) Electroporation in biological cell and tissue: an overview. Food Engineering Series. pp 1–37.
33. Arps JJ (1953) The effect of temperature on the density and electrical resistivity of sodium chloride solutions. Petroleum Transactions 198: 327–330.
34. Minkowycz WJ, Sparrow EM, Murthy JY (2006) Numerical Bio-Heat Transfer in *Handbook of Numerical Heat Transfer* John Wiley & Sons Inc.
35. Mazzoleni AP, Sisken BF, Kahler RL (1986) Conductivity values of tissue culture medium from 20°C to 40°C. Bioelectromagnetics 7: 95–99.
36. Kaatze U (1989) Complex permittivity of water as a function of frequency and temperature. J Chem Eng Data 34.
37. Ingebritsen SE, Sanford WE (1998) Groundwater in Geologic Processes Cambridge University Press.
38. Miklavcic D, Semrov D, Mekid H, Mir LM (2000) A validated model of in vivo electric field distribution in tissues for electrochemotherapy and for DNA electrotransfer for gene therapy. Biochim Biophys Acta 1523: 73–83.
39. Diaz-Rivera RE (2000) Micro and nano scale bioelectronics in cell micro-electroporation. PhD Doctoral Dissertation, UC Berkeley.
40. Edd JF, Ivorra A, Horowitz L, Rubinsky B (2008) Imaging cryosurgery with EIT: tracking the ice front and post-thaw tissue viability. Physiological Measurement 29.
41. Lee EW, Thai S, Kee ST (2010) Irreversible electroporation: a novel image-guided cancer therapy. Gut Liver 4: S99–S104.
42. Ball C, Thomson K, Kavnoudias H (2010) Irreversible electroporation: a new challenge in "out of operating theater." Anesth Analg 110: 1305–1309.

14

Efficacy Evaluation of Subtotal and Total Gastrectomies in Robotic Surgery for Gastric Cancer Compared with that in Open and Laparoscopic Resections

Liang Zong[1]•, Yasuyuki Seto[1*•], Susumu Aikou[1], Takamasa Takahashi[2]

1 Department of Gastrointestinal Surgery, Graduate School of Medicine, University of Tokyo, Tokyo, Japan, 2 Division of Surgical Oncology, Department of Surgery, Nagoya University Graduate School of Medicine, Nagoya, Japan

Abstract

Purposes: Robotic gastrectomy (RG), as an innovation of minimally invasive surgical method, is developing rapidly for gastric cancer. But there is still no consensus on its comparative merit in either subtotal or total gastrectomy compared with laparoscopic and open resections.

Methods: Literature searches of PubMed, Embase and Cochrane Library were performed. We combined the data of four studies for RG *versus* open gastrectomy (OG), and 11 studies for robotic RG *versus* laparoscopic gastrectomy (LG). Moreover, subgroup analyses of subtotal and total gastrectomies were performed in both RG *vs.* OG and RG *vs.* LG.

Results: Totally 12 studies involving 8493 patients met the criteria. RG, similar with LG, significantly reduced the intraoperative blood loss than OG. But the duration of surgery is longer in RG than in both OG and LG. The number of lymph nodes retrieved in RG was close to that in OG and LG (WMD = −0.78 and 95% CI, −2.15−0.59; WMD = 0.63 and 95% CI, −2.24−3.51). And RG did not increase morbidity and mortality in comparison with OG and LG (OR = 0.92 and 95% CI, 0.69−1.23; OR = 0.72 and 95% CI, 0.25−2.06) and (OR = 1.06 and 95% CI, 0.84−1.34; OR = 1.55 and 95% CI, 0.49−4.94). Moreover, subgroup analysis of subtotal and total gastrectomies in both RG *vs.* OG and RG *vs.* LG revealed that the scope of surgical dissection was not a positive factor to influence the comparative results of RG *vs.* OG or LG in surgery time, blood loss, hospital stay, lymph node harvest, morbidity, and mortality.

Conclusions: This meta-analysis highlights that robotic gastrectomy may be a technically feasible alternative for gastric cancer because of its affirmative role in both subtotal and total gastrectomies compared with laparoscopic and open resections.

Editor: Jose Luis Hernández, Clínica Universidad de Navarra, Spain

Funding: The authors have no funding or support to report.

Competing Interests: The authors have declared that no competing interests exist.

* Email: seto-tky@umin.ac.jp

• These authors contributed equally to this work.

Introduction

Gastric cancer is the fourth most common malignancy and second leading cause of cancer death in the world [1]. Surgical resection remains the only curative treatment option and open gastrectomy with lymphadenectomy took a leading position in the treatment of gastric cancer for a long time. Kitano *et al.* firstly reported the laparoscopy-assisted distal gastrectomy for gastric cancer in 1994 [2]. Since then, LG has been gradually spread worldwide [3–5].

Minimally invasive surgery represents a developing trend for its unique characteristics. However, conventional laparoscopic surgery itself, accompanied by some limitations such as instrument movement, amplification of hand tremor, two-dimensional imaging, and ergonomic discomfort for the surgeons. Robotic surgery, an emerging technology, was invented to overcome the disadvantages of conventional laparoscopic surgery in 1997 [6]. For robotic surgery, several robotic devices have been developed, but only the Da Vinci Surgical System was widely used [7]. To date, robotic surgery has been maturely adopted in many fields of advanced surgical procedures worldwide, especially for prostate cancer [8]. In the field of gastric cancer, robotic gastrectomy (RG) has been reported to be beneficial for patients, with less injury and also with compatible short-term oncologic outcomes to open gastrectomy (OG) or laparoscopic gastrectomy (LG) [9–20].

However, sample size, a single institution design and different appraise system of complications limited these studies to conclude objective result. To overcome these limitations, a meta-analysis of RG *vs*. OG or LG for gastric cancer was performed to determine the relative merits of RG for gastric cancer.

Methods

Publication Search

Three electronic databases (PubMed, EMBASE, and Cochrane Library) were searched (last search was updated on 01 June 2013, using the search terms: robotics OR robot PLUS gastrectomy PLUS cancer OR carcinoma OR adenocarcinoma OR malignancy PLUS open OR laparoscope). Article language was limited to English. All eligible studies were retrieved, and their bibliographies were checked for other relevant publications. Review articles and bibliographies of other relevant studies identified were hand-searched to identify additional eligible studies. Only published studies with full-text articles were included. When the same patient population was included in several publications, only the most recent or complete study was used in this meta-analysis.

Inclusion Criteria

The inclusion criteria were as follows: (a) controlled studies of RG *vs*. LG or RG *vs*. OG for gastric cancer; (b) report on at least one of the outcome measures mentioned below; and (c) sufficient published data to estimate an odds ratio (OR) with 95% confidence interval (CI).

Exclusion criteria

Abstracts, letters, editorials and expert opinions, reviews without original data, case reports and studies lacking control groups were excluded. The following studies or data were also excluded: (1) they reported on gastric surgery for benign lesions and gastrointestinal stromal tumor (GIST) and did not contain a distinct group of patients with gastric cancer, (2) the outcomes and parameters of patients were not clearly reported; (3) it was impossible to extract the appropriate data from the published results; and (4) there was overlap between authors or centers in the published literature.

Quality Assessment

The methodological quality of the studies included was assessed. Jadad Scale and MINORS were usually used to assess the quality of RCTs and non-RCTs, respectively [21,22].

Data Extraction

Information was carefully extracted from all eligible studies by two of the authors (Zong L and Seto Y), according to the inclusion criteria listed above. The following information were collected from each study: first author's surname, publication date, district, resection extent, reconstruction method, BMI index, TNM stage, study type, and total number of patients in RG group and OG group or LG group, respectively. We did not define a minimum number of patients for inclusion in our meta-analysis.

Statistical Analysis

Odd ratios with 95% CI were used for the comparisons of dichotomous variables (e.g., morbidity, and mortality) between surgical methods according to the method of Woolf. Heterogeneity assumption was confirmed by the X^2-based Q-test. A P-value greater than 0.10 for the Q-test indicated a lack of heterogeneity among the studies, therefore, the OR estimate for each study was calculated by the fixed-effects model (the Mantel-Haenszel method). Otherwise, the random-effects model (the DerSimonian and Laird method) was used. The significance of the pooled OR was determined by the Z-test and $P>0.05$ was considered statistically significant. Weighted mean difference (WMD) with 95% confidence intervals (95% CI) was calculated for continuous variables (e.g., operation time, and blood loss). WMD was pooled by using the inverse variance model. Sensitivity analyses were carried out to determine if modification of the inclusion criteria for this meta-analysis affected the final results. An estimate of potential publication bias was carried out using the funnel plot, in which the OR for each study was plotted against its log (OR). An asymmetric plot suggested possible publication bias. Funnel plot asymmetry was assessed using Egger's linear regression test, a linear regression approach to measure funnel plot asymmetry on the natural logarithm scale of the OR. The significance of the intercept was determined by the t-test, as suggested by Egger ($P<0.05$ was considered representative of statistically significant publication bias). All statistical tests were performed with Review Manager Version 5.0 (The Cochrane Collaboration, Oxford, England).

Results

Study Characteristics

Of the 14 published pieces of literature [9–20,23], 12 studies were eligible in this meta-analysis. Two studies published by the same team from the same institute within the same study interval were regarded as 1 trial, but both studies were included and shared the same study number because some separately published data was complementary [17,23]. Hence, a total of 12 studies including 8493 patients were used in the pooled analyses. Table 1 lists the studies identified and their main characteristics. Of the 12 groups, sample size ranged from 39 to 5839 (Figure 1).

Robotic gastrectomy versus open gastrectomy

The mean operation time of RG was 68.47 minutes longer than OG, but intraoperative blood loss and hospital stay were significantly reduced by RG (WMD = 68.47 and 95% CI, 63.40−73.54; WMD = −106.63 and 95% CI, −163.13−−50.13; WMD = −2.49 and 95% CI, −3.72−−1.27). The difference of lymph node harvest between RG and OG was not statistically significant (WMD = −0.78 and 95% CI, −2.15−0.59). Moreover, Meta-analyses on morbidity and mortality indicated that there was no significant differences between RG and OG (OR = 0.92 and 95% CI, 0.69−1.23; OR = 0.72 and 95% CI, 0.25−2.06). Also, specifically for anastomotic leakage, no difference was observed between two groups (OR = 1.72 and 95% CI, 0.97−3.07). Subgroup analysis of subtotal gastrectomy, and subtotal and total gastrectomies for above parameters all showed a similar trend with the combined results (Table 2) (Figure 2).

Robotic gastrectomy versus Laparoscopic gastrectomy

Operation time was significantly longer in RG compared with LG (WMD = 57.15 and 95% CI, 42.26−72.05). Both as the minimally invasive surgery, RG did not showed a priority in intraoperative blood loss (WMD = −28.59 and 95% CI, −56.57−−0.62). As for postoperative hospital stay, there was no significant difference (WMD = −0.16 and 95% CI, −0.87−0.55). In analysis of lymph node harvest, it did not attain statistical significance between RG and LG (WMD = 0.63 and 95% CI, −2.24−3.51). Further analysis revealed that RG did not carry additional postoperative morbidity, as well as anastomotic leakage, and mortality when compared with LG (OR = 1.06 and 95% CI, 0.84−1.34; OR = 1.10 and 95% CI, 0.66−1.82; OR = 1.55 and 95% CI, 0.49−4.94) (Table 3) (Figure 3). However, Meta-analysis

Table 1. Main characteristics of all studies included in the meta-analysis.

Study	Study Period	District	Size	Study Group	Resection extent	Reconstruction method	BMI	Stage	Study type
Caruso *et al*	2011	Italy	149	RG/OG	Total/Subtotal 12/17;37/83	NA	27±3/28±4	NA	Controlled
Eom *et al*	2012	Korea	92	RG/LG	Subtotal 30;62	NA	24.2/24.1	81/9/2	Controlled
Huang *et al*	2012	Taiwan	689	RG/LG/OG	Total/Subtotal 7/32;7/57; 179/407	B-I/B-II/Roux-en-Y	24.2±3.7/24. ±3.3/23±3.6	282/122/285	Controlled
Hyun *et al*	2012	Korea	121	RG/LG	Total/Subtotal 9/29; 18/65	B-I/B-II/Roux-en-Y	23.8±2.6/23.8±2.9	97/14/10	Controlled
Kang *et al*	2012	Korea	382	RG/LG	Total/Subtotal 16/84;37/245	B-I/B-II/Roux-en-Y	23.7±3.7/23.6±3.5	NA	Controlled
Kim *et al*	2010	Korea	39	RG/LG/OG	Subtotal 12;11;16	NA	21.3±3.4/25.3±2.5/25.2±1.9	27/9/3	Controlled
Kim *et al*	2012	Korea	5839	RG/LG/OG	Total/Subtotal 109/158/1232; 327/703/3309	B-I/B-II/Roux-en-Y	23.6±3.1/23.5±2.8/23.3±8.0	NA	Controlled
Park *et al*	2012	Korea	150	RG/LG	Subtotal 30;120	NA	NA	NA	Controlled
Pugliese *et al*	2010	Italy	64	RG/LG	Subtotal 16;48	NA	NA	NA	Controlled
Song *et al*	2009	Korea	40	RG/LG	Subtotal 20;20	NA	23.4±2.1/22.4±2.1	39/1/0	Controlled
Woo *et al*	2011	Korea	827	RG/LG	Total/Subtotal 62/172; 108/481	B-I/B-II/Roux-en-Y	23.5±3/23.5±3	NA	Controlled
Yoon *et al*	2012	Korea	101	RG/LG	Total 36;65	NA	23.2±2.5/23.6±3.4	84/14/3	Controlled

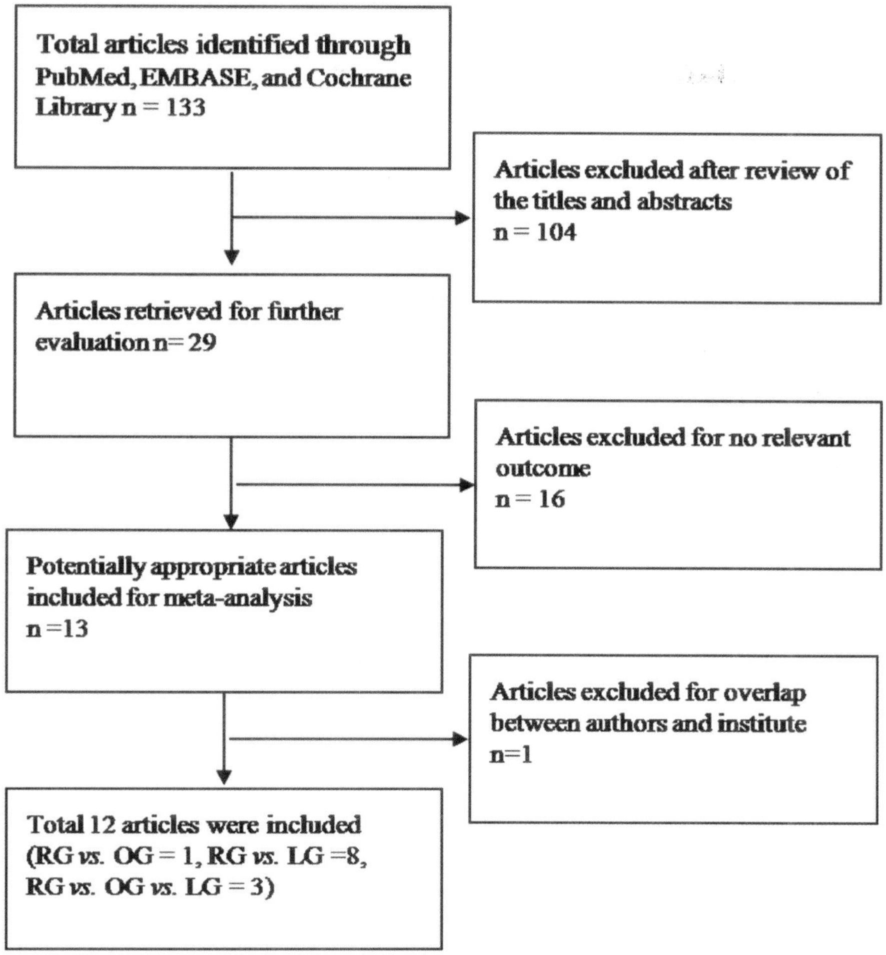

Figure 1. Flow chart of literature selection.

on another surgical outcome evaluation system with Clavien-Dindo grades also did not show significant differences in any subdivided grade. Subgroup analysis of subtotal gastrectomy, total gastrectomy, and subtotal and total gastrectomies was also performed for above parameters and no single subgroup showed a heterogeneous result with the combined one (Table 3) (Figure 4).

Publication Bias

Begg's funnel plot was performed to assess publication bias. The heterogeneity tests for comparing the 12 combined studies showed heterogeneity in some analyses such as operation time, blood loss and so on; however, when significant heterogeneity occurred among the studies, random-effects model was used.

Discussion

Radical gastrectomy with lymphadenectomy has been widely applied in open surgery as standard surgical treatment for gastric cancer. Although minimally invasive surgery improves quality of life, it should be ensured that this technique does not increase morbidity and mortality [24]. With the developing of technique, minimally invasive surgery has gained a revolutionized application in general surgery from last century. But for gastric cancer, minimally invasive surgery experienced a controversy focusing on morbidity and mortality for a long time. Laparoscopic gastrectomy with limited lymphadenectomy is rapidly increasing and quickly admitted in early gastric cancer because of the mass and individual screening in Japan [25]. But the data was still incomplete to support the widespread use of laparoscopic gastrectomy for advanced gastric cancer in last decade [26].

Open gastrectomy with D2 lymphadenectomy is a technically demanding operation for advanced gastric cancer compared with D1, although there is the potential for appreciable morbidity and mortality [27,28]. Therefore, the assessment in favor of D2 lymphadenectomy makes it an integral part of laparoscopic surgery for advanced gastric cancer. Recently strong evidence from a multi-center retrospective study of laparoscopic surgery over open surgery confirmed the therapeutic role of Laparoscopic gastrectomy in advanced gastric cancer [29].

Robotic surgery, as an innovation of laparoscopic surgery, might be a simpler way to expand the indications of minimally invasive surgery for gastric cancer. However, controlled prospective studies are needed to evaluate the role of robotics in the management of gastric cancer. Some studies have demonstrated that robotic total and subtotal gastrectomies with D2-lymphadenectomy are technically feasible and safe, with acceptable surgical and oncological short-term results [15,30–32]. It is particularly notable that only a few reports have examined the technical feasibility of robotic surgery for gastric cancer till 2011 [9,14,17–19], and the number of patients included in these studies was too

Table 2. Meta-analyses results for robotic gastrectomy vs. open gastrectomy.

Parameters	Studies	Sample Size		Heterogeneity	OR or WMD	Effect 95% CI	P
Operation time	3	481	4674	P = 0.74, I^2 = 0%	68.47	63.40–73.54	P<0.00001
Subgroup of SG	1	16	12	NA	77.20	54.75–99.65	P<0.00001
Subgroup of SG and TG	2	465	4662	P = 1.00, I^2 = 0%	68.00	62.79–73.21	P<0.00001
Intraoperative blood loss	3	481	4674	P = 0.003, I^2 = 83%	−106.63	−163.13– −50.13	P = 0.0002
Subgroup of SG	1	16	12	NA	−48.50	−91.07– −5.93	P = 0.03
Subgroup of SG and TG	2	465	4662	P = 0.04, I^2 = 77%	−139.05	−217.08– −61.02	P = 0.0005
Hospital stay	3	481	4674	P = 0.06, I^2 = 64%	−2.49	−3.72– −1.27	P<0.0001
Subgroup of SG	1	16	12	NA	−1.60	−2.41– −0.79	P<0.0001
Subgroup of SG and TG	2	465	4662	P = 0.34, I^2 = 0%	−3.07	−4.14– −2.01	P<0.00001
Lymph node harvest	4	520	5260	P = 0.55, I^2 = 0%	−0.78	−2.15–0.59	P = 0.27
Subgroup of SG	1	16	12	NA	−2.20	−10.15–5.75	P = 0.59
Subgroup of SG and TG	3	504	5248	P = 0.37, I^2 = 0%	−0.73	−2.13–0.66	P = 0.30
Anastomotic leakage	4	520	5260	P = 0.53, I^2 = 0%	1.72	0.97–3.07	P = 0.06
Subgroup of SG	1	16	12	NA	NE	NE	NA
Subgroup of SG and TG	3	504	5248	P = 0.53, I^2 = 0%	1.72	0.97–3.07	P = 0.06
Morbidity	4	520	5260	P = 0.65, I^2 = 0%	0.92	0.69–1.23	P = 0.59
Subgroup of SG	1	16	12	NA	0.13	0.01–2.92	P = 0.20
Subgroup of SG and TG	3	504	5248	P = 0.97, I^2 = 0%	0.95	0.71–1.27	P = 0.72
Mortality	4	520	5260	P = 0.52, I^2 = 0%	0.72	0.25–2.06	P = 0.54
Subgroup of SG	1	16	12	NA	0.13	0.01–2.92	P = 0.20
Subgroup of SG and TG	3	504	5248	P = 0.72, I^2 = 0%	0.98	0.32–2.96	P = 0.97

SG, subtotal gastrectomy; TG, total gastrectomy; NA, not applicable; NE, not estimable; OR, odds ratio; WED, weighted mean difference; CI, confidence interval.

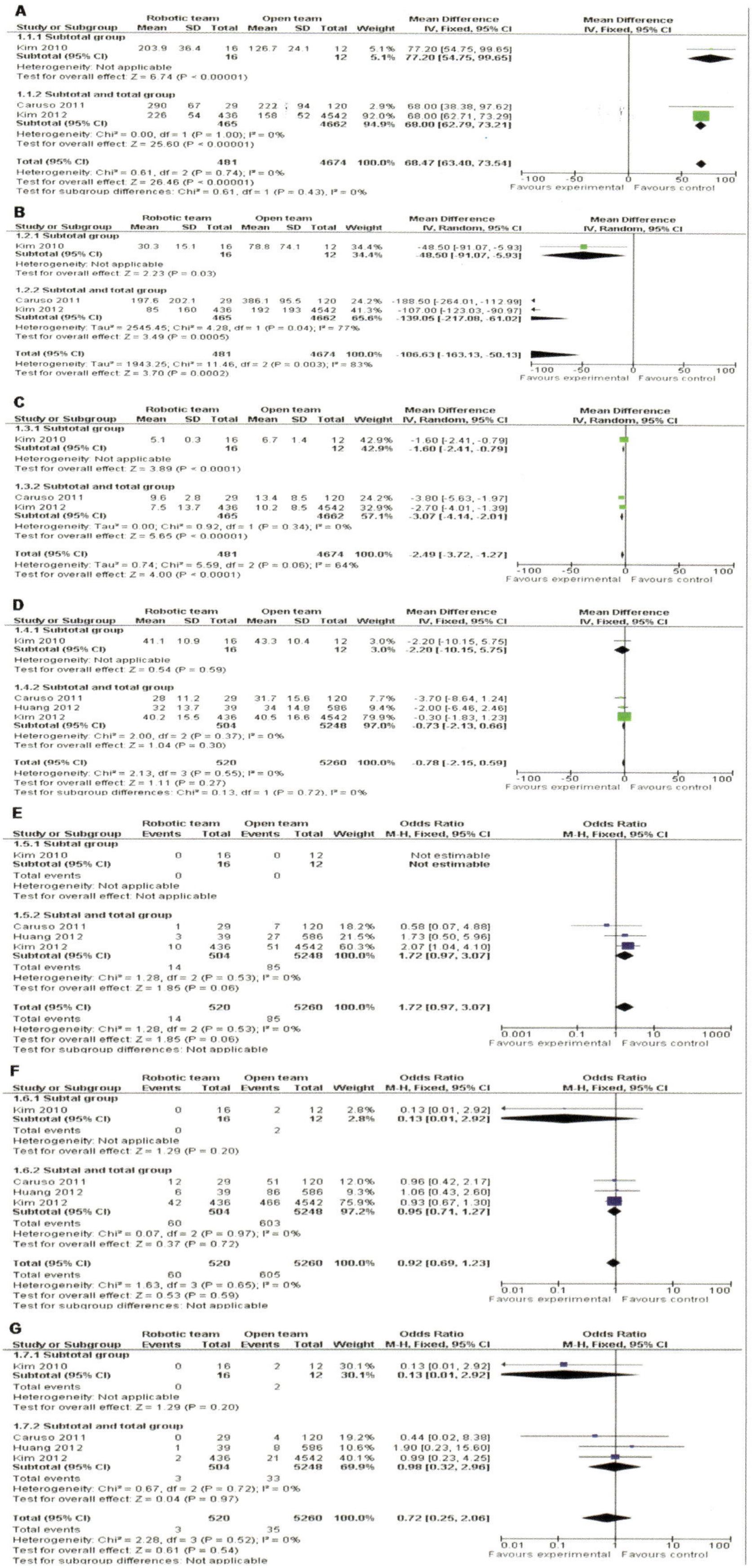

Figure 2. RG *vs.* OG: a) Operation time; b) Intraoperative blood loss; c) Hospital stay; d) Lymph node harvest; e) Anastomotic leakage; f) Morbidity; g) Mortality.

Table 3. Meta-analyses results for robotic gastrectomy vs. laparoscopic gastrectomy.

Parameters	Studies	Sample Size		Heterogeneity	OR or WMD	Effect 95% CI	P
Operation time	8	898	1961	$P<0.00001$, $I^2=88\%$	57.15	42.26−72.05	$P<0.00001$
Subgroup of SG	3	52	79	$P=0.03$, $I^2=72\%$	86.73	56.61−116.84	$P<0.00001$
Subgroup of TG	1	36	65	NA	95.60	55.26−135.94	$P<0.00001$
Subgroup of SG and TG	4	810	1817	$P=0.0002$, $I^2=85\%$	38.09	25.44−50.74	$P<0.00001$
Intraoperative blood loss	7	862	1896	$P<0.00001$, $I^2=92\%$	−28.59	−56.57−−0.62	$P=0.05$
Subgroup of SG	3	52	79	$P=0.0007$, $I^2=86\%$	−11.00	−61.25−39.26	$P=0.67$
Subgroup of SG and TG	4	810	1817	$P<0.00001$, $I^2=95\%$	−39.54	−79.71−0.63	$P=0.05$
Hospital stay	7	882	1950	$P=0.59$, $I^2=0\%$	−0.16	−0.87−0.55	$P=0.65$
Subgroup of SG	2	36	68	$P=0.65$, $I^2=0\%$	−0.29	−1.36−0.79	$P=0.60$
Subgroup of TG	1	36	65	NA	−1.50	−4.34−1.34	$P=0.30$
Subgroup of SG and TG	4	810	1817	$P=0.35$, $I^2=8\%$	−0.11	−0.89−1.11	$P=0.83$
Lymph node harvest	8	837	1743	$P<0.0001$, $I^2=78\%$	0.63	−2.24−3.51	$P=0.67$
Subgroup of SG	3	52	79	$P=0.07$, $I^2=62\%$	−3.77	−9.63−2.09	$P=0.21$
Subgroup of TG	1	36	65	NA	3.40	−1.87−8.67	$P=0.21$
Subgroup of SG and TG	4	749	1599	$P=0.39$, $I^2=0\%$	2.33	1.05−3.62	$P=0.0004$
Anastomotic leakage	11	997	2207	$P=0.96$, $I^2=0\%$	1.10	0.66−1.82	$P=0.71$
Subgroup of SG	5	112	261	NA	2.03	0.18−23.22	$P=0.57$
Subgroup of TG	1	36	65	NA	0.24	0.01−4.87	$P=0.36$
Subgroup of SG and TG	5	849	1881	$P=0.99$, $I^2=0\%$	1.16	0.68−1.96	$P=0.59$
Morbidity	11	997	2207	$P=0.65$, $I^2=0\%$	1.06	0.84−1.34	$P=0.60$
Subgroup of SG	5	112	261	$P=0.37$, $I^2=7\%$	1.29	0.61−2.72	$P=0.51$
Subgroup of TG	1	36	65	NA	1.10	0.36−3.32	$P=0.87$
Subgroup of SG and TG	5	849	1881	$P=0.57$, $I^2=0\%$	1.04	0.81−1.34	$P=0.76$
Mortality	11	997	2207	$P=0.96$, $I^2=0\%$	1.55	0.49−4.94	$P=0.45$
Subgroup of SG	5	112	261	NA	3.13	0.18−53.21	$P=0.43$
Subgroup of TG	1	36	65	NA	NE	NE	NA
Subgroup of SG and TG	5	849	1881	$P=0.99$, $I^2=0\%$	1.36	0.38−4.88	$P=0.63$
Clavien-Dindo grade							
I+II	9	965	2148	$P=0.22$, $I^2=26\%$	1.15	0.86−1.53	$P=0.35$
Subgroup of SG	3	80	202	$P=0.50$, $I^2=0\%$	1.77	0.69−4.54	$P=0.23$
Subgroup of TG	1	36	65	NA	2.46	0.62−9.82	$P=0.20$
Subgroup of SG and TG	5	849	1881	$P=0.13$, $I^2=43\%$	1.06	0.77−1.44	$P=0.73$
III	9	965	2148	$P=0.82$, $I^2=0\%$	1.07	0.72−1.60	$P=0.73$
Subgroup of SG	3	80	202	$P=0.99$, $I^2=0\%$	2.07	0.33−13.01	$P=0.44$
Subgroup of TG	1	36	65	NA	0.28	0.03−2.43	$P=0.25$

Table 3. Cont.

Parameters	Studies	Sample Size		Heterogeneity	OR or WMD	Effect 95% CI	P
Subgroup of SG and TG	5	849	1881	P = 0.81, I^2 = 0%	1.12	0.74–1.70	P = 0.60
IV	9	965	2148	P = 0.85, I^2 = 0%	0.70	0.34–1.43	P = 0.32
Subgroup of SG	3	80	202	NA	NE	NE	NA
Subgroup of TG	1	36	65	NA	NE	NE	NA
Subgroup of SG and TG	5	849	1881	P = 0.85, I^2 = 0%	0.70	0.34–1.43	P = 0.32
V	9	965	2148	P = 0.99, I^2 = 0%	1.36	0.38–4.88	P = 0.63
Subgroup of SG	3	80	202	NA	NE	NE	NA
Subgroup of TG	1	36	65	NA	NE	NE	NA
Subgroup of SG and TG	5	849	1881	P = 0.99, I^2 = 0%	1.36	0.38–4.88	P = 0.63

SG, subtotal gastrectomy; TG, total gastrectomy; NA, not applicable; NE, not estimable; OR, odds ratio; WED, weighted mean difference; CI, confidence interval.

small to generalize its application for gastric cancer [14,17,18]. Recently some large sized studies have been conducted to evaluate the efficacy and safety of robotic gastrectomy for gastric cancer [11,13,15,19]. But single comparison and conflict results limited them to conclude persuasible conclusions. However, those examined in the present study allowed meta-analyses to be performed, providing a better view of the safety and efficacy of RG in gastric cancer. In reality, it is difficult to conduct a high-quality RCT to evaluate a new surgical intervention because of some obstacles such as learning curve effects, ethical and culture resistance, and urgent or unexpected conditions during operation in surgical treatment. For these reasons, to include non-RCTs is an appropriate strategy to extend the source of evidence [33].

In the first part of RG versus OG, our analyses highlighted the advantage of RG in minimal injury because less intraoperative blood loss and shorter postoperative hospital stay were observed. But its complication in technique correspondently brought RG significantly longer operation time than OG. Further analyses of lymph node harvest, anastomotic leakage, morbidity, and mortality between RG and OG did not show significant differences. Although no controlled study for single total gastrectomy was included in subgroup analysis, we deduced that RG was feasible and safe in either subtotal gastrectomy or total gastrectomy compared with OG by similar evidences in subtotal and total mixed group and subtotal single group.

Continually, in comparison of RG and LG, we found it was similar in surgical injury for these two methods because of no significant difference in intraoperative blood loss. The disadvantage of longer surgical duration was also observed in RG, although significant heterogeneity existed. The heterogeneity might be caused by surgeons' experience. However, it is important to stress that surgeons had got considerable experience of LG before RG, which helped them adapt quickly to the robotic procedure. Therefore, the effect of learning curve was limited in RG. Also, higher BMI might be another important factor to increase operation time and several reports described the association between gender and BMI as increased operation time [34,35]. But Park *et al* thought that this factor could be overcome by surgeon's expertise [36]. To explore the influence of BMI to our study, we made comparisons of BMI among three groups and no significant difference was observed (data not shown). Importantly, for analyses of lymph node harvest, anastomotic leakage, morbidity, and mortality, similar results were achieved between RG and LG in either subtotal gastrectomy or total gastrectomy. We also make a pooled analyses using Clavien-Dindo (C–D) classification. Still, no significant difference was observed. What's far more important to limit the application of RG is the higher cost compared with LG. Due to the limited published study, meta-analysis for cost evaluation was not performed. But nevertheless, recent study by Park *et al* showed the total cost for RG was significantly higher than LG with a difference of €3189 [16].

In summary, we found that Robotic subtotal and total gastrectomies combined with lymphadenectomy are technically feasible and safe for gastric cancer, and can produce satisfying short-term postoperative outcomes. However, a weakness of present study was lack of randomized controlled studies included and significant heterogeneity was observed in operative time, intraoperative blood loss, length of hospital stay and lymph node harvest. In addition, total and subtotal gastrectomy was pooled together in most of included studies, which limited us to make a more precise conclusion. Also, economic value and long-term survival outcome are the mandatory appraisal index. Importantly, high-quality randomized controlled studies should be conducted to evaluate the role of robotic surgery for gastric cancer in future.

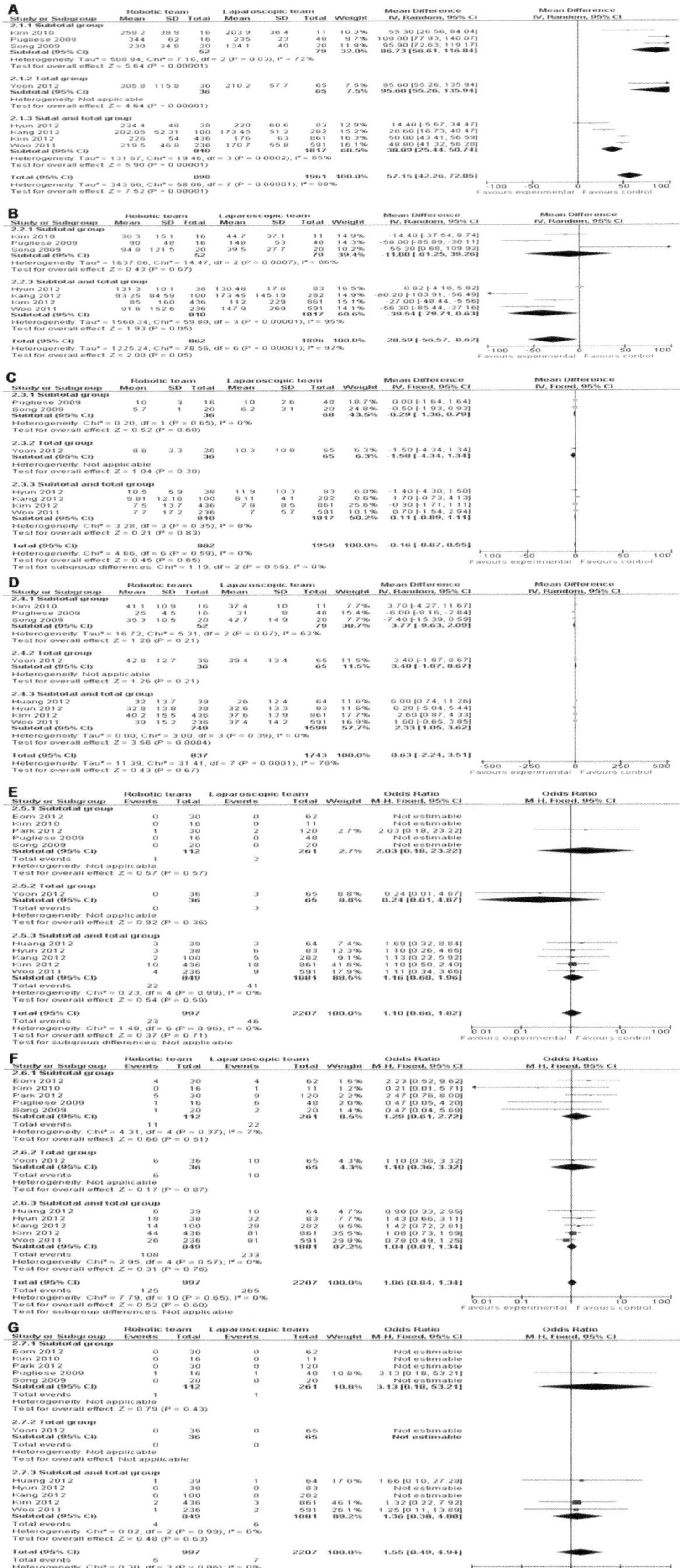

Figure 3. RG *vs.* LG: a) Operation time; b) Intraoperative blood loss; c) Hospital stay; d) Lymph node harvest; e) Anastomotic leakage; f) Morbidity; g) Mortality.

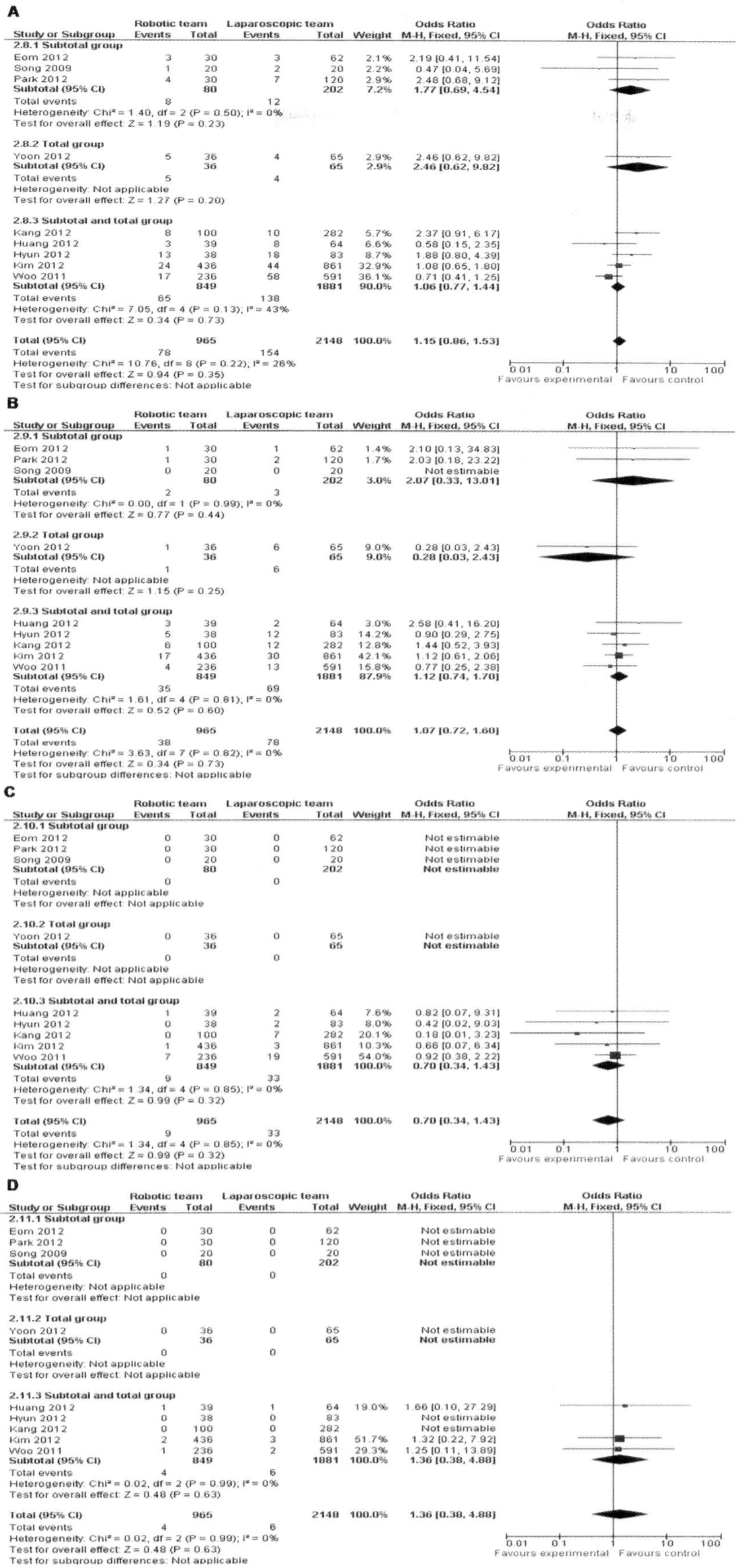

Figure 4. RG *vs.* LG: a) Clavien-Dindo grade I and II; b) Clavien-Dindo grade III; c) Clavien-Dindo grade IV; d) Clavien-Dindo grade V.

Author Contributions

Conceived and designed the experiments: LZ. Performed the experiments: LZ. Analyzed the data: LZ SA. Contributed reagents/materials/analysis tools: LZ TT. Contributed to the writing of the manuscript: LZ YS. Revised the manuscript: LZ YS.

References

1. Hohenberger P, Gretschel S (2003) Gastric cancer. Lancet 362: 305–315.
2. Kitano S, Iso Y, Moriyama M, Sugimachi K (1994) Laparoscopy-assisted Billroth I gastrectomy. Surg Laparosc Endosc 4: 146–148.
3. (1993) National Institutes of Health Consensus Development Conference Statement on Gallstones and Laparoscopic Cholecystectomy. Am J Surg 165: 390–398.
4. Adachi Y, Suematsu T, Shiraishi N, Katsuta T, Morimoto A, et al. (1999) Quality of life after laparoscopy-assisted Billroth I gastrectomy. Ann Surg 229: 49–54.
5. Kim MC, Kim KH, Kim HH, Jung GJ (2005) Comparison of laparoscopy-assisted by conventional open distal gastrectomy and extraperigastric lymph node dissection in early gastric cancer. J Surg Oncol 91: 90–94.
6. Cadière GB, Himpens J, Germay O, Izizaw R, Degueldre M, et al. (2001) Feasibility of robotic laparoscopic surgery: 146 cases. World J Surg 25: 1467–1477.
7. Tooher R, Pham C (2004) The da Vinci Surgical Robotics System: Technology Overview ASERNIP-S Report No. 45. Adelaide, South Australia: ASERNIP-S ISBN: 0909844658.
8. Atug F, Castle EP, Woods M, Davis R, Thomas R (2006) Robotics in urologic surgery: an evolving new technology. Int J Urol 13: 857–863
9. Caruso S, Patriti A, Marrelli D, Ceccarelli G, Ceribelli C, et al. (2011) Open vs robot-assisted laparoscopic gastric resection with D2 lymph node dissection for adenocarcinoma: a case-control study. Int J Med Robot 7: 452–458.
10. Eom BW, Yoon HM, Ryu KW, Lee JH, Cho SJ, et al. (2012) Comparison of surgical performance and short-term clinical outcomes between laparoscopic and robotic surgery in distal gastric cancer. Eur J Surg Oncol 38: 57–63.
11. Huang KH, Lan YT, Fang WL, Chen JH, Lo SS, et al. (2012) Initial Experience of Robotic Gastrectomy and Comparison with Open and Laparoscopic Gastrectomy for Gastric Cancer. J Gastrointest Surg 16: 1303–1310.
12. Hyun MH, Lee CH, Kwon YJ, Cho SI, Jang YJ, et al. (2013) Robot versus laparoscopic gastrectomy for cancer by an experienced surgeon: comparisons of surgery, complications, and surgical stress. Ann Surg Oncol 20: 1258–1265.
13. Kang BH, Xuan Y, Hur H, Ahn CW, Cho YK, et al. (2012) Comparison of Surgical Outcomes between Robotic and Laparoscopic Gastrectomy for Gastric Cancer: The Learning Curve of Robotic Surgery. J Gastric Cancer 12: 156–163.
14. Kim MC, Heo GU, Jung GJ (2010) Robotic gastrectomy for gastric cancer: surgical techniques and clinical merits. Surg Endosc 24: 610–615.
15. Kim KM, An JY, Kim HI, Cheong JH, Hyung WJ, et al. (2012) Major early complications following open, laparoscopic and robotic gastrectomy. Br J Surg 99: 1681–1687.
16. Park JY, Jo MJ, Nam BH, Kim Y, Eom BW, et al. (2012) Surgical stress after robot-assisted distal gastrectomy and its economic implications. Br J Surg 99: 1554–61.
17. Pugliese R, Maggioni D, Sansonna F, Costanzi A, Ferrari GC, et al. (2010) Subtotal gastrectomy with D2 dissection by minimally invasive surgery for distal adenocarcinoma of the stomach: results and 5-year survival. Surg Endosc 24: 2594–2602.
18. Song J, Kang WH, Oh SJ, Hyung WJ, Choi SH, et al. (2009) Role of robotic gastrectomy using da Vinci system compared with laparoscopic gastrectomy: initial experience of 20 consecutive cases. Surg Endosc 23: 1204–1211.
19. Woo Y, Hyung WJ, Pak KH, Inaba K, Obama K, et al. (2011) Robotic gastrectomy as an oncologically sound alternative to laparoscopic resections for the treatment of early-stage gastric cancers. Arch Surg 146: 1086–1092.
20. Yoon HM, Kim YW, Lee JH, Ryu KW, Eom BW, et al. (2012) Robot-assisted total gastrectomy is comparable with laparoscopically assisted total gastrectomy for early gastric cancer. Surg Endosc 26: 1377–81.
21. Jadad AR, Moore RA, Carroll D, Jenkinson C, Reynolds DJ, et al. (1996) Assessing the quality of reports of randomized clinical trials: is blinding necessary? Control Clin Trials.; 17: 1–12.
22. Slim K, Nini E, Forestier D, Kwiatkowski F, Panis Y, et al. (2003) Methodological index for non-randomized studies (MINORS): development and validation of a new instrument. ANZ J Surg 73: 712–716.
23. Pugliese R, Maggioni D, Sansonna F, Ferrari GC, Forgione A, et al. (2009) Outcomes and survival after laparoscopic gastrectomy for adenocarcinoma. Analysis on 65 patients operated on by conventional or robot-assisted minimal access procedures. Eur J Surg Oncol 35: 281–288.
24. Zeng YK, Yang ZL, Peng JS, Lin HS, Cai L (2012) Laparoscopy-assisted versus open distal gastrectomy for early gastric cancer: evidence from randomized and nonrandomized clinical Trials. Ann Surg 256: 39–52.
25. Shimizu S, Uchiyama A, Mizumoto K, Morisaki T, Nakamura K, et al. (2000) Laparoscopically assisted distal gastrectomy for early gastric cancer: is it superior to open surgery? Surg Endosc 14: 27–31.
26. Katsios GC, Baltogiannis G, Roukos DH (2010) Laparoscopic surgery for gastric cancer: comparative-effectiveness research and future trends. Expert Rev Anticancer Ther 10: 473–476.
27. Cuschieri A, Fayers P, Fielding J, Craven J, Bancewicz J, et al. (1996) Postoperative morbidity and mortality after D1 and D2 resections for gastric cancer: preliminary results of the MRC randomised controlled trial. The Surgical Cooperative Group. Lancet 347: 995–9.
28. Songun I, Putter H, Kranenbarg EM, Sasako M, van de Velde CJ (2010) Surgical treatment of gastric cancer: 15-year follow-up results of the randomised nationwide Dutch D1D2 trial. Lancet Oncol 11: 439–449
29. Park do J, Han SU, Hyung WJ, Kim MC, Kim W, et al. (2012) Long-term outcomes after laparoscopy-assisted gastrectomy for advanced gastric cancer: a large-scale multicenter retrospective study. Surg Endosc 26: 1548–53.
30. Patriti A, Ceccarelli G, Bellochi R, Bartoli A, Spaziani A, et al. (2008) Robot-assisted laparoscopic total and partial gastric resection with D2 lymph node dissection for adenocarcinoma. Surg Endosc 22: 2753–60.
31. D'Annibale A, Pende V, Pernazza G, Monsellato I, Mazzocchi P, et al. (2011) Full robotic gastrectomy with extended (D2) lymphadenectomy for gastric cancer: surgical technique and preliminary results. J Surg Res 166: e113–20.
32. Uyama I, Kanaya S, Ishida Y, Inaba K, Suda K, et al. (2012) Novel integrated robotic approach for suprapancreatic D2 nodal dissection for treating gastric cancer: technique and initial experience. World J Surg 36: 331–337.
33. McCulloch P, Taylor I, Sasako M, Lovett B, Griffin D (2002) Randomised trials in surgery: problems and possible solutions. BMJ 324: 1448–1451.
34. Kim KH, Kim MC, Jung GJ, Kim HH (2006) The impact of obesity on LADG for early gastric cancer. Gastric Cancer 9: 303–307
35. Lee HJ, Kim HH, Kim MC, Ryu SY, Kim W, et al. (2009) The impact of a high body mass index on laparoscopy assisted gastrectomy for gastric cancer. Surg Endosc 23: 2473–2479.
36. Park SS, Kim MC, Park MS, Hyung WJ (2012) Rapid adaption of robotic gastrectomy for gastric cancer by experienced laparoscopic surgeons. Surg Endosc 26: 60–67.

15

Treatment Results in the Different Surgery of Intradural Extramedullary Tumor of 122 Cases

Shaohui Zong[1], Gaofeng Zeng[2], Li Du[1], Ye Fang[1], Taihang Gao[1], Jingmin Zhao[3]*

1 Department of Spine Osteopathia, the First Affiliated Hospital of Guangxi Medical University, Nanning, Guangxi, P.R. China, **2** College of Public Hygiene of Guangxi Medical University, Nanning, Guangxi, P.R. China, **3** Department of Orthopaedics Trauma and Hand Surgery, the First Affiliated Hospital of Guangxi Medical University, Nanning, Guangxi, P.R. China

Abstract

Study Design: A retrospective study of intradural extramedullary tumor.

Objective: To compare the treatment results in the different surgeries of spinal intradural extramedullary tumor.

Methods: The study retrospectively reviewed 122 patients. The minimally invasive surgery (MIS) group was divided into Group A (hemilaminectomy + tumor microscopic excision) and Group B (laminectomy + tumor microscopic excision + pedicle screw fixation). Meanwhile, the non-MIS group was divided into Group C (hemilaminectomy + tumor excision), Group D (laminectomy + tumor excision), and Group E (laminectomy + tumor excision + pedicle screw fixation). In order to study postoperative spinal stability, we simultaneously divided all of the subjects into three categories, namely Group HE: hemilaminectomy + tumor excision; Group LE: laminectomy + tumor excision; and Group LEPSF: laminectomy + tumor excision + pedicle screw fixation.

Results: The MIS group exhibited fewer postoperative complications ($p<0.05$), better short-term clinical efficacy ($p<0.05$) and less non-surgical cost ($p<0.05$) than in non-MIS group. The rate of postoperative spinal instability in hemilaminectomy was lower than in laminectomy in a single spinal segment ($p<0.05$). The rate of postoperative spinal instability in laminectomy + pedicle screw fixation was lower than in hemilaminectomy and laminectomy in two or more spinal segments ($p<0.05$).

Conclusion: In the case of appropriate surgical indications, minimally invasive surgery for intradural extramedullary tumor is a useful method that can successfully produce good clinical results and reduce non-surgical cost. In addition, pedicle screw fixation helps avoid spinal postoperative instability.

Editor: Zachary A. Smith, Northwestern University, United States of America

Funding: The authors acknowledge support from the Guangxi Science and Technology Plan Fund, Gui Ke Gong 1298003-5-1. The funders had no role in study design, data collection and analysis, decision to publish, or preparation of the manuscript.

Competing Interests: The authors have declared that no competing interests exist.

* Email: zhaojingmin3008@sina.com

Introduction

Intradural extramedullary tumors are very common in the osteopathic departments, accounting for approximately two-thirds of all primary intraspinal neoplasms [1]. As the tumors grow larger, the main outcome may be the compression of the spinal cord, which can cause back pain and worsening sensory and motor loss. The analyses of data from 25 cases revealed that the remaining spinal canal area was decreased to 20–30% of the normal spinal canal [2]. Therefore, the primary goal of the therapy for spinal intradural tumors is to decompress the spinal cord and remove it thoroughly without recurrence.

Nowadays, surgery is the effective approach for benign intradural extramedullary tumors [3]. For older people, minimally invasive surgery for benign intradural extramedullary tumor removal still represents the best therapeutic option [4,5]. Although a conventional approach without a microscope can have a good curative effect, several drawbacks still exist, including greater intraoperative blood loss and a higher risk of injury to the spinal cord or nerve roots. With the development of technology, manipulation with a microscope could avoid these problems as far as possible. When removing spinal intradural extramedullary tumors by MIS or non-MIS, the damage to the anatomical structure of the posterior column of the spine will affects postoperative spinal stability.

This study reviewed a series of 53 consecutive patients with spinal intradural extramedullary tumors who underwent MIS and 69 consecutive patients with spinal intradural extramedullary tumors who underwent non-MIS. The purpose of this retrospective study is to compare the treatment results between MIS and non-MIS in these cases of spinal intradural extramedullary tumor and to analyze the postoperative spinal stability and health economics arising from the different surgical techniques.

Table 1. Summary of baseline characteristics of intradural extramedullary tumor patients.

Groups	N	Age (year)	Male/Female	Course of disease (mouth)
MIS group	53	41.15±14.73	29/24	32.45±6.81
Non-MIS group	69	43.25±16.42	37/32	30.67±5.28
Group A	19	42.84±11.25	11/8	28.25±8.14
Group B	34	41.42±13.47	16/18	29.53±8.75
Group C	24	40.26±15.08	14/10	33.67±7.99
Group D	18	43.71±12.23	10/8	30.73±7.43
Group E	27	43.54±14.67	15/12	31.84±6.58
Group HE	43	40.87±12.54	21/22	29.72±4.73
Group LE	18	41.62±13.75	10/8	34.91±7.54
Group LESPF	61	43.92±15.68	35/26	33.14±9.36

There was no significant difference between the MIS group and Non-MIS group ($p>0.05$). This was the same among the five groups (Group A, Group B, Group C, Group D, Group E; $p>0.05$) and among the three groups (Group HE, Group LE, Group LESPF; $p>0.05$). Data are expressed as the mean ± standard deviation.

Materials and Methods

Ethical statement

All study procedures were reviewed and approved by the Institutional Ethics Review Board at the First Affiliated Hospital of Guangxi Medical University and conducted according to the principles expressed in the Declaration of Helsinki. Informed consent was exempted by the board due to the retrospective nature of this research.

Patient characteristics

122 patients who underwent surgical resection of intradural extramedullary tumors were retrospectively analyzed from January 2010 to June 2012. Data were obtained from the departments of surgery of six hospitals in the south of China. The ages of patients ranged from 15 to 82 years, with a mean age of 42 years. Symptom duration before surgery ranged from 2 months to 9 years, with a mean symptom duration of 31.2 months. The following inclusion criteria were used: 1) all of the subjects had intradural extramedullary tumor; 2) all of the subjects exhibited integrity of the spine and spinal stability before surgery; 3) clinical diagnosis was determined by physical examination, magnetic resonance imaging (MRI), and pathology; and 4) clinical and radiological follow-up was carried out for 12–60 months (average 28 months). Patients who underwent surgery again because of the recurrence of intraspinal tumor were excluded. The spinal levels of intradural extramedullary tumor were cervical vertebrae in 36 cases, cervicothoracic vertebrae in 2 cases, thoracic vertebrae in 39 cases, thoracolumbar vertebrae in 3 cases, and lumbosacral vertebrae in 42 cases.

Surgical methods

All the patients were placed in the prone position under general anesthesia and a posterior median approach was chosen. The choice of surgical procedure depended on the location and size of the tumor. Hemilaminectomy was adopted when the tumor was small or located laterally or dorsolaterally to the spinal cord. Laminectomy was adopted when the tumor was large or located ventrally to the spinal cord. Pedicle screw fixation was required after multilevel laminectomy. Based on the spinal level of tumor, we inserted the pedicle screws in above 1-below 1. The subjects were divided into two groups according to the type of differential surgery, namely the MIS group (53 cases) and the non-MIS group (69 cases). The MIS group was subdivided into two groups, as follows:

- Group A: hemilaminectomy + tumor microscopic excision, 19 cases; and
- Group B: laminectomy + tumor microscopic excision + pedicle screw fixation, 34 cases.

Table 2. Summary of the results for operating time, intraoperative blood loss, resection rate, duration of hospital stay, and complications.

Groups	N	Operating time (min)	Intraoperative blood loss (ml)	Resection rate (%)	Duration of hospital stay (d)	Complications
MIS group	53	270.00±147.99★	307.14±185.13★	77.36▲	21.88±10.15★	2★
Non-MIS group	69	173.26±81.36	540.08±282.15	72.46	26.42±11.60	12

This table shows the results for operating time, intraoperative blood loss, resection rate, duration of hospital stay, and complications in the MIS and Non-MIS group. "Resection rate" means the percentage of the cases of total resection of tumor. Data are expressed as the mean ± standard deviation.

★$p<0.05$ vs. MIS group;

▲$p>0.05$ vs. Non-MIS group.

Table 3. Analysis of short-term and long-term clinical efficacy.

Groups	N	Short-term clinical efficacy			Long-term clinical efficacy		
		Effectivity	Nullity	Rate of effectivity (%)	Effectivity	Nullity	Rate of effectivity (%)
MIS group	53	52	1	98.11*	51	2	96.22▲
Non-MIS group	69	59	10	85.50	64	5	92.75

This table shows the results for short-term and long-term clinical efficacy in the MIS and Non-MIS groups.
*$p<0.05$ vs. Non-MIS group;
▲$p>0.05$ vs. Non-MIS group.

Meanwhile, the non-MIS group was subdivided into the following three groups:

- Group C: hemilaminectomy + tumor excision, 24 cases;
- Group D: laminectomy + tumor excision, 18 cases;
- Group E: laminectomy + tumor excision + pedicle screw fixation, 27 cases.

In order to study postoperative spinal stability, 122 patients were simultaneously divided into three categories, as follows:

- Group HE: hemilaminectomy + tumor excision, 43 cases;
- Group LE: laminectomy + tumor excision, 18 cases; and
- Group LEPSF: laminectomy + tumor excision + pedicle screw fixation, 61 cases.

Clinical outcome evaluation

The preoperative neurological status and neurological status at the time of discharge were evaluated in terms of back pain, dysesthesia, dyskinesia, and sphincter disturbance. Each category was divided into three grades, namely improved, unchanged, and deteriorative. In the postoperative evaluation of recent clinical efficacy, improvement and no change in neurological status were regarded as effectivity and deterioration of neurological status was regarded as nullity.

The evaluation of the long-term clinical efficacy was carried out using the American Spinal Injury Association classification (ASIA) [6]. In the evaluation of long-term clinical efficacy at the time of final follow-up (12–60 months, average 28 months), improvement was regarded as effectivity, while no change and deterioration were regarded as nullity.

All of the patients underwent examination of lateral roentgenograms during follow-up every 6 months. A spinal instability was diagnosed when either of the following conditions was observed [7]: 1. Abnormal mobility: abnormal segmental motion of a vertebral body of more than 15°; and 2. abnormal slide: anterior or posterior slide of a vertebral body of more than 3 mm.

Health economics analysis

The total costs of hospitalization included surgical and non-surgical costs. Internal fixation device cost was included in surgical cost. Non-surgical cost included drug cost and hospital bed cost. Because the patients were from different socioeconomic backgrounds, an accurate estimation of work loss-related costs was not possible and this item was excluded from the cost analysis.

Statistical analysis

All data are presented as the mean ± standard error of the mean (SEM). The statistical analysis was performed using SPSS 16.0 (SPSS, Inc., Chicago, IL, USA). Enumeration data were tested by the chi-squared test. Measurement data were tested by analysis of variance and t tests. A value of $p<0.05$ (two-tailed) was considered statistically significant.

Results

There was no significant difference in age, gender or the course of disease between the MIS group and non-MIS group ($p>0.05$; Table 1). This was the same among the five groups (Group A, Group B, Group C, Group D, Group E; $p>0.05$; Table 1) and among the three groups (Group HE, Group LE, Group LESPF; $p>0.05$; Table 1).

Table 4. Summary of results of duration of hospital stay, recovery time, loss of working time.

Groups	N	Duration of hospital stay (d)	Recovery time (d)	Loss of working time (d)
A	19	21.42±10.36	19.29±8.92	50.13±15.76
B	34	22.35±9.83	31.12±7.79	59.98±12.83
C	24	24.76±7.81★	22.31±6.78★	52.69±10.33★
D	18	25.29±11.92•	42.72±7.25▲	75.38±15.22▲
E	27	28.73±13.47▲	34.18±9.6•	71.81±17.19▲

This table shows the results for the duration of hospital stay, recovery times, and loss of working time in five groups (Group A, Group B, Group C, Group D, Group E). "Recovery time" means the postoperative activity time. "Duration of hospital stay" means the postoperative days in hospital. "Loss of working time" represents the duration from admission to the start of work after hospital discharge. Data are expressed as the mean ± standard deviation.
★$p>0.05$ vs. Group A;
▲$p<0.05$ vs. Group B;
•$p>0.05$ vs. Group B.

Clinical results

In the MIS group (53 cases), postoperative pathologies showed schwannoma in 26 cases, meningioma in 12, dermoid cyst in 4, hemangioma in 3, and lipoma in 2. Among these, 41 tumors were totally removed, 10 were subtotally removed, and 2 were partially removed. Two complications were observed in the MIS group, including one case of infection and one case of myasthenia. Meanwhile, in the non-MIS group (69 cases), postoperative

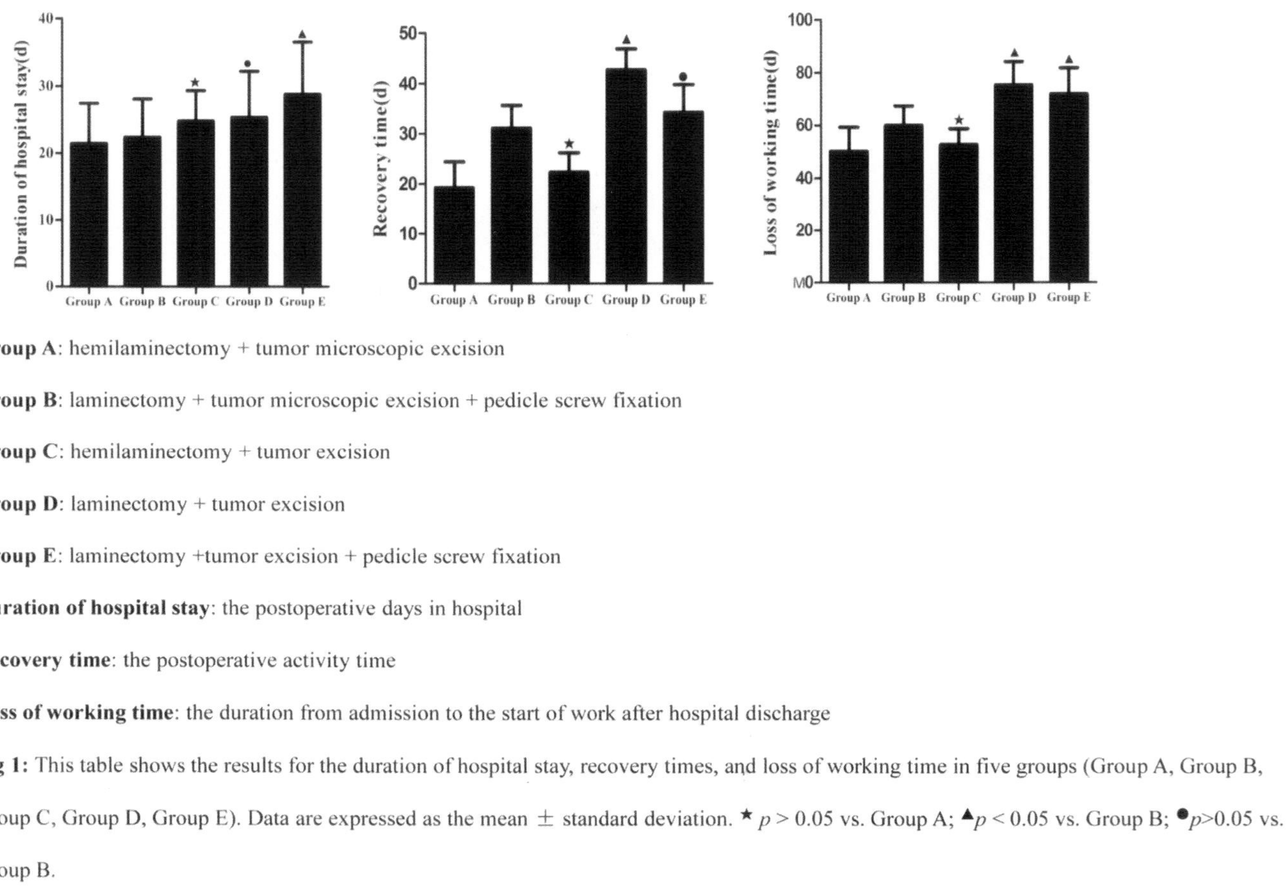

Figure 1. This table shows the results for the duration of hospital stay, recovery times, and loss of working time in five groups (Group A, Group B, Group C, Group D, Group E). Data are expressed as the mean ± standard deviation. ★$p>0.05$ vs. Group A; ▲$p<0.05$ vs. Group B; ●$p>0.05$ vs. Group B. Group A: hemilaminectomy + tumor microscopic excision. Group B: laminectomy + tumor microscopic excision + pedicle screw fixation. Group C: hemilaminectomy + tumor excision. Group D: laminectomy + tumor excision. Group E: laminectomy + tumor excision + pedicle screw fixation. Duration of hospital stay: the postoperative days in hospital. Recovery time: the postoperative activity time. Loss of working time: the duration from admission to the start of work after hospital discharge.

Table 5. Summary of various expenses.

Groups	N	Surgical cost (CNY)	Non-surgical cost (CNY)	Cost of hospitalization (CNY)
A	19	13467±7682	7782±3129	20971±12318
B	34	29314±12854	6459±2743	34354±13214
C	24	10525±9078★	10974±5607▲	21509±8842★
D	18	11628±7216˙	11691±8329˙	22319±11327˙
E	27	27612±10722■	9621±6031˙	37234±11999■

This table shows the analysis of health economics for the five surgical approaches. Data are expressed as the mean ± standard deviation.
★$p>0.05$ vs. Group A;
▲$p<0.05$ vs. Group A;
˙$p<0.05$ vs. Group B;
■$p>0.05$ vs. Group B.

pathologies showed schwannoma in 29 cases, meningioma in 15, dermoid cyst in 12, arachnoid cyst in 9, enterogenous cyst in 3, and hemangioma in 1. Among these, 50 tumors were totally removed, 15 were subtotally removed, and 4 were partially removed. Twelve complications were observed in the non-MIS group, including six cases of leakage of cerebrospinal fluid, three cases of infection, two cases of myasthenia, and one case of localized pain.

There was no significant difference in the rate of tumor resection between the MIS group and non-MIS group (p>0.05). The estimated blood loss and hospital stay durations observed in the MIS group were significantly less than in the non-MIS group (p<0.05). The operating time observed in the MIS group was significantly longer than in the non-MIS (p<0.05). The rate of postoperative complication in the MIS group was lower than in the non-MIS group (p<0.05) (Table 2).

As the neurological status was reevaluated at the time of discharge, the results were as follows: In the MIS group, postoperative neurological status improved or remained unchanged in 52 cases and worsened in 1 case (dysesthesia). In the non-MIS group, postoperative neurological status improved or remained unchanged in 59 cases and worsened in 10 cases (4 cases of back pain, 3 cases of dysesthesia, 2 cases of dyskinesia, 1 case of sphincter disturbance). Based on the results above, the short-term clinical efficacy in the MIS group was superior to that in the non-MIS group (p<0.05; Table 3).

According to ASIA, the results of the long-term clinical efficacy were observed as follows: In the MIS group, as the neurological status was reevaluated at the time of the final follow-up (12–60 months, average 28 months), neurological status improved in 51 cases and remained unchanged in 2 cases. In the non-MIS group, as the neurological status was reevaluated at the time of the final follow-up (12–60 months, average 28 months), neurological status improved in 65 cases, remained unchanged in 4 cases, and worsened in 1 case. Based on the results, there was no statistically significant difference between the MIS group and non-MIS group in terms of long-term clinical efficacy (p>0.05; Table 3).

Health economics analysis

There were no significant differences in the hospital stay durations, recovery times, or loss of working time between Group A and Group C (p>0.05). The hospital stay durations and loss of working time observed in Group B were significantly less than in Group E (p<0.05). There was no significant difference in recovery times between Group B and Group E (p>0.05). The recovery times and loss of working time in Group B were significantly less than in Group D (p<0.05). There was no significant difference in hospital stay durations between Group B and Group D (p>0.05; Table 4; Figure 1).

In terms of the costs of surgery, there is no significant difference between Group A and Group C (p>0.05), which was same between Group B and Group E (p>0.05). Group B was significantly higher than Group D (p<0.05). Meanwhile, in relation to non-surgical costs, those in Group A were significantly less than those in Group C (p<0.05). In addition, those of Group B were significantly less than those of Group E (p<0.05), while those of Group B were significantly less than those of Group D (p<0.05). Regarding the total costs of hospitalization, the total costs of hospitalization between Group A and Group C showed no significant difference (p>0.05), which was same between Group B and Group E (p>0.05). On the other hand, those of Group D were significantly less than those of Group B (p<0.05) (Table 5).

Study of postoperative spinal stability

The rate of postoperative spinal instability in Group HE and Group LEPSF were significantly lower than that in Group LE in a single spinal segment (p<0.05). The rate of postoperative spinal instability between Group HE and Group LEPSF showed no significant difference in a single operative segment. The rate of postoperative spinal instability in Group LEPSF was significantly lower than those in Group HE and Group LE in two or more spinal operative segments (p<0.05). The rate of postoperative spinal instability between Group HE and Group LE showed no significant difference in two or more operative segments (p>0.05; Table 6).

Discussion

Intradural extramedullary tumors account for two-thirds of primary spinal tumors [8]. Most intradural extramedullary tumors are benign, and they exhibit no specific symptoms. Radicular pain and worsening sensory and motor loss are common manifestations. Therefore, most of the patients are wrongly diagnosed with cervical spondylopathy or intervertebral disk herniation. MRI is very crucial to confirm the diagnosis of intradural extramedullary tumors. Once the diagnosis is confirmed, the best treatment for nonmalignant intradural extramedullary tumor is surgery. The goal of surgery is complete surgical resection while preserving spinal stability, without worsening the preoperative neurological status.

All the processes of conventional surgical tumor resection are carried out without using microscope, which may lead to a greater likelihood of incomplete tumor resection, as well as more damage to the spinal cord and vessels surrounding the spinal canal. With

Table 6. Summary of postoperative spinal stability in different segments.

Groups	1 segment			2 segments			>2 segments		
	stable	instable	Rate of stability (%)	stable	instable	Rate of stability (%)	stable	instable	Rate of stability (%)
HE	21	0	100.00	8	5	61.54	3	6	33.33
LE	4	2	66.67★	3	3	50.00·	1	5	16.67·
LEPSF	22	1	95.65▲·	26	2	92.86★▲	9	1	90.00★▲

This table shows the results of postoperative spinal stability of various surgical approaches in different segments. Abbreviations: HE: hemilaminectomy + tumor excision; LE: laminectomy + tumor excision; LEPSF: laminectomy + tumor excision + pedicle screw fixation.

★ $p<0.05$ vs. Group HE;
▲ $p<0.05$ vs. Group LE;
· $p>0.05$ vs. Group HE.

the improvement of medical devices, surgeons are increasingly using microscopy to perform surgical tumor resection. MIS can provide a clearer visual operative field and more delicate operative maneuvers, which can avoid the damage to the spinal cord and peripheral nerves as far as possible, reduce intraoperative blood loss and postoperative complications, and increase the rate of complete removal of tumors. It was reported that MIS allowed removal of the tumor with minimal impairment from cutting of nerve fibers at the nerve root [9]. Regarding intramedullary tumors, MIS made it possible to reduce postoperative mortality from 38.5 to 4.5%, exclude various complications (postoperative liquorrhea, meningitis), restore the disturbed functions of the spinal cord fully, and prolong postoperative remission and the patient's survival [10]. After total resection, restoration of full spinal cord function can happen in limited numbers of cases.

In our present study, the MIS group had the advantages of less estimated blood loss, shorter hospital stays, and fewer postoperative complications than those were observed in the non-MIS group ($p<0.05$). The short-term clinical efficacy of the MIS group was superior to that of the non-MIS group ($p<0.05$). However, there was no significant difference in the resection rates of tumors or long-term clinical efficacy between the MIS group and non-MIS group ($p>0.05$). Micromanipulation achieved less intraoperative blood loss than in the non-MIS group through avoiding accidental injury of epidural and spinal cord vessels as much as possible and precisely intercepting arteries supplying the tumor. In the MIS group, micromanipulation prevented as many complications as possible, such as postoperative infection and cerebrospinal leakage; this is because micromanipulation could reduce intraoperative blood loss and trauma to tissues around surgical site. What's more, a small mount of intraoperative blood loss has modesty impact on patient's body immunity and the duration before functional exercises on limb function, which is helpful to reduce postoperative infection effectively. Although non-MIS manipulation did not directly damage the anatomical structure of the spinal cord, it increased the damage to the vessels supplying the spinal cord than in the MIS group, which could lead to less-than-ideal postoperative spinal function recovery and short-term clinical efficacy.

Although we cannot use health economics analysis to determine the best treatment for any particular disease, we can get some useful references for surgical options. In this study, the non-surgical cost in MIS is less than in non-MIS ($p<0.05$), this is because MIS can result in the less intraoperative blood loss, lower postoperative complications, shorter durations of hospital stay and better short-term clinical efficiency. As surgical cost takes a great proportion in the total cost of hospitalization, the total costs of hospitalization between Group A (hemilaminectomy + tumor microscopic excision) and Group C (hemilaminectomy + tumor excision) showed no significant difference, which was same between Group B (laminectomy + tumor microscopic excision + pedicle screw fixation) and Group E (laminectomy + tumor excision + pedicle screw fixation). Because the costs of the internal fixation device must be taken into consideration, the total cost of hospitalization in Group B (laminectomy + tumor microscopic excision + pedicle screw fixation) is not less than in Group D (laminectomy + tumor excision). The health economics analysis was based on data from six hospitals, and therefore, may not be representative of costs at other hospitals.

In our study, we found that hemilaminectomy for intradural extramedullary tumor had better postoperative spinal stability than laminectomy with a single spinal segment. However, conventional laminectomy is still widely used for the surgical removal of spinal intradural extramedullary tumor, which can offer more familiar exposure and a wider view of the surgical field to surgeons than in hemilaminectomy. In contrast, some serious drawbacks of laminectomy still exist, such as spinal instability, epidural fibrosis, the absence of osseous protection for the spinal cord, and postoperative dorsal pain [11,12].

The removal of the posterior lamina, spinous process, paravertebral muscles, supraspinous ligament, interspinous ligament, and ligamentum flavum is needed in the surgical corridor of laminectomy, which causes great damage to the posterior column of the spine, in turn jeopardizing spinal stability [13,14,15,16]. In an effort to maintain spinal stability, hemilaminectomy avoids damage to the posterior structure of the vertebral column by preserving the supraspinous ligament, interspinous ligament, and paravertebral muscle of the opposite side. Therefore, hemilaminectomy has less impact on spinal biomechanics [17,18]. On the other hand, the disadvantage of hemilaminectomy is the narrow surgical corridor, which increases the risk of injury to spinal cord [19]. In our study, there was no statistical difference about spinal stability between hemilaminectomy and laminectomy in two or more operative segments of spine. Another result was that laminectomy + pedicle screw fixation showed better postoperative spinal stability than hemilaminectomy and laminectomy in two or more spinal operative segments. It is generally known that pedicle screw fixation offers a significant biomechanical advantage [20], and is superior to other techniques regarding the promotion of mechanical strength [21,22]. As a result, great internal stability is observed.

In this study, we have found that MIS is advantageous in the removal of intradural extramedullary tumor, this is because MIS can reduce intraoperative blood loss, duration of hospital stay, postoperative complications, non-surgical cost and have better short-term clinical efficacy compared with non-MIS. In addition, in two or more spinal operative segments, pedicle screw fixation helps avoid spinal postoperative instability. However, we have not investigated if the MIS is helpful to postoperative stability in this study. Besides that, the follow-up time and preoperative radiographic assessment of spinal stability need to be further improved in our future study. In summary, the study provides some insight to help surgeons choose the appropriate surgical method for intradural extramedullary tumor.

Author Contributions

Conceived and designed the experiments: JZ SZ. Performed the experiments: GZ LD. Analyzed the data: YF TG. Contributed to the writing of the manuscript: LD SZ GZ.

References

1. Albanese V, Platania N (2002) Spinal intradural extramedullary tumors. Personal experience. Journal of neurosurgical sciences. 46(1): 18–24.
2. Yeo DK, Im SB, Park KW, Shin DS, Kim BT, et al. (2011) Profiles of spinal cord tumors removed through a unilateral hemilaminectomy. Journal of Korean Neurosurgical Society. 50(3): 195–200.
3. Sachdev S, Dodd RL, Chang SD, Soltys SG, Adler JR, et al. (2011) Stereotactic radiosurgery yields long-term control for benign intradural, extramedullary spinal tumors. Neurosurgery. 69(3): 533–539.
4. Postalci L, Tugcu B, Gungor A, Guclu G (2010) Spinal meningiomas: recurrence in ventrally located individuals on long-term follow-up; a review of 46 operated cases. Turkish neurosurgery. 21(4): 449–453.
5. Sun Z, Sun L, Li T, Ma X, Zhang Z (2011) Intraosseous trigeminal schwannoma of mandible with intracranial extension. The Journal of Laryngology & Otology. 125(04): 418–422.
6. Kirshblum SC, Memmo P, Kim N, Campagnolo D, Millis S, et al. (2002) Comparison of the revised 2000 American Spinal Injury Association classification standards with the 1996 guidelines. American journal of physical medicine & rehabilitation. 81(7): 502–505.
7. Lida Y, Kataoka O, Sho T, Sumi M, Hirose T, et al. (1990) Postoperative lumbar spinal instability occurring or progressing secondary to laminectomy. Spine. 15(11): 1186–1189.
8. Helseth A, Mørk SJ (1989) Primary intraspinal neoplasms in Norway, 1955 to 1986: a population-based survey of 467 patients. Journal of neurosurgery. 71(6): 842–845.
9. Kobayashi S, Uchida K, Kokubo Y, Yayama T, Nakajima H, et al. (2007) A schwannoma of the S1 dural sleeve was resected while the intact nerve fibers were preserved using a microscope. Report of a case with early MRI findings. Minimal Invasive Neurosurgery. 50(2): 120–123.
10. Starodubtsev AI (1984) Surgical treatment of intramedullary tumors. Zhurnal voprosy neirokhirurgii imeni NN Burdenko. (4): 22–25.
11. Mayfield FH (1976) Complications of laminectomy. Clinical neurosurgery. 23: 435–439.
12. Yasuoka S, Peterson HA, MacCarty CS (1982) Incidence of spinal column deformity after multilevel laminectomy in children and adults. Journal of neurosurgery. 57(4): 441–445.
13. Smith ZA, Vastardis GA, Carandang G, Havey RM, Hannon S, et al. (2014) Biomechanical Effects of a Unilateral Approach to Minimally Invasive Lumbar Decompression. PloS one. 9(3): e92611.
14. Canbay S, Hasturk AE, Basmaci M, Erten F, Harman F (2012) Management of thoracal and lumbar schwannomas using a unilateral approach without instability: an analysis of 15 cases. Asian spine journal. 6(1): 43–49.
15. Iacoangeli M, Gladi M, Di Rienzo A, Dobran M, Alvaro L, et al. (2012) Minimally invasive surgery for benign intradural extramedullary spinal meningiomas: experience of a single institution in a cohort of elderly patients and review of the literature. Clinical interventions in aging. 7: 557–564.
16. Zong S, Zeng G, Xiong C, Wei B (2013) Treatment Results in the Differential Surgery of Intradural Extramedullary Schwannoma of 110 Cases. PloS one. 8(5): e63867.
17. Panjabi MM, White AA 3rd (1980) Basic biomechanics of the spine. Neurosurgery. 7(1): 76–93.
18. Ogden AT, Bresnahan L, Smith JS, Natarajan R, Fessler RG (2009) Biomechanical comparison of traditional and minimally invasive intradural tumor exposures using finite element analysis. Clinical Biomechanics. 24(2): 143–147.
19. Guidetti B (1974) Removal of extramedullary benign spinal cord tumours. In: Advances and technical standards in neurosurgery. Springer Vienna. 173–197.
20. Mazel C, Hoffmann E, Antonietti P, Grunenwald D, Henry M, et al. (2004) Posterior cervicothoracic instrumentation in spine tumors. Spine. 29(11): 1246–1253.
21. Kotani Y, Cunningham BW, Abumi K, McAfee PC (1994) Biomechanical analysis of cervical stabilization systems: an assessment of transpedicular screw fixation in the cervical spine[J]. Spine. 19(22): 2529–2539.
22. Kothe R, Rüther W, Schneider E, Linke B (2004) Biomechanical analysis of transpedicular screw fixation in the subaxial cervical spine. Spine. 29(17): 1869–1875.

Digitalized Design of Extraforaminal Lumbar Interbody Fusion: A Computer-Based Simulation and Cadaveric Study

Mingjie Yang¶, Cheng Zeng¶, Song Guo¶, Jie Pan, Yingchao Han, Zeqing Li, Lijun Li*, Jun Tan*

Department of Spine Surgery, Shanghai East Hospital, Tongji University School of Medicine, Shanghai, People's Republic of China

Abstract

Purpose: This study aims to investigate the feasibility of a novel lumbar approach named extraforaminal lumbar interbody fusion (ELIF), a newly emerging minimally invasive technique for treating degenerative lumbar disorders, using a digitalized simulation and a cadaveric study.

Methods: The ELIF surgical procedure was simulated using the Mimics surgical simulator and included dissection of the superior articular process, dilation of the vertebral foramen, and placement of pedicle screws and a cage. ELIF anatomical measures were documented using a digitalized technique and subsequently validated on fresh cadavers.

Results: The use of the Mimics allowed for the vivid simulation of ELIF surgical procedures, while the cadaveric study proved the feasibility of this novel approach. ELIF had a relatively lateral access approach that was located 8–9 cm lateral to the median line with an access depth of approximately 9 cm through the intermuscular space. Dissection of the superior articular processes could fully expose the target intervertebral discs and facilitate a more inclined placement of the pedicle screws and cage with robust enhancement.

Conclusions: According to the computer-based simulation and cadaveric study, it is feasible to perform ELIF. Further research including biomechanical study is needed to prove ELIF has a superior ability to preserve the posterior tension bands of the spinal column, with similar effects on spinal decompression, fixation, and fusion, and if it can enhance post-fusion spinal stability and expedites postoperative recovery.

Editor: Paul Park, University of Michigan, United States of America

Funding: This study was supported by grants from Discipline leader plan of the health ministry of pudong area, Shanghai, China. Program number PWRD 2011-2. The funders had no role in study design, data collection and analysis, decision to publish, or preparation of the manuscript.

Competing Interests: The authors have declared that no competing interests exist.

* Email: jesoy@126.com (LL); dr.tan@139.com (JT)

¶ These authors are co-first authors on this work.

Introduction

Lumbar interbody fusion (LIF), such as posterior lumbar interbody fusion (PLIF) and transforaminal lumbar interbody fusion (TLIF), is the mainstay surgical treatment for degenerative lumbar disease, lumbar instability, and intervertebral disc disorders. Spinal surgeons are always attempting to modify the surgical approaches to LIF in more minimal invasive ways. These newly emerging modifications include anterior LIF, with a trans- or extraperitoneal approach anterior to the lumbar vertebrae [1], extreme lateral LIF, with a trans-psoas-major-muscle approach that is lateral to the lumbar vertebrae [2], and axial LIF, with a presacral approach [3]. However, these modified techniques are subject to some limitations including a steep learning curve, technical difficulty of manipulation, and high risk of procedural complications such as retrograde ejaculation, vascular or ureteral injury, and compromised lumbosacral plexus or genitofemoral nerve function [4,5]. Therefore, conventional PLIF and TLIF are still preferred in current practice [6].

Inspired by the conception of transforaminal endoscopy (the Tessys technique), we developed a modified TLIF technique, namely extreme lateral TLIF (ELIF) [7]. ELIF has a more lateral access approach than TLIF, avoiding the inferior articular process and allowing for full exposure of the superior counterpart, which causes the nerve compression-associated symptoms. ELIF also facilitates the decompression of the lateral vertebral canal and the fusion of vertebral bodies in a "safety triangle."

The primary objective of this study was to assess the feasibility of ELIF using a computer-based simulation and to validate the digitalized anatomic measurements using a cadaveric model.

Materials and Methods

Ethics Statement

This study has been reviewed and approved by ethics committee of Shanghai East Hospital, Tongji University school of medcine before the study began. And the ethic statement form has been upload in the attach files.

In this study we use DICOM data of a patient, and the patient's written informed consent was provided.

Our research also involved the use of two fresh lumbar cadaveric specimens which were provided by the Department of Anatomy, Shanghai Medical college, Fudan University. This department is also a donation centre with the URL:http://www.redcross-sha.org/view.aspx?id = 5199. And the written informed consent from the donor were obtained for use of this sample in research.

Three-dimensional modeling and simulated ELIF

A 26-year-old man (height, 172 cm; weight, 67 kg; body mass index, 22.6 kg/m^2) diagnosed with an $L_{4/5}$ lumbar disc herniation was recruited for a lumbar computed tomography (CT) scan preoperatively from the T_{12} level to the entrance of the pelvis using a dual source scanner (SOMATOM Definition Flash; Siemens Medical Solutions Inc., Forchheim, Germany). The scanning parameters were as follows: tube current = 250 mA, tube voltage = 120 kV, scanning slice thickness = 1.0 mm, and reconstruction slice thickness = 1.0 mm. Digital imaging and communications in medicine (DICOM) data obtained from the scanning were imported into the Mimics V14.0 system (Materialise NV, Leuven, Belgium) for image post-processing. The region of interest was selected and reconstructed using the automatic reconstruction module. The bone tissue threshold was also automatically set to clearly visualize the anatomy in the region of interest and produce the mask of the target tissue. The region growing technique was used to acquire the masks for the femoral head, pelvis, sacrum, and five lumbar vertebrae, each of which was independently processed and individually colored. The masks were selected for further three-dimensional (3D) reconstruction and smoothing to generate the 3D solid model for the bony pelvis, including the lumbar and sacral vertebrae.

The L_5 vertebral body was separately extracted, and the superior articular processes were partially (approximately 3/4) dissected using the simulated cutter with an appropriate angle. The processed L_5 vertebral body was restored to the original spinal column. The bases of the superior articular process residuals were shown to partially articulate with the inferior articular processes; however, the intervertebral foramen was dilated roughly 30% compared to prior to the operation. This enlarged foramen allowed the surgeon to perform lateral recess decompression, intervertebral space dissection, and cage placement. A sterolithography (STL) file was imported to this model to simulate the instrumentation of the body fusion cage and pedicle screws into an appropriate location.

Digitalized measurement of the ELIF anatomical indices

Lumbar CT scanning data were obtained from 60 adult outpatients, including 30 males and 30 females aged 18–55 years, none of whom had a known lumbar tumor, inflammation, scoliosis, spondylolisthesis, or congenital spinal malformation. All patients were placed in the supine position, and a 64-detector spiral CT scanner equipped with a SYNGO workstation (SOMATOM Sensation) was used for the lumbar CT scan. The scanning parameters were as follows: tube current = 250 mA; tube voltage = 120 kV; scanning slice thickness = 1.0 mm; and reconstruction slice thickness = 1.0 mm. The scanning levels included the vertebrae from the T_{12} level to the S_3 level and the neighboring structures. The DICOM data were imported to Mimics 14.0 equipped with a multifunctional 3D image measurement module to produce axial, sagittal, and coronal two-dimensional (2D) multi-planar rendering (MPR) images. These MPR images were combined with the 3D reconstructed solid images for the measurement of anatomical indices of ELIF at the L_{3-4} and L_{4-5} levels, respectively. These indices included the distance of the incision to the median line, the depth of the access approach, the angle and length of the screw placement, and the length of the instrumented cage (Figure 1). These indices can be obtained by measurement system in Mimics 14.0.

Mock ELIF on cadaver

Our use of the cadaveric specimens complied with the institutional and national regulations. Two fresh lumbar cadaveric specimens from male donors were provided by the Department of Anatomy, Shanghai Medical College, Fudan University. A longitudinal right paramedian incision (3–5 cm) was made parallel to L_{4-5} and 8–9 cm distant to the median line. The subcutaneous tissue and thoracolumbar fascia were sequentially incised and the intermuscular space was bluntly dissected. The transverse process of the L_5 vertebra was palpable though an approximate 45° angle. The L_{4-5} facet joint was dissected along the transverse process toward the median line. The vertebral body was exposed along the convergence of the superior process and the transverse process base and slightly toward the ventral side. Upon palpation of the infrapedicular notch, the vertebral body was further dissected toward the ventral side to expose the L_{4-5} disc. The superior part of the intervertebral space was slightly dissected along the orientation of the nerve root to expose the L_4 nerve root. A Φ2.0-mm orthopedic grinder or boning knife was used to resect ¾ of the superior articular process to fully expose the entire intervertebral foramen, nerve root orientation and exit, and lateral spinal dural sac. The nerve root was well preserved and the intervertebral disc was dissected through the dilated foramen. Following the dissection of the intervertebral space, the interbody fusion cage was instrumented. The convergence of the L_{4-5} superior and transverse processes was drilled and threaded for the placement of the pedicle screws. In the placement of the pedicle screw, the inner wall of the pedicle was explored using a nerve hook, while the nerve root was retracted and well preserved. The connect rod was placed and the screws were tightened. A repeated exploration was performed to ensure good preservation of the nerve root and stability of the internal fixation system prior to ELIF completion.

Statistical analysis

All data were processed using the SPSS statistical software package (version 20.0; SPSS Inc., Chicago, IL, USA) and expressed as mean ± SD. The means were compared using one-way analysis of variance and the independent samples were compared using Student's t test. P values<0.05 were considered statistically significantly.

Results

The use of the Mimics system enabled 3D solid simulation and vivid preoperative planning for ELIF (Figure 2). The removal of the superior articular process allowed for decompression of the spinal lateral recess and dilation of the foramen, which facilitated further dissection of the intervertebral space and cage placement.

Use of the Mimics also allowed a whole-3D crossover measurement of the target point, line, and plane on a 3D object, which helped the determination of the spatial location and angle. Tables 1 and 2 show the ELIF anatomical measures on the axial, sagittal, and coronal planes in combination with the reconstructed 3D solid model images. The ELIF incision was located approximately 8–9 cm lateral to the median line; the access approach was roughly 8–9 cm; the pedicle screw was 1 cm longer than that used

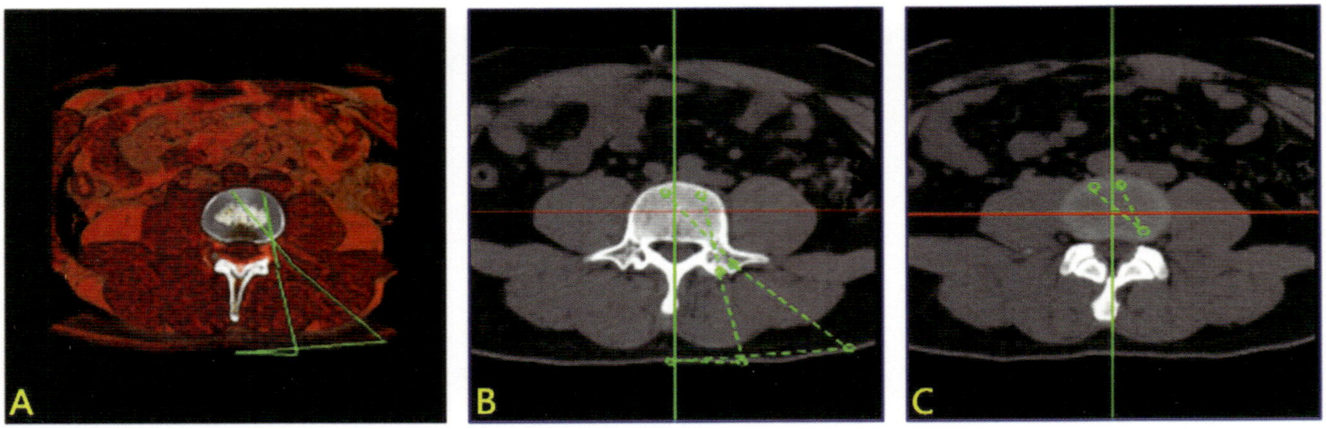

Figure 1. Mimics measurement of anatomical indices on two-dimensional extraforaminal lumbar interbody fusion (ELIF) and TLIF multi-planar rendered images. (A) transverse view of a three-dimensional image; (B) measurement of the distance of the incision to the median line, the depth of the access approach, and the length of the pedicle screw; and (C) measurement of the length of the interbody fusion cage.

in TLIF; the angle of the screw placement was more inclined, at approximately 40°; and the cage length was approximately 30 mm. Compared to TLIF, ELIF had a more lateral incision that avoided the inferior articular process and allowed for direct access to the hypertrophic, compressed superior articular process through a lateroposterior approach, and the pedicle screw and cage were implanted in a more inclined angle and with a significantly greater length ($P<0.01$).

It was feasible to achieve a digitally designed surgical approach, procedure, and decompression on the cadaveric specimens with good consistency with the preoperative planning (Figure 3). Digitalized operative planning showed good accuracy, safety, and stability. The present digitalization technology could not accurately reconstruct images of the minute vascular vessels and nerves, and the mock cadaveric operation was not identical to the actual operation. For example, it was highly risky to access the para- and intraspinal venous plexuses.

Discussion

Digital medicine is a newly emerging technique which incorporates information technology into clinical medicine. This technique uses a laser scanner, CT, magnetic resonance (MR), and other digital equipment to acquire human body tomographic data. After further integrating these data, spinal digitalized 3D reconstruction can demonstrate the morphology of the spinal column from multiple angles and directions, which allows a clear and full visualization of the disease in whole and in detail. Furthermore, this technique can be used for the selection of surgical approach, the assessment of surgical risk and outcome, and preoperative planning on the digitalized model, for instance, simulating implantation of the cage [8–9].

In this study, we used Mimics 14.0 software, which is highly integrated and user-friendly for 3D image production and editing. The Mimics surgical simulation module is a surgical simulation platform for the data analysis of the human regional anatomy and the planning of the skin incision, dissection, and implantation.

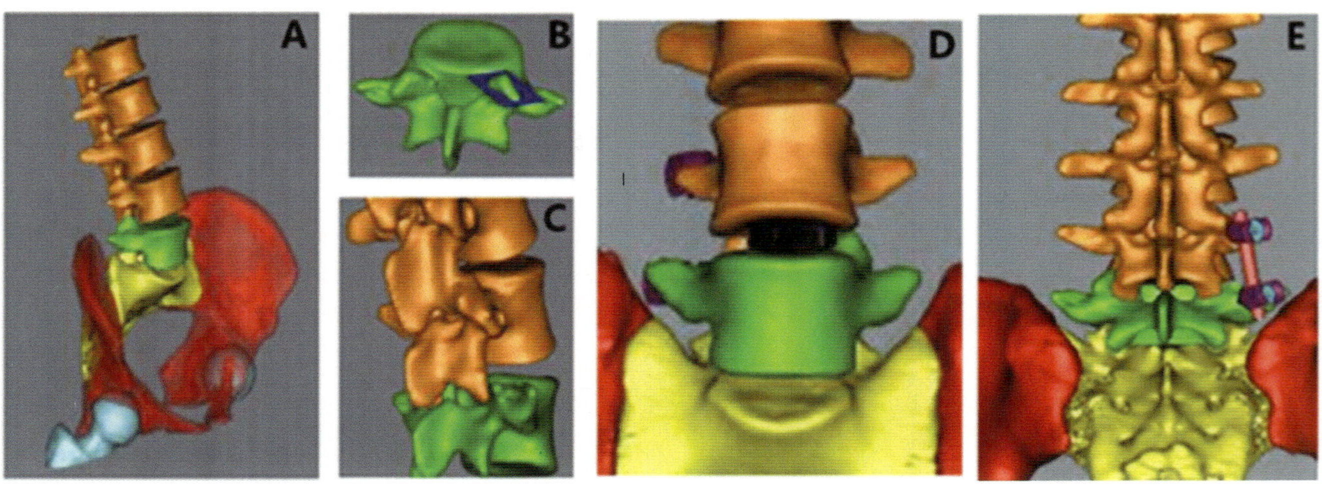

Figure 2. Mimics simulation of extraforaminal lumbar interbody fusion. (A) Three-dimensional reconstruction of the spinal column; (B) extraction of the L_5 vertebral body and resection of the superior articular process; (C) exposure of the intervertebral space following resection of the superior articular process; (D) placement of the cage through the intervertebral foramen; (E) implantation of the pedicle screws.

Table 1. L_{3-4} ELIF and TLIF anatomical measures.

		Distance of incision to the central line (mm)	Depth of access approach (mm)	Cage length (mm)	Pedicle screw length (mm)		Pedicle screw inclination (°)	
					L_3	L_4	L_3	L_4
ETLIF	M	87.0±4.1	85.1±7.4	32.0±1.9	55.2±1.5	55.8±3.0	40.4±2.1	39.1±3.5
	F	83.3±4.0	81.7±6.8	29.8±1.8	51.6±3.5	52.2±2.4	37.7±1.3	37.6±3.2
TLIF	M	38.5±4.4	57.9±4.5	28.4±2.0	47.9±2.1	48.8±3.4	13.8±4.2	11.5±3.6
	F	35.3±4.2	54.3±5.2	26.5±2.1	45.1±4.1	46.0±3.1	12.1±1.6	10.2±3.3

Table 2. L_{4-5} ELIF and TLIF anatomical measures.

		Distance of incision to the central line (mm)	Depth of access approach (mm)	Cage length (mm)	Pedicle screw length (mm)		Pedicle screw inclination (°)	
					L_4	L_5	L_4	L_5
ETLIF	M	87.6±3.8	86.9±4.5	32.2±2.2	55.8±3.0	57.2±1.3	39.1±3.5	39.1±3.5
	F	81.3±3.4	83.0±4.2	30.3±2.0	52.2±2.4	54.4±2.2	37.6±3.2	37.6±3.2
TLIF	M	37.0±4.1	56.4±5.2	28.5±2.2	48.8±3.4	51.3±5.1	11.5±3.6	11.5±3.6
	F	32.9±2.7	54.0±4.9	26.8±2.1	46.0±3.1	48.7±1.2	10.2±3.3	10.2±3.3

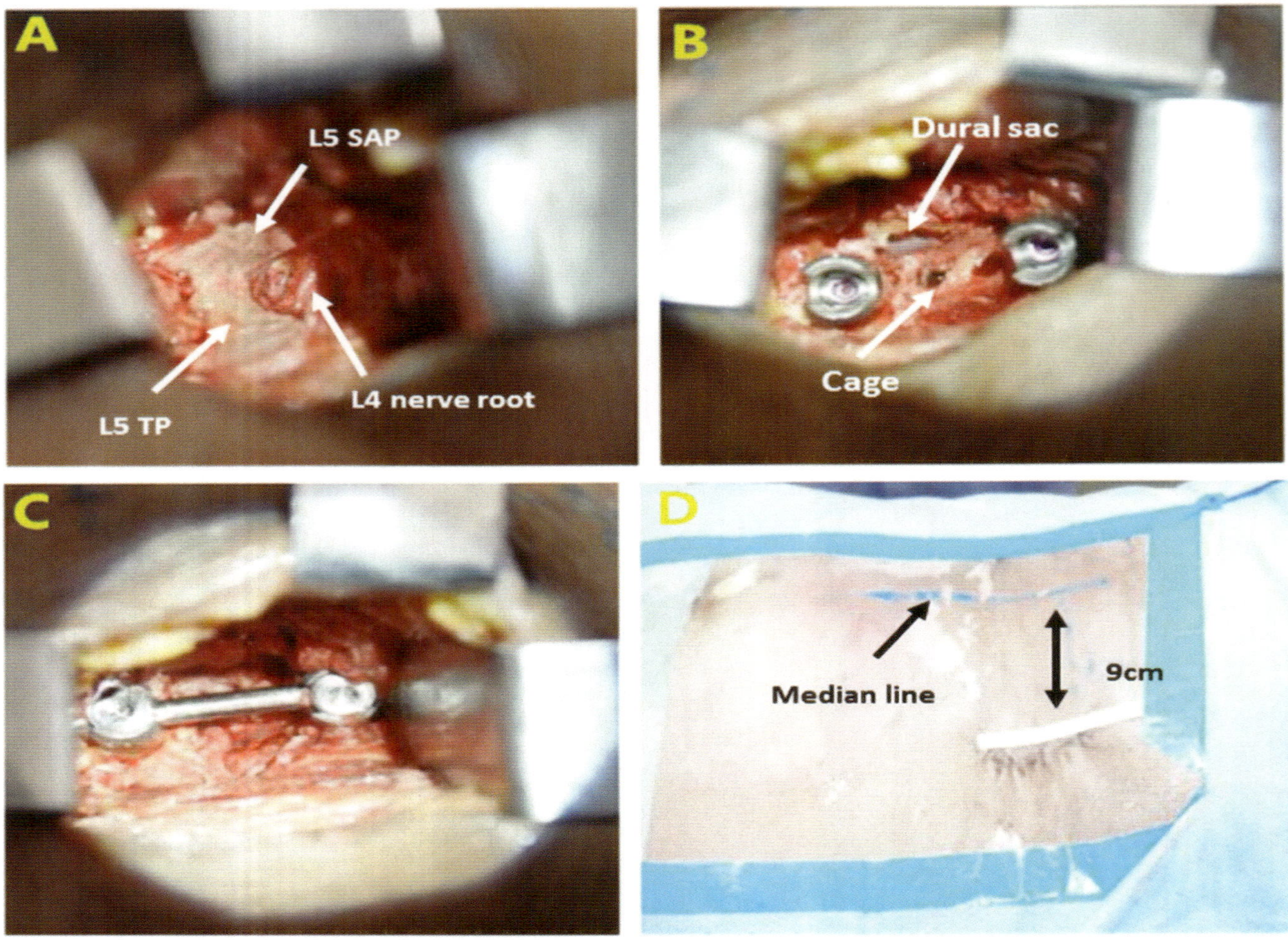

Figure 3. Mock L_{4-5} extraforaminal lumbar interbody fusion on cadaveric specimen. (A) palpation of the L_5 transverse process and exposure of the superior articular process toward the medial side with preservation of the L_4 nerve root; (B) resection of the superior articular process, dissection of the intervertebral space, and implantation of the cage and pedicle screws; (C) assembly and fixation of the connect rod; and (D) closure of the incision.

Compared to conventional gross anatomy measurements and solid operative presentations, 3D reconstruction technology can accurately reproduce the anatomical features of the target structure. The digitalized anatomical model can allow for a 3D dynamic and visualized manipulation in the computer system, which saves materials and time and improves the accuracy of the examination result. In this study, we used multiple digital techniques to simulate key ELIF procedures such as resection of the superior articular process, dissection of the intervertebral space, placement of the cage and pedicle screws, and acquisition of the relevant anatomical measures. All of these results were further validated by the results of the mock operation performed on the cadaveric specimens.

Harms et al. [10] reported a modified TLIF in 1982, which had a more lateral access approach and allowed for lumbar interbody fusion from the posterolateral foramen and the preservation of posterior tension structures such as the supraspinous and interspinous ligaments and laminal attachment of the sacrospinous muscle. Therefore, this modified TLIF has a minimal effect on the mechanical load distribution of the spinal column. Additionally, this modified procedure avoids excessive retraction of the dural sac and nerve roots and reduces the risk of intraspinal venous plexus bleeding and nerve root injury. As a major development in the concept of minimally invasive spinal surgery, Holly et al. [11] innovated a minimally invasive TLIF based on conventional TLIF, which had an access approach through the intermuscular space between the multifidus muscle and the longissimus dorsi muscle. TLIF procedures could be completed inside the catheter and minimize operative injuries. Compared to PLIF, TLIF preserves the spinous process and lamina that are not causative of neurological symptoms, while only the symptomatic lateral spinal canal is specifically decompressed with a great emphasis on the maximized preservation of the lumbar muscles and bony structure [12]. As the inferior articular process overlies the dorsal side of the superior articular process, TLIF requires the preceding resection of the inferior and superior articular process for nerve root decompression and intervertebral space dissection. However, the inferior articular process is not the etiological cause in most cases, but it is sacrificed for the establishment of the access approach and the surgical field [13]. As inspired by the development of Joimax foraminal endoscopy, we designed a more lateral approach than TLIF, namely ELIF. This approach passes through the intermuscular space between the multifidus muscle and the longissimus dorsi muscle and avoids the inferior articular process. It also allows for the direct exposure and resection of the superior articular process that causes neurological symptoms and enables the decompression of the lateral spinal canal and interbody fusion in the safety angle. ELIF is even more minimally invasive since it preserves the posterior tension structures including the inferior articular process, lamina, and attaching ligaments and muscles. The superior articular process is partially resected, and the residual portion can still articulate with and support the inferior articular process. The more inclined approach in ELIF results in a more inclined (45° or even coronal) cage implantation compared to that in TLIF. Therefore, a lengthened cage needs to be placed since it can increase the bone grafting bed area, prevent cage subsidence, and improve the fusion rate. Moreover, the use of more inclined and longer pedicle screws can penetrate the three columns of the vertebral bodies, which enhances the mechanical strength and results in good stability with unilateral fixation [14,15]. Our digital anatomical measurement results confirmed that ELIF had a more inclined placement of pedicle screws using longer pedicle screws and a longer cage compared to TLIF. Furthermore, ELIF can make direct decompression in lateral and even part of central canal which is totally different in ALIF and X/DLIF. But ELIF also has some potential shortcomings compared to TLIF. The more lateral incision of ELIF make the approach much deeper than TLIF, so this places a greater burden on lighting in operation site and surgical skills. And we can't make reduction because the inferior facet joint is left intact, so it's difficult to treat spondylolisthesis with ELIF.

We used the simulated ELIF to determine the anatomical indices in the mock ELIF on the cadaveric specimens. The incision was made 9 cm distal to the median line, and the approach passes the intermuscular space and reaches the transverse process. Further dissection along the transverse process toward the mediosuperior side was made to fully expose the superior articular process and reach the intervertebral foramen. The exit nerve is located on the ventral side of the inter-transverse-process ligament as a leg of the safety triangle, and the ligament is appropriately dissected to identify the nerve root. It is essential to locate the nerve root in a retrograde manner and preserve the nerve root during placement of the superior pedicle screw [16,17]. Resection of the superior articular process can fully expose the intervertebral foramen, which is located distal to the dural sac and the inferior nerve root. The exit nerve root should be properly preserved during intervertebral space decompression and cage placement. In the placement of the pedicle screw, the inner wall of the pedicle is explored using a nerve hook and adjustment of the inclining angle (approximately 40°) while avoiding the entrance to the spinal canal.

According to the computer-based simulation and cadaveric study, it is feasible to perform ELIF. In conclusion, ELIF is a more inclined approach than TLIF and the lateral resection of the symptomatic superior articular process allows for better disc dissection and cage placement. Further research including biomechanical study is needed to prove ELIF has a superior ability to preserve the posterior tension bands of the spinal column, with similar effects on spinal decompression, fixation, and fusion, and it can enhance post-fusion spinal stability and expedites postoperative recovery. However, this approach also has some disadvantages such as the intervertebral foramen area has abundant venous plexuses and is at high risk of bleeding and nerve injury, it is also difficult to decompress centrally and need a steep learning curve to perform ELIF.

Author Contributions

Conceived and designed the experiments: JT LJL MJY. Performed the experiments: CZ YCH SG ZQL. Analyzed the data: MJY CZ JP. Contributed reagents/materials/analysis tools: CZ YCH SG. Wrote the paper: MJY LJL CZ.

References

1. Hsieh PC, Koski TR, O'Shaughnessy BA, Sugrue P, Salehi S, et al. (2007) Anterior lumbar interbody fusion in comparison with transforaminal lumbar interbody fusion: implications for the restoration of foraminal height, local disc angle, lumbar lordosis, and sagittal balance. J Neurosurg Spine, 7:379–86.
2. Rodgers WB, Gerber EJ, Patterson J (2011) Intraoperative and early postoperative complications in extreme lateral interbody fusion: an analysis of 600 cases. Spine, 36:26–32.
3. Lindley EM, McCullough MA, Burger EL, Brown CW, Patel VV (2011) Complications of axial lumbar interbody fusion. J Neurosurg Spine, 15:273–9.
4. Tobler WD, Ferrara LA (2011) The presacral retroperitoneal approach for axial lumbar interbody fusion: a prospective study of clinical outcomes, complications and fusion rates at a follow-up of two years in 26 patients. J Bone Joint Surg Br, 93:955–60.
5. Cahill KS, Martinez JL, Wang MY, Vanni S, Levi AD (2012) Motor nerve injuries following the minimally invasive lateral transpsoas approach. J Neurosurg Spine, 17:227–31.
6. Hey HW, Hee HT (2010) Lumbar degenerative spinal deformity: Surgical options of PLIF, TLIF and MI-TLIF. Indian J Orthop, 44:159–62.
7. Di Paola CP, Molinari RW (2008) Posterior lumbar interbody fusion. J Am Acad Orthop Surg, 16:130–9.
8. Kadoury S, Labelle H (2012) Classification of three-dimensional thoracic deformities in adolescent idiopathic scoliosis from a multivariate analysis. Eur Spine J, 21:40–9.
9. Hong JY, Suh SW, Easwar TR, Modi HN, Yang JH, et al. (2011) Evaluation of the three-dimensional deformities in scoliosis surgery with computed tomography: efficacy and relationship with clinical outcomes. Spine, 36:1259–65.
10. Rosenberg WS, Mummaneni PV (2001) Transforaminal lumbar interbody fusion: technique, complications, and early results. Neurosurgery, 48:569–74.
11. Holly LT, Schwender JD, Rouben DP, Foley KT (2006) Minimally invasive transforaminal lumbar interbody fusion: indications, technique, and complications. Neurosurg Focus, 20:E6.
12. Lee KH, Yue WM, Yeo W, Soeharno H, Tan SB (2012) Clinical and radiological outcomes of open versus minimally invasive transforaminal lumbar interbody fusion. Eur Spine J, 21:2265–70.
13. Mura PP, Costaglioli M, Piredda M, Caboni S, Casula S (2011) TLIF for symptomatic disc degeneration: a retrospective study of 100 patients. Eur Spine J, 20, Suppl 1:57–60.
14. Feng ZZ, Cao YW, Jiang C, Jiang XX (2011) Short-term outcome of bilateral decompression via a unilateral paramedian approach for transforaminal lumbar interbody fusion with unilateral pedicle screw fixation. Orthopedics, 34:364.
15. Xiao YX, Chen QX, Li FC (2009) Unilateral transforaminal lumbar interbody fusion: a review of the technique, indications and graft materials. J Int Med Res, 37:908–17.
16. Lau D, Lee JG, Han SJ, Lu DC, Chou D (2011) Complications and perioperative factors associated with learning the technique of minimally invasive transforaminal lumbar interbody fusion (TLIF). J Clin Neurosci, 18:624–7.
17. Lee DH, Kim NH, Park JB, Hwang CJ, Lee CS, et al. (2011) CT scan assessment of the pathway of the true lateral approach for transforaminal endoscopic lumbar discectomy: is It possible? J Bone Joint Surg Br. 93:1395–9.

17

Stereotactic Aspiration versus Craniotomy for Primary Intracerebral Hemorrhage

Jia-Wei Wang, Jin-Ping Li, Ying-Lun Song, Ke Tan, Yu Wang, Tao Li, Peng Guo, Xiong Li, Yan Wang, Qi-Huang Zhao*

Department of neurosurgery, Beijing Chao-Yang Hospital, Capital Medical University, Beijing, P. R. China

Abstract

Background: A wealth of evidence based on the randomized controlled trials (RCTs) has indicated that surgery may be a better choice in the management of primary intracerebral hemorrhage (ICH) compared to conservative treatment. However, there is considerable controversy over selecting appropriate surgical procedures for ICH. Thus, this meta-analysis was performed to assess the effects of stereotactic aspiration compared to craniotomy in patients with ICH.

Methods: According to the study strategy, we searched PUBMED, EMBASE and Cochrane Central Register of Controlled Trials. Other sources such as the internet-based clinical trial registries, relevant journals and the lists of references were also searched. After literature searching, two investigators independently performed literature screening, assessment of quality of the included trials and data extraction. The outcome measures included death or dependence, total risk of complication, and the risk of rebleeding, gastrointestinal hemorrhage and systematic infection.

Results: Four RCTs with 2996 participants were included. The quality of the included trials was acceptable. Stereotactic aspiration significantly decreased the odds of death or dependence at the final follow-up (odds ratio (OR): 0.80, 95% confidence interval (CI): 0.69–0.93; P = 0.004) and the risk of intracerebral rebleeding (OR: 0.44, 95% CI: 0.26–0.74; P = 0.002) compared to craniotomy with no significant heterogeneity among the study results.

Conclusions: The present meta-analysis provides evidence that the stereotactic aspiration may be associated with a reduction in the odds of being dead or dependent in primary ICH, which should be interpreted with caution. Further trials are needed to identify those patients most likely to benefit from the stereotactic aspiration.

Editor: Damir Janigro, Cleveland Clinic, United States of America

Funding: This work was supported by the grant from Beijing Chao-Yang Hospital, Capital Medical University (No.YQ201314). The funders had no role in study design, data collection and analysis, decision to publish, or preparation of the manuscript.

Competing Interests: The authors have declared that no competing interests exist.

* Email: chaoyanghospital@126.com

Introduction

As a leading cause of mortality and morbidity worldwide, spontaneous intracerebral hemorrhage (ICH) has received considerable attention in the clinical practice [1]. It is estimated that 10–30 cases per 100,000 persons are affected annually, with many suffering fatal or permanently disabled injuries [2,3]. Unfortunately, despite the well-known deleterious effects of ICH, medical and surgical interventions remain limited, and advancements in treatment have been relatively non-existent [2,4].

Current mainstay for the management of ICH consists of conservative treatment and surgical evacuation [2]. Generally, conservative treatment is mainly applied to the patients with small hematomas and absence of neurological deficits, while the surgery tends to be used in those with large hemorrhage and progressive neurological deterioration [5,6]. A recent systematic review of 15 randomized controlled trials comparing surgical evacuation with conservative treatment in the management of ICH indicates a significant advantage for surgical evacuation with an odds ratio (OR) of 0.74 ($P<0.0001$) in patients with ICH [7]. However, the effect is not very robust (95% CI: 0.64–0.86) and there is heterogeneity because these trials involve several types of surgical procedures such as craniotomy and stereotactic aspiration. Therefore, these issues have led to increasing enthusiasm in identifying which type of surgical procedures can benefit most in the ICH treatment.

In recent years, minimally invasive neurosurgical technique such as stereotactic aspiration appear to be a promising alternative approach to treat ICH, which is different from the commonly used craniotomy [8,9]. A number of large case series have reported the efficiency of stereotactic aspiration in the patients with ICH [10,11]. It is believed that stereotactic aspiration can relieve the mass effect resulting from the hematoma with reduced intervention in body homeostasis and decrease the injury of brain tissue, which is beneficial to improve the outcome of patients with ICH [12]. However, to our knowledge, it is still uncertain about the effects of stereotactic aspiration in the treatment of ICH compared to craniotomy. With the publication of recent literatures involving stereotactic aspiration and craniotomy [13,14,15,16], it is possible for us to further compare the effects of stereotactic aspiration with the one of craniotomy in the management of ICH.

The present meta-analysis was performed to determine whether stereotactic aspiration was effective in decreasing the risk of death or dependence and reducing the complication rates compared to craniotomy in the treatment of ICH.

Materials and Methods

Study identification

We performed a systematic review of the published literatures to identify all the clinical randomized controlled trials (RCTs), in which stereotactic aspiration had been compared to craniotomy in the treatment of the patients with primary spontaneous ICH that was confirmed by computed tomography (CT) scanning. The craniotomy treatment included both the conventionally open craniotomy with large bone flap and the key-hole craniotomy with small bone flap. Studies that were either not randomized controlled trials or that did not directly involve the effects of stereotactic aspiration on the treatment of patients with primary ICH were eliminated.

Search strategy

Based on the text words or MeSH terms such as "Stereotaxic Techniques", "Stereotactic", "Craniotomy", "Intracerebral hemorrhage" and "Intracranial Hemorrhage, Hypertensive", an electronic search for relevant articles was conducted on PUBMED(- present), EMBASE(- present) and the Cochrane Central Register of Controlled Trials (CENTRAL, - present) without language limitation. The internet-based clinical trial registries such as ClinicalTrials.gov, Stroke Trials Registry, International Clinical Trials Registry Platform (ICTRP) and International Standard Randomized Controlled Trial Number Register (ISRCTN) were also searched for suitable studies. Abstracts and conference proceedings from the International Stroke Conference were searched where available. In addition, the journals such as Stroke, Neurosurgery and Journal of Neurosurgery were searched for further studies. And we also complemented this by using the *Related Articles* function on PUBMED and searching the reference lists of relevant articles. For full details of the search strategy, see *Search strategy S1*. The search was performed independently by two investigators and was completed on February 2014.

Literature screening

After literature search, two investigators independently reviewed the titles and abstracts of all studies identified and excluded those that were obviously irrelevant. Then the full articles of the remaining studies were retrieved and independently reviewed by them using a structured form to determine eligibility and extract data. Disagreements were resolved by consensus or by a third investigator if needed. We contacted study authors for clarifications and further information when necessary.

Quality assessment

The quality of eligible studies was formally evaluated by using the Cochrane Collaboration's tool for assessing the risk of bias in randomized trials. Specifically, studies were judged on the following items: adequacy of the random sequence generation ("yes" = 2, "unclear" = 1 and "no" = 0); allocation concealment and blinding ("yes" = 2, "unclear" = 1 and "no" = 0); the completeness of outcome data ("yes" = 2, "unclear" = 1 and "no" = 0); the possibility of selective outcome reporting ("yes" = 0 and "unclear" = 1 and "no" = 2). Studies with a total score of <2 were considered as low-quality literatures.

Data extraction

We extracted the following data from each study: baseline characteristics, the design and objective, number of patients, timing of measurements, main results of the study, and follow-up results. The primary outcome was the composite outcome of death or dependence for help from other people for their activities of daily living (ADL) at the end of follow-up. The secondary outcomes included death at the end of follow-up and post-operative complication rates (such as re-bleeding, gastrointestinal (GI) hemorrhage and systemic infection). In the present study, the cut-off points for the various scales to define dependence in ADL were score 60 or less for the Barthel Index (BI) and grade 3 or less for the Glasgow Outcome Scale (GOS) [17,18].

Statistical analysis

A heterogeneity-based method of meta-analysis was performed using Review Manager for Windows (version 5.2, Cochrane Collaboration and Update Software) for prospective RCTs. Heterogeneity between studies was assessed by means of the standard Cochran Q statistic and I^2 statistic. And heterogeneity was pre-specified as $P<0.10$ or $I^2>50\%$ in the present study. The summary odds ratio (OR) was used as the effect parameter for the meta- analysis and the 95% confidence interval (CI) was used to interpret the results. A fixed-effect model was used to merge the values of OR to estimate the overall effect size when the heterogeneity between studies was not reached. Otherwise, a random-effect model was used in the statistics. Considering the possibility that effectiveness may differ according to the surgical technique used, subgroup analyses were performed according to the types of craniotomy. All tests were 2-sided, and statistical significance was defined as a probability value of <0.05 if not specially stated.

Results

Characteristics of included studies

In total, 88 articles were initially identified, of which 84 articles were excluded, leaving 4 studies for final analysis. Figure 1 described the flow diagram of search results and study selection. PRISMA checklist was listed in *checklist S1*.

All the four included studies were prospective randomized controlled trials [13,14,15,16]. A total of 2996 participants were enrolled in the four trials, among which 1695 (56.6%) patients were included in the group with stereotactic aspiration treatment. All the included trials had distinct inclusion criteria and exclusion criteria. The trials, in which hemorrhage was caused by aneurysm, vascular malformations, tumor apoplexy, trauma, cerebral infarction or disturbance of blood coagulation, were excluded. Each trial described the baseline characteristics of the enrolled participants, and there were no significant differences in the baseline characteristics of participants between groups in these trials other than the Zhao study. Table 1 summarized the baseline data of the four included trials.

The intervention group in the four included trials was treated with stereotactic aspiration that was guided by the preoperative

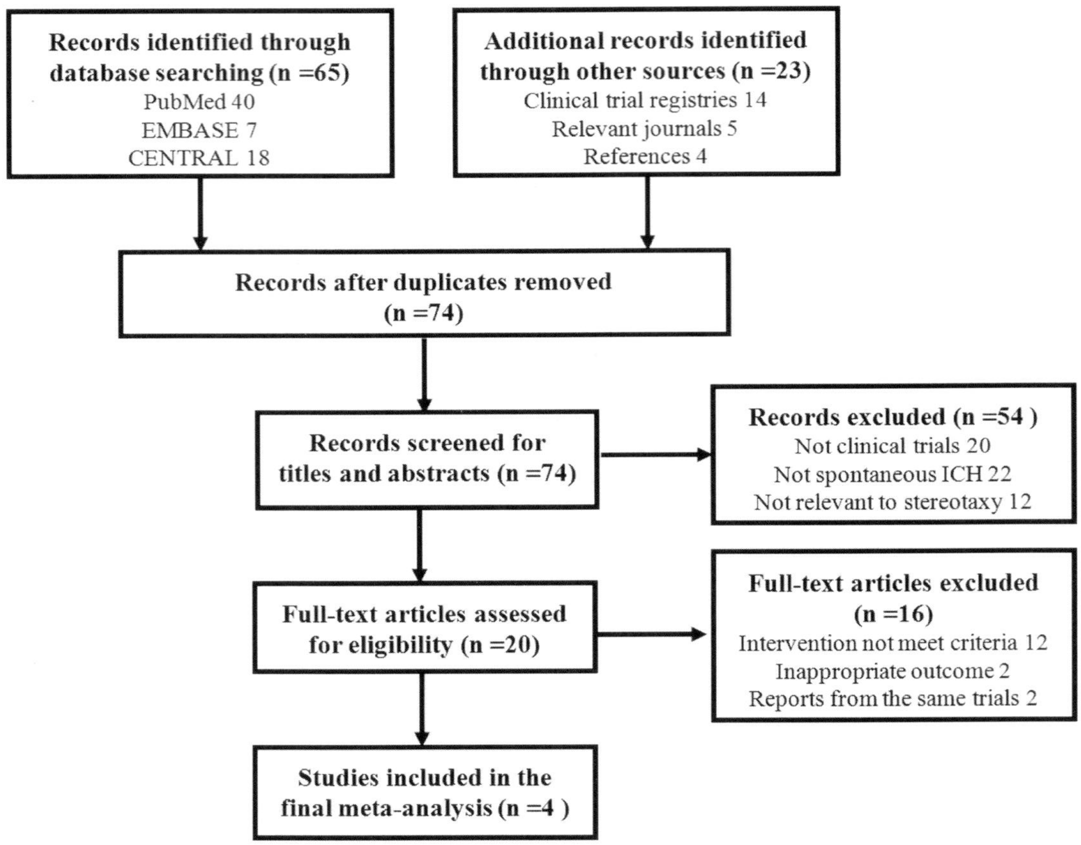

Figure 1. Flow chart of study inclusion in the present meta-analysis.

CT scanning while the control group was treated with either the conventional open craniotomy with large bone flap or the key-hole craniotomy with small bone flap. One study among these trials had three treatment arms: stereotactic aspiration, conventional open craniotomy and key-hole craniotomy [15]. And the type of craniotomy in the Cho trial was uncertain [13]. In addition, the best medical treatment was provided to all the participants in these trials. The duration of follow-up was three months for three studies [13,14,15] or twelve months for one study [16].

Risk of bias in included studies

The risk of bias within the studies was graded according to the criteria described in the Cochrane Collaboration's tool for assessing the risk of bias in randomized trials. Although the blinding of outcome assessment was not mandatory in the present study considering it was difficult in the studies of surgical intervention, there were two studies reporting that blinding was performed[14,15]. There was no loss to follow up in three trials [13,15,16] and only one trial reported one patient lost to follow-up[14]. As described in Table 1, the score of each study in every item was listed and the total scores of the four studies ranged from 4 to 6. Overall, the quality of the four included studies was acceptable.

Effect of stereotactic aspiration on death or dependence at the end of follow-up

As shown in Figure 2, there were two studies reporting the effect of stereotactic aspiration on death or dependence at the end of follow-up [14,15]. Data indicated stereotactic aspiration could significantly decrease the odds of being dead or dependent at the final follow-up in comparison with craniotomy (OR: 0.80, 95% CI: 0.69–0.93; $P = 0.004$), which was associated with statistically non-significant heterogeneity ($P = 0.68$, $I^2 = 0\%$) (Figure 2A). Furthermore, subgroup analysis based on the type of craniotomy was performed (Figure 2B and 2C), which demonstrated that there was a significant reduction in death or dependence in stereotactic aspiration compared to conventional open craniotomy ($P = 0.001$) while the difference was not significant between stereotactic aspiration and key-hole craniotomy ($P = 0.28$). When sensitivity analysis excluding Zhao study was performed, there was only one trial reporting both death and dependence at the end of follow-up, in which the number of patients in death or dependence was 90 in 159 patients treated with stereotactic aspiration while the one was 93 in 145 patients treated with craniotomy.

Effect of stereotactic aspiration on death at the end of follow-up

Data on the effect of stereotactic aspiration on death at the end of follow-up was available in each included studies (Figure 3). The pooled OR of death at the end of follow-up using stereotactic aspiration compared to craniotomy was 0.85 (95% CI: 0.72–1.02, $P = 0.08$), indicating that there was no significant difference in death between the groups treated with either stereotactic aspiration or craniotomy (Figure 3A). However, further subgroup analysis based on the type of craniotomy indicated stereotactic aspiration was associated with a statistical reduction in death

Table 1. Characteristics of the participants and quality assessment of the included trials.

Study	Baseline characteristics					Timing of surgery	Thrombolysis	Types of craniotomy in Group control	Quality assessment				
	Age (year)	Sex (M/F)	Total patients	GCS	Volume (ml)				Randomized generation	Allocation concealment	Complete outcome data	Selective reporting	Total score
Cho 2006[13]	30–70	41/19	60	9–13	≥25	<24 h	Yes	n/a	1	1	1	1	4
Sun 2010[14]	40–75	196/108	304	n/a	30–80	<72 h	Yes	Keyhole	2	2	1	1	6
Zhao 2005[15]	14–75	n/a	2464	≥5	≥30	<24 h	No	Conventional, Keyhole	1	1	1	1	4
Zhou 2011[16]	40–75	109/59	168	4–15	30–100	<24 h	Yes	Conventional	2	1	1	1	5

GCS: Glasgow coma scale; n/a: not available.

compared to conventional open craniotomy (P = 0.03, Figure 3B) while the difference was not significant when compared to key-hole craniotomy (P = 0.64, Figure 3C). Moreover, sensitivity analysis excluding Zhao study was performed to rule out the risk of selective bias. The results of sensitivity analysis demonstrated stereotactic aspiration still significantly decreased the odds of death at the final follow-up compared to craniotomy (OR: 0.58, 95% CI: 0.37–0.89; P = 0.01).

Effect of stereotactic aspiration on the total risk of complication

As described in Figure 4, each included study reported the effect of stereotactic aspiration on the total risk of complication. Data in Figure 4A indicated the pooled OR of total risk of complication using stereotactic aspiration compared to craniotomy was 0.45 (95% CI: 0.20–1.03, P = 0.06), indicating that there was no significant difference in the risk of complication between the groups treated with either stereotactic aspiration or craniotomy. However, there was statistically significant heterogeneity in the results among the studies ($P<0.00001$, $I^2 = 90\%$), which was the reason that the random-effect model was used in the statistics. Further subgroup analysis based on the type of craniotomy (Figure 4B and 4C) also showed there was no significant difference in the risk of complication between the subgroups.

Effect of stereotactic aspiration on the risks of rebleeding, GI hemorrhage and systematic infection

For the risk of intracerebral rebleeding, data was available in three included studies [13,14,16] (Figure 5). Our results indicated stereotactic aspiration could significantly decrease the odds of risk of intracerebral rebleeding in comparison with craniotomy (OR: 0.44, 95% CI: 0.26–0.74; P = 0.002), which was associated with statistically non-significant heterogeneity (P = 0.60, $I^2 = 0\%$). Furthermore, subgroup analysis based on the type of craniotomy demonstrated that there was a significant reduction in risk of rebleeding in the group treated with stereotactic aspiration compared to key-hole craniotomy (P = 0.003) while the difference was not significant when compared to other subgroups.

As shown in Figure 6, there were two trials reporting the effect of stereotactic aspiration on the risk of GI hemorrhage [14,16]. Considering that there was statistically significant heterogeneity in the results among the studies (P = 0.004, $I^2 = 88\%$), the random-effect model was used in the statistics. The pooled OR of risk of GI hemorrhage using stereotactic aspiration compared to craniotomy was 0.66 (95% CI: 0.17–2.60, P = 0.56), indicating that there was no significant difference in the risk of GI hemorrhage between the groups with different treatment (Figure 6). However, further subgroup analysis based on the type of craniotomy showed stereotactic aspiration reduced the risk of GI hemorrhage compared to conventional open craniotomy (P = 0.002).

Data on the effect of stereotactic aspiration on the systematic infection was available in three included studies [13,14,16] (Figure7). Our results indicated there was no significant difference in the risk of systematic infection between the groups treated with either stereotactic aspiration or craniotomy (OR: 1.09, 95% CI: 0.68–1.76; P = 0.72), which was associated with statistically non-significant heterogeneity (P = 0.77, $I^2 = 0\%$). Further subgroup analysis based on the type of craniotomy showed the same results.

Discussion

In the present meta-analysis of four RCTs, we investigated the effects of stereotactic aspiration on the death or dependence and the risk of complication compared to craniotomy in patients with

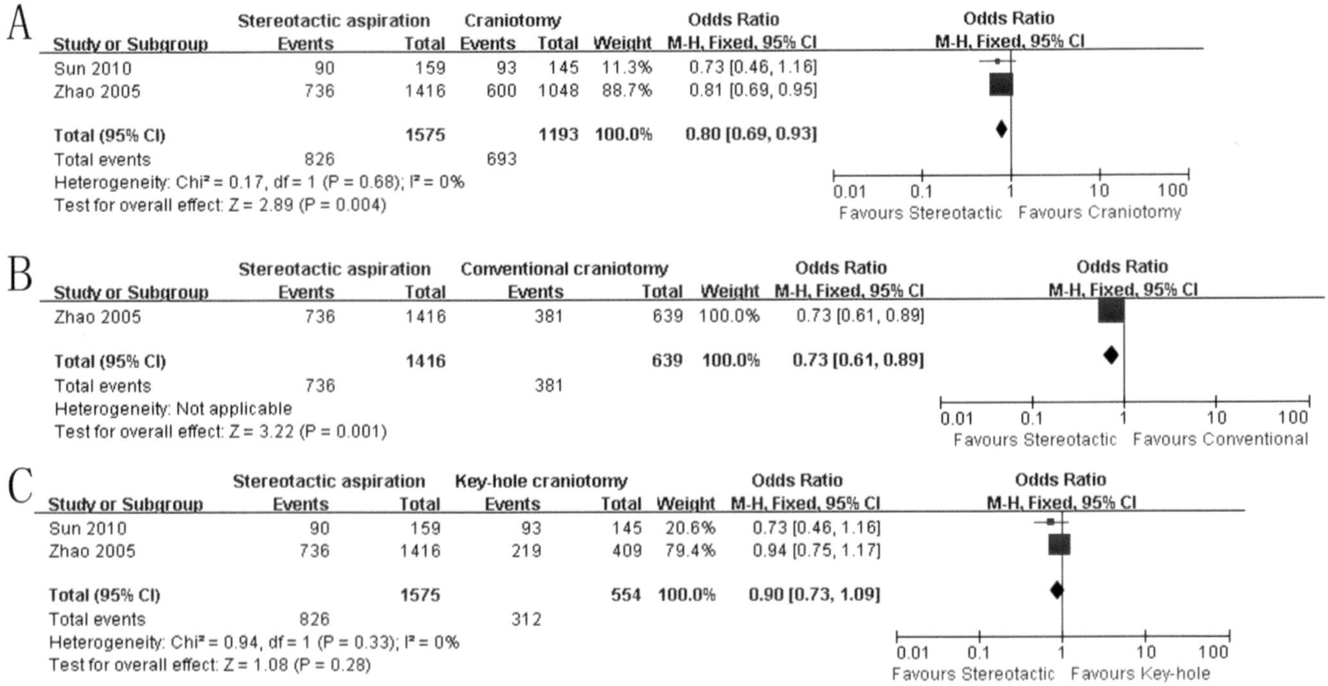

A

Study or Subgroup	Stereotactic aspiration Events	Total	Craniotomy Events	Total	Weight	Odds Ratio M-H, Fixed, 95% CI
Sun 2010	90	159	93	145	11.3%	0.73 [0.46, 1.16]
Zhao 2005	736	1416	600	1048	88.7%	0.81 [0.69, 0.95]
Total (95% CI)		**1575**		**1193**	**100.0%**	**0.80 [0.69, 0.93]**
Total events	826		693			

Heterogeneity: Chi² = 0.17, df = 1 (P = 0.68); I² = 0%
Test for overall effect: Z = 2.89 (P = 0.004)

B

Study or Subgroup	Stereotactic aspiration Events	Total	Conventional craniotomy Events	Total	Weight	Odds Ratio M-H, Fixed, 95% CI
Zhao 2005	736	1416	381	639	100.0%	0.73 [0.61, 0.89]
Total (95% CI)		**1416**		**639**	**100.0%**	**0.73 [0.61, 0.89]**
Total events	736		381			

Heterogeneity: Not applicable
Test for overall effect: Z = 3.22 (P = 0.001)

C

Study or Subgroup	Stereotactic aspiration Events	Total	Key-hole craniotomy Events	Total	Weight	Odds Ratio M-H, Fixed, 95% CI
Sun 2010	90	159	93	145	20.6%	0.73 [0.46, 1.16]
Zhao 2005	736	1416	219	409	79.4%	0.94 [0.75, 1.17]
Total (95% CI)		**1575**		**554**	**100.0%**	**0.90 [0.73, 1.09]**
Total events	826		312			

Heterogeneity: Chi² = 0.94, df = 1 (P = 0.33); I² = 0%
Test for overall effect: Z = 1.08 (P = 0.28)

Figure 2. Death or dependence between the groups. A: stereotactic aspiration versus craniotomy; B: stereotactic aspiration versus conventional open craniotomy; C: stereotactic aspiration versus key-hole craniotomy. M-H: Mantel-Haenszel.

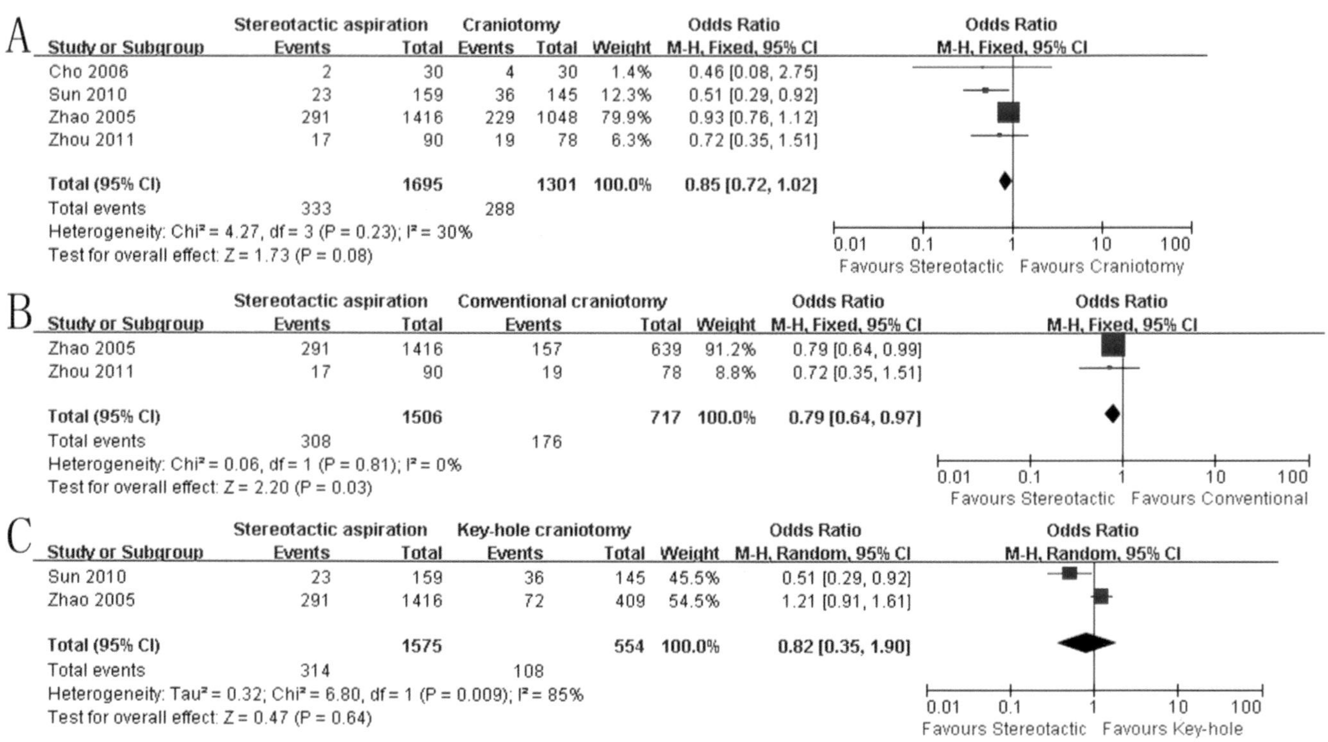

A

Study or Subgroup	Stereotactic aspiration Events	Total	Craniotomy Events	Total	Weight	Odds Ratio M-H, Fixed, 95% CI
Cho 2006	2	30	4	30	1.4%	0.46 [0.08, 2.75]
Sun 2010	23	159	36	145	12.3%	0.51 [0.29, 0.92]
Zhao 2005	291	1416	229	1048	79.9%	0.93 [0.76, 1.12]
Zhou 2011	17	90	19	78	6.3%	0.72 [0.35, 1.51]
Total (95% CI)		**1695**		**1301**	**100.0%**	**0.85 [0.72, 1.02]**
Total events	333		288			

Heterogeneity: Chi² = 4.27, df = 3 (P = 0.23); I² = 30%
Test for overall effect: Z = 1.73 (P = 0.08)

B

Study or Subgroup	Stereotactic aspiration Events	Total	Conventional craniotomy Events	Total	Weight	Odds Ratio M-H, Fixed, 95% CI
Zhao 2005	291	1416	157	639	91.2%	0.79 [0.64, 0.99]
Zhou 2011	17	90	19	78	8.8%	0.72 [0.35, 1.51]
Total (95% CI)		**1506**		**717**	**100.0%**	**0.79 [0.64, 0.97]**
Total events	308		176			

Heterogeneity: Chi² = 0.06, df = 1 (P = 0.81); I² = 0%
Test for overall effect: Z = 2.20 (P = 0.03)

C

Study or Subgroup	Stereotactic aspiration Events	Total	Key-hole craniotomy Events	Total	Weight	Odds Ratio M-H, Random, 95% CI
Sun 2010	23	159	36	145	45.5%	0.51 [0.29, 0.92]
Zhao 2005	291	1416	72	409	54.5%	1.21 [0.91, 1.61]
Total (95% CI)		**1575**		**554**	**100.0%**	**0.82 [0.35, 1.90]**
Total events	314		108			

Heterogeneity: Tau² = 0.32; Chi² = 6.80, df = 1 (P = 0.009); I² = 85%
Test for overall effect: Z = 0.47 (P = 0.64)

Figure 3. Death between the groups. A: stereotactic aspiration versus craniotomy; B: stereotactic aspiration versus conventional open craniotomy; C: stereotactic aspiration versus key-hole craniotomy. M-H: Mantel-Haenszel.

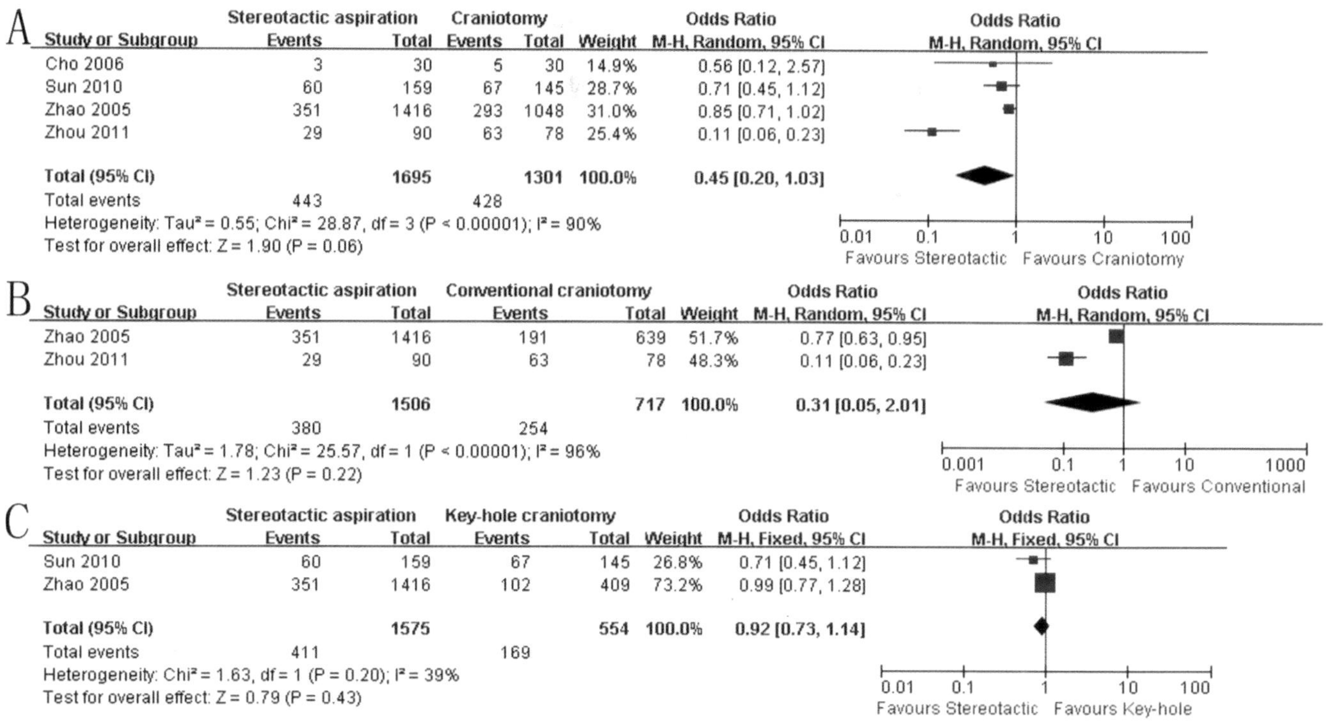

Figure 4. Total risk of complication between the groups. A: stereotactic aspiration versus craniotomy; B: stereotactic aspiration versus conventional open craniotomy; C: stereotactic aspiration versus key-hole craniotomy. M-H: Mantel-Haenszel.

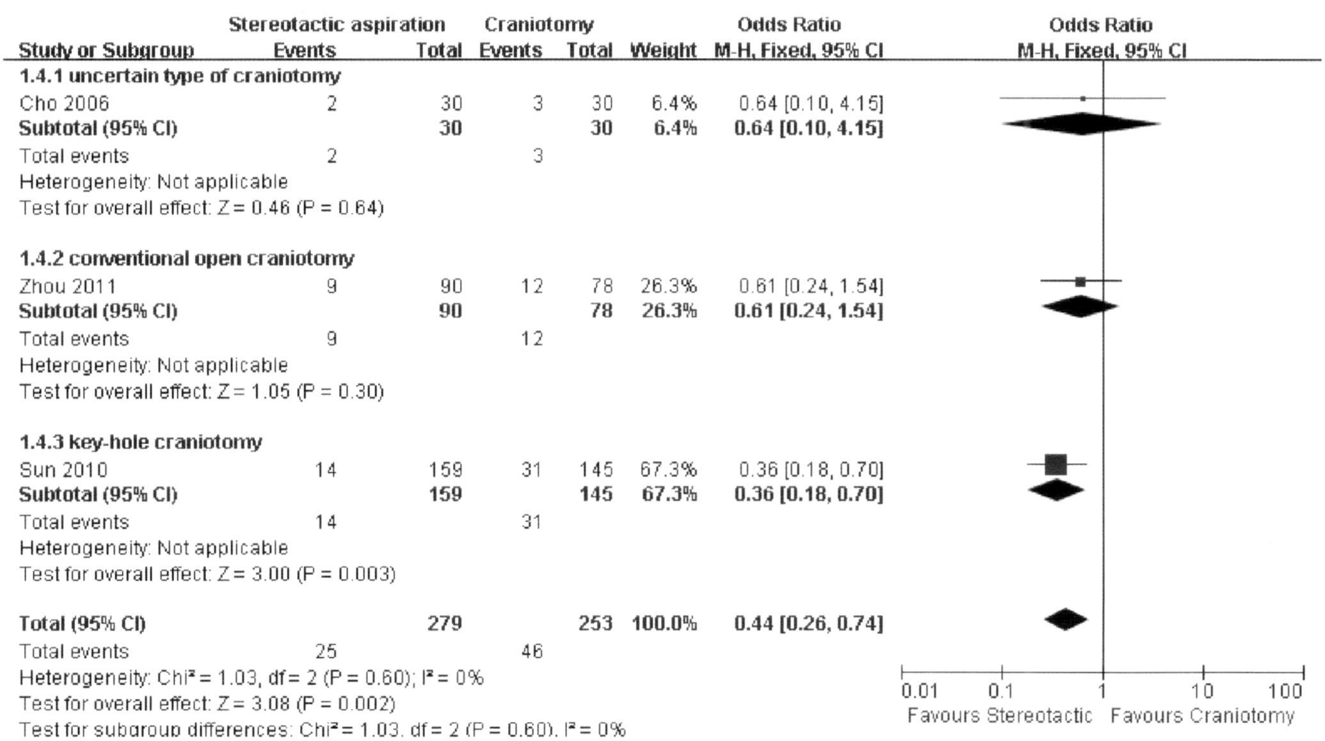

Figure 5. Risk of rebleeding between the groups based on the type of craniotomy. M-H: Mantel-Haenszel.

Study or Subgroup	Stereotactic aspiration Events	Stereotactic aspiration Total	Craniotomy Events	Craniotomy Total	Weight	Odds Ratio M-H, Random, 95% CI
1.5.1 conventional open craniotomy						
Zhou 2011	16	90	31	78	49.2%	0.33 [0.16, 0.66]
Subtotal (95% CI)		**90**		**78**	**49.2%**	**0.33 [0.16, 0.66]**
Total events	16		31			
Heterogeneity: Not applicable						
Test for overall effect: Z = 3.10 (P = 0.002)						
1.5.2 key-hole craniotomy						
Sun 2010	29	159	21	145	50.8%	1.32 [0.71, 2.43]
Subtotal (95% CI)		**159**		**145**	**50.8%**	**1.32 [0.71, 2.43]**
Total events	29		21			
Heterogeneity: Not applicable						
Test for overall effect: Z = 0.88 (P = 0.38)						
Total (95% CI)		**249**		**223**	**100.0%**	**0.66 [0.17, 2.60]**
Total events	45		52			
Heterogeneity: Tau² = 0.85; Chi² = 8.51, df = 1 (P = 0.004); I² = 88%						
Test for overall effect: Z = 0.59 (P = 0.56)						
Test for subgroup differences: Chi² = 8.51, df = 1 (P = 0.004), I² = 88.2%						

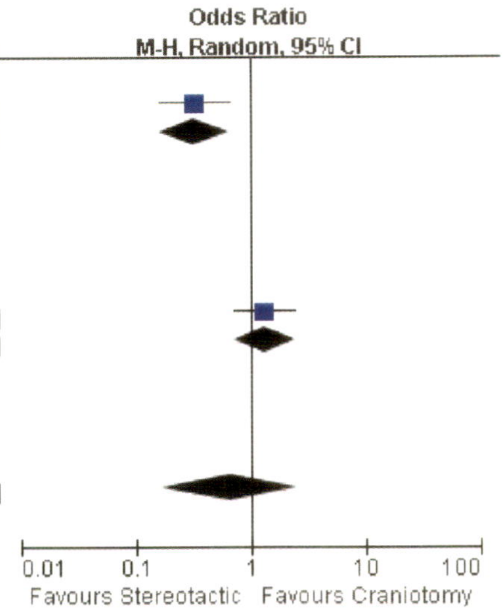

Figure 6. Risk of gastrointestinal hemorrhage between the groups based on the type of craniotomy. M-H: Mantel-Haenszel.

primary ICH. The main findings are as follows: (1) Stereotactic aspiration significantly decreased the odds of being dead or dependent in patients with primary ICH. (2) There was no significant difference in the total risk of complication between the groups with either stereotactic aspiration or craniotomy treatment. (3) The OR of the risk of rebleeding was significantly reduced by stereotactic aspiration in comparison with craniotomy. (4) Subgroup analysis based on the type of craniotomy indicated stereotactic aspiration could significantly reduce the risk of death/dependence, death and GI hemorrhage compared to conventional open craniotomy, which was also associated with the significantly decreased risk of rebleeding compared to key-hole craniotomy.

Although previous systematic reviews have reported surgical evacuation for patients with ICH is associated with a significant decrease in OR of unfavorable outcome compared to conservative treatment [7,19]. However, its evidence is not very robust and there may be a best type of surgical procedures by which patients can benefit most. Moreover, to our knowledge, previous studies

Study or Subgroup	Stereotactic aspiration Events	Stereotactic aspiration Total	Craniotomy Events	Craniotomy Total	Weight	Odds Ratio M-H, Fixed, 95% CI
1.6.1 uncertain type of craniotomy						
Cho 2006	1	30	2	30	6.0%	0.48 [0.04, 5.63]
Subtotal (95% CI)		**30**		**30**	**6.0%**	**0.48 [0.04, 5.63]**
Total events	1		2			
Heterogeneity: Not applicable						
Test for overall effect: Z = 0.58 (P = 0.56)						
1.6.2 conventional open craniotomy						
Zhou 2011	8	90	7	78	21.2%	0.99 [0.34, 2.86]
Subtotal (95% CI)		**90**		**78**	**21.2%**	**0.99 [0.34, 2.86]**
Total events	8		7			
Heterogeneity: Not applicable						
Test for overall effect: Z = 0.02 (P = 0.98)						
1.6.3 key-hole craniotomy						
Sun 2010	36	159	29	145	72.8%	1.17 [0.67, 2.03]
Subtotal (95% CI)		**159**		**145**	**72.8%**	**1.17 [0.67, 2.03]**
Total events	36		29			
Heterogeneity: Not applicable						
Test for overall effect: Z = 0.56 (P = 0.57)						
Total (95% CI)		**279**		**253**	**100.0%**	**1.09 [0.68, 1.76]**
Total events	45		38			
Heterogeneity: Chi² = 0.52, df = 2 (P = 0.77); I² = 0%						
Test for overall effect: Z = 0.36 (P = 0.72)						
Test for subgroup differences: Chi² = 0.52, df = 2 (P = 0.77), I² = 0%						

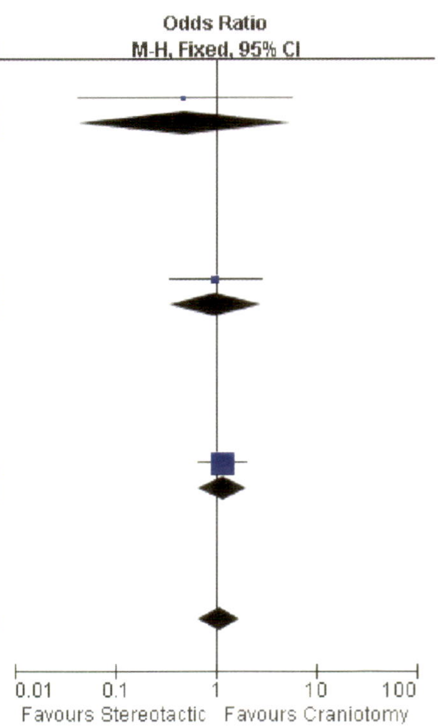

Figure 7. Risk of systematic infection between the groups based on the type of craniotomy. M-H: Mantel-Haenszel.

about the stereotactic aspiration are mainly compared with conservative treatment [8,20]. There is little known about the difference in the treatment benefit between the stereotactic aspiration and craniotomy that are the two commonly used surgical procedures in the treatment of ICH. Thus, our study provides a timely and substantial evidence for the clinicians in the selection of appropriate procedures.

Death or dependence for help from other people in ADLs was chosen as the primary outcome measure in the present meta-analysis for several reasons. First, in the context of critical illness such as ICH, death or dependence is a clinically relevant outcome that is of immediate importance to patients, and data on death or dependence is reported in many of the studies. Furthermore, considering clinicians would like to know whether survivors are functionally dependent or independent in ADLs and death alone may be inadequate, thus death or dependence instead of death alone is used. Finally, we may expect data on death or dependence in ADLs would be less prone to measurement error or biased reporting compared to the data on pathophysiological outcomes. The pathophysiological end-points are usually used as surrogates for the adverse outcome because we may assume a direct relationship between them. However, assumption may sometimes be inappropriate. And when trials collect data on a number of physiological end-points, there is the potential for bias due to the selective publication of end-points showing striking treatment effects [21].

This review includes the larger number of patients and the internal validity of the results, which are the main strengths of this review. There is non-significant heterogeneity ($P = 0.68$, $I^2 = 0\%$) between the studies for the primary outcome of death or dependence. Although data on dependence were lacked in the Cho and Zhou study in the present meta-analysis, functional status based on scales such as Barthel Index (BI) at the end of follow-up was reported, which indicated stereotactic aspiration could significant improve the BI compared to the craniotomy. Moreover, data on death in both studies also showed there was a decrease in mortality in the groups treated with stereotactic aspiration compared to the craniotomy. Therefore, we have reason to expect that the primary outcome in the Cho and Zhou study was statistically better in the stereotactic aspiration group than the one in the craniotomy group, which is consistent with the conclusion of this review.

As we all know, adverse effects are as important as the efficacy of the interventions in clinical trials. Thus, we also compared the complications in our meta-analysis to enable clinicians to use our results to make fully informed choices. Our data indicated there was no significant difference in the total risk of complication between the groups with either stereotactic aspiration or craniotomy treatment. However, further analysis based on the type of complication revealed stereotactic aspiration could significant reduce the risk of re-bleeding compared to craniotomy. Moreover, previous studies have demonstrated that rebleeding can significantly increase the risk of unfavorable outcomes in patients with ICH [22], which is compatible with our data showing that reduced risk of rebleeding with stereotactic aspiration treatment is associated with decreased risk of death or dependence. In addition, we should keep in mind that the intervention time from onset of hemorrhage to surgery is also an important factor in rebleeding because the acute stage after ICH onset is prone to rebleeding [23]. As described in Table 1, the intervention time in the four included trials is within 24 h or 72 h and we are lack of the individual patient data. Thus the analysis based on the intervention time is not performed in the present meta-analysis, which may be beneficial to understand the role of intervention time in the risk of rebleeding.

There are some limitations in the present study. First, although we have attempted to bring together all relevant RCTs in this meta-analysis and a total of 2996 participants have been enrolled in the four trials, a few unpublished studies may be missed. Second, there are differences in the admission GCS and the age of patients between groups in the Zhao study, which are the potential factors of the outcome for ICH. In the present study, in order to rule out the risk of bias from the inclusion of the Zhao study, sensitivity analysis excluding Zhao study was further performed. And the results of sensitivity analysis demonstrated stereotactic aspiration still significantly decreased the odds of death at the final follow-up compared to craniotomy. In addition, there are other reported adverse effects such as seizure, which are not described and analyzed in detail in this article considering these adverse effects are not commonly reported and the data are relatively lack.

In conclusion, the present meta-analysis provides evidence that the stereotactic aspiration may be associated with a reduction in the odds of being dead or dependent compared to craniotomy in primary spontaneous intracerebral hemorrhage, which should be interpreted with caution. Further trials are needed to identify those patients most likely to benefit from the stereotactic aspiration.

Author Contributions

Conceived and designed the experiments: JWW QHZ. Performed the experiments: JWW JPL YLS KT Yu Wang TL PG XL Yan Wang. Analyzed the data: JWW JPL YLS KT Yu Wang TL PG XL Yan Wang. Contributed reagents/materials/analysis tools: JWW. Wrote the paper: JWW QHZ.

References

1. van Asch CJ, Luitse MJ, Rinkel GJ, van der Tweel I, Algra A, et al. (2010) Incidence, case fatality, and functional outcome of intracerebral haemorrhage over time, according to age, sex, and ethnic origin: a systematic review and meta-analysis. Lancet Neurol 9: 167–176.
2. Morgenstern LB, Hemphill JR, Anderson C, Becker K, Broderick JP, et al. (2010) Guidelines for the management of spontaneous intracerebral hemorrhage: a guideline for healthcare professionals from the American Heart Association/American Stroke Association. Stroke 41: 2108–2129.
3. Sacco S, Marini C, Toni D, Olivieri L, Carolei A (2009) Incidence and 10-year survival of intracerebral hemorrhage in a population-based registry. Stroke 40: 394–399.
4. Adeoye O, Broderick JP (2010) Advances in the management of intracerebral hemorrhage. Nature Reviews Neurology 6: 593–601.
5. Rincon F, Mayer SA (2008) Clinical review: Critical care management of spontaneous intracerebral hemorrhage. Crit Care 12: 237.
6. Kelly ML, Sulmasy DP, Weil RJ (2013) Spontaneous intracerebral hemorrhage and the challenge of surgical decision making: a review. Neurosurg Focus 34: E1.
7. Mendelow AD, Gregson BA, Rowan EN, Murray GD, Gholkar A, et al. (2013) Early surgery versus initial conservative treatment in patients with spontaneous supratentorial lobar intracerebral haematomas (STICH II): a randomised trial. Lancet 382: 397–408.
8. Ramanan M, Shankar A (2013) Minimally invasive surgery for primary supratentorial intracerebral haemorrhage. J Clin Neurosci 20: 1650–1658.
9. Staykov D, Huttner HB, Kohrmann M, Bardutzky J, Schellinger PD (2010) Novel approaches to the treatment of intracerebral haemorrhage. Int J Stroke 5: 457–465.

10. Umebayashi D, Mandai A, Osaka Y, Nakahara Y, Tenjin H (2010) Effects and complications of stereotactic aspiration for spontaneous intracerebral hemorrhage. Neurol Med Chir (Tokyo) 50: 538–544.
11. Carhuapoma JR, Barrett RJ, Keyl PM, Hanley DF, Johnson RR (2008) Stereotactic aspiration-thrombolysis of intracerebral hemorrhage and its impact on perihematoma brain edema. Neurocrit Care 8: 322–329.
12. Gaab MR (2011) Intracerebral hemorrhage (ICH) and intraventricular hemorrhage (IVH): improvement of bad prognosis by minimally invasive neurosurgery. World Neurosurg 75: 206–208.
13. Cho DY, Chen CC, Chang CS, Lee WY, Tso M (2006) Endoscopic surgery for spontaneous basal ganglia hemorrhage: comparing endoscopic surgery, stereotactic aspiration, and craniotomy in noncomatose patients. Surg Neurol 65: 547–556.
14. Sun H, Liu H, Li D, Liu L, Yang J, et al. (2010) An effective treatment for cerebral hemorrhage: minimally invasive craniopuncture combined with urokinase infusion therapy. Neurol Res 32: 371–377.
15. Zhao JZ, Zhou DB, Zhou LF, Wang RZ, Wang DJ, et al. (2005) The efficacy of three different approaches in treatment of hypertensive intracerebral hemorrhage: a multi-center single-blind study of 2464 patients. Zhonghua Yi Xue Za Zhi 85: 2238–2242.
16. Zhou H, Zhang Y, Liu L, Han X, Tao Y, et al. (2011) A prospective controlled study: minimally invasive stereotactic puncture therapy versus conventional craniotomy in the treatment of acute intracerebral hemorrhage. BMC Neurol 11: 76.
17. Shih MM, Rogers JC, Skidmore ER, Irrgang JJ, Holm MB (2009) Measuring stroke survivors' functional status independence: five perspectives. Am J Occup Ther 63: 600–608.
18. Balu S (2009) Differences in psychometric properties, cut-off scores, and outcomes between the Barthel Index and Modified Rankin Scale in pharmacotherapy-based stroke trials: systematic literature review. Curr Med Res Opin 25: 1329–1341.
19. Prasad K, Mendelow AD, Gregson B (2008) Surgery for primary supratentorial intracerebral haemorrhage. Cochrane Database Syst Rev: D200.
20. Zhou X, Chen J, Li Q, Ren G, Yao G, et al. (2012) Minimally invasive surgery for spontaneous supratentorial intracerebral hemorrhage: a meta-analysis of randomized controlled trials. Stroke 43: 2923–2930.
21. Bunn F, Roberts I, Tasker R, Akpa E (2004) Hypertonic versus near isotonic crystalloid for fluid resuscitation in critically ill patients. Cochrane Database Syst Rev: D2045.
22. Wang KW, Cho CL, Chen HJ, Liang CL, Liliang PC, et al. (2011) Molecular biomarker of inflammatory response is associated with rebleeding in spontaneous intracerebral hemorrhage. Eur Neurol 66: 322–327.
23. Ovesen C, Christensen AF, Krieger DW, Rosenbaum S, Havsteen I, et al. (2014) Time course of early postadmission hematoma expansion in spontaneous intracerebral hemorrhage. Stroke 45: 994–999.

18

Comparison of Robotic Surgery with Laparoscopy and Laparotomy for Treatment of Endometrial Cancer

Longke Ran[1,2], Jing Jin[1], Yan Xu[3], Youquan Bu[2], Fangzhou Song[2]*

1 Department of Bioinformatics, Chongqing Medical University, Chongqing, China, **2** Molecular Medicine and Cancer Research Center, Chongqing Medical University, Chongqing, China, **3** Department of Obstetrics and Gynecology, Southwest Hospital, Third Military Medical University, Chongqing, China

Abstract

Purpose: To compare the relative merits among robotic surgery, laparoscopy, and laparotomy for patients with endometrial cancer by conducting a meta-analysis.

Methods: The MEDLINE, Embase, PubMed, Web of Science, and Cochrane Library databases were searched. Studies clearly documenting a comparison between robotic surgery and laparoscopy or between robotic surgery and laparotomy for endometrial cancer were selected. The outcome measures included operating time (OT), number of complications, length of hospital stay (LOHS), estimated blood loss (EBL), number of transfusions, total lymph nodes harvested (TLNH), and number of conversions. Pooled odds ratios and weighted mean differences with 95% confidence intervals were calculated using either a fixed-effects or random-effects model.

Results: Twenty-two studies were included in the meta-analysis. These studies involved a total of 4420 patients, 3403 of whom underwent both robotic surgery and laparoscopy and 1017 of whom underwent both robotic surgery and laparotomy. The EBL ($p = 0.01$) and number of conversions ($p = 0.0008$) were significantly lower and the number of complications ($p < 0.0001$) was significantly higher in robotic surgery than in laparoscopy. The OT, LOHS, number of transfusions, and TLNH showed no significant differences between robotic surgery and laparoscopy. The number of complications ($p < 0.00001$), LOHS ($p < 0.00001$), EBL ($p < 0.00001$), and number of transfusions ($p = 0.03$) were significantly lower and the OT ($p < 0.00001$) was significantly longer in robotic surgery than in laparotomy. The TLNH showed no significant difference between robotic surgery and laparotomy.

Conclusions: Robotic surgery is generally safer and more reliable than laparoscopy and laparotomy for patients with endometrial cancer. Robotic surgery is associated with significantly lower EBL than both laparoscopy and laparotomy; fewer conversions but more complications than laparoscopy; and shorter LOHS, fewer complications, and fewer transfusions but a longer OT than laparoscopy. Further studies are required.

Editor: Shannon M. Hawkins, Baylor College of Medicine, United States of America

Funding: This work was supported by grants from the National Natural Science Foundation of China (Nos. 81101994 and 81072125). The funders had no role in study design, data collection and analysis, decision to publish, or preparation of the manuscript.

Competing Interests: The authors have declared that no competing interests exist.

* Email: fzsongcq@126.com

Introduction

Endometrial carcinoma is the most common female genital tract malignancy in Western countries [1]. It is also the most common gynecologic cancer overall; 1 of every 40 women worldwide will develop endometrial cancer. Surgery is a major component of the diagnosis and treatment of endometrial cancer. Endometrial cancer is increasingly being treated with more minimally invasive approaches, including laparoscopy [2]. However, these minimally invasive approaches to the treatment of endometrial cancer have been limited due to long operation times (OTs), safety considerations, and other factors [3–5]. Thus, robotic surgery, the most novel minimally invasive technique, was developed to help overcome the technical limitations of laparoscopy and laparotomy. This technique enables surgeons to more easily perform complex procedures through improved visualization, more accurate instrument control, and improved ease of use of instruments [3]. Reza *et al.* [4] found that robot-assisted hysterectomy was associated with a longer OT but shorter length of hospital stay (LOHS), lower estimated blood loss (EBL), and fewer transfusions and complications than was open surgery. O'Neill *et al.* [5] showed that robot-assisted hysterectomy offers benefits with respect to a shorter LOHS and fewer blood transfusions than seen with open surgery.

However, the laparoscopic approach is reportedly a feasible alternative to conventional surgical treatment in patients with endometrial carcinoma [6]. Whether robotic surgery is superior to laparoscopy or laparotomy remains unclear. Therefore, the present meta-analysis compared the outcomes of the three currently used surgical approaches in patients with endometrial cancer: robotic surgery, laparoscopy, and laparotomy.

Materials and Methods

Literature search

The electronic databases of PubMed, MEDLINE, EMBASE, Web of Science, and the Cochrane Library were searched to identify eligible English-language publications (from January 1990 to September 2013). The following text and key words were used in the search: "laparoscopy and laparotomy," "robotic-assisted with laparotomy," "robotic versus open," "robotic versus laparoscopic," "robotics versus laparoscopy," "robotics or laparoscopy," "robotics and laparotomy," "robotic versus laparotomy," and "robotic-assisted laparoscopy, laparoscopy, and laparotomy" in combination with "endometrial cancer." Logical combinations of these and related terms were used to maximize sensitivity. Finally, additional relevant articles were identified by searching the references of eligible articles.

Selection criteria

The inclusion criteria for this meta-analysis were analysis of either a retrospective or prospective cohort; comparison of robotic surgery with laparoscopy or laparotomy for treatment of endometrial cancer; evaluation of the following six outcomes: OT, number of complications, LOHS, EBL, number of transfusions, total lymph nodes harvested (TLNH), and number of conversions; and clear documentation of the surgical techniques being compared (either "robotic" and "laparoscopy" or "robotic" and "laparotomy"). When the same institution reported more than one study, either the higher-quality or most recent publication was included in the analysis to avoid including the same patients.

The exclusion criteria for this meta-analysis were as follows: the above-mentioned outcomes of interest were not reported for the two techniques or it was impossible to calculate these outcomes from the published results, it was impossible to extract the appropriate data from the published results, neither the surgical outcomes nor patient parameters were clearly reported, and patients with endometrial cancer were not evaluated.

Data extraction and quality assessment

Data extraction was carried out by two reviewers (L.R. and J.J.), and quality assessment was performed by another two reviewers (Y.X. and F.S.). Any disagreements were resolved by discussion between the reviewers. For continuous variables, the sample size, mean, and standard deviation (SD) were calculated. For dichotomous variables, the total number of patients in each group and the number of patients with each outcome of interest were calculated. Some studies reported median rather than mean values and range or interquartile range rather than SD; in such cases, the mean and SD were estimated [7]. Studies that gave no information on the SD or range were excluded from the meta-analysis. The study quality was assessed using the criteria developed by the Newcastle–Ottawa Scale (NOS) for quality assessment [8].

Statistical analysis

The meta-analysis was performed using Review Manager (version 5.1.4; Copenhagen: The Nordic Cochrane Centre, The Cochrane Collaboration, 2008) and Stata (version 11.2; StataCorp LP; College Station, TX, USA) software. All test results were considered to be statistically significant at $p<0.05$. We analyzed dichotomous variables by estimating odds ratios with their 95% confidence interval (95% CI) and continuous variables using the weighted mean difference (WMD) with the 95% CI. The pooled effect was calculated using either a random-effects or fixed-effects model. Heterogeneity was evaluated with χ^2 and I^2 values. We considered significant heterogeneity to be present when χ^2 was within the 10% level of significance ($p<0.10$) and the I^2 statistic was>50%. If the I^2 statistic was>50%, indicating significant heterogeneity, the random-effects model was used. Otherwise, the fixed-effects model was used. Possible publication bias was assessed by Begg's funnel plots and Egger's regression test.

Results

In total, 540 studies were identified and screened for retrieval using the above-described strategy. After screening the title or abstract, 475 studies were excluded and 79 were retrieved and evaluated in detail. Fifty-seven of these studies met the exclusion criteria, and 22 satisfied the selection criteria and were included in this meta-analysis (Fig. 1).

The patients' demographic and clinical characteristics are depicted in Table 1. The majority of studies (16/22, 72%) were carried out in the United States; there was one study each from Switzerland, Korea, Turkey, Spain, France, and Italy. Of all 22 studies, 8 compared robotic surgery and laparoscopy [9–16], 6 compared robotic surgery and laparotomy [17–22], and 8 compared robotic surgery, laparoscopy, and laparotomy [2,19,21,23–27]. The 8 studies that compared robotic surgery and laparoscopy included 3403 participants (1822 who underwent robotic surgery and 1581 who underwent laparoscopy). The 6 studies that compared robotic surgery and laparotomy included 1017 participants (445 who underwent robotic surgery and 572 who underwent laparotomy).

Quality assessment

The present review evaluated no randomized controlled trials; all included studies were retrospective or prospective studies. The study characteristics and participant features are given in Table 1. The main characteristics of the 22 studies were assessed using the NOS. All studies scored moderately well on the NOS. A score of 7

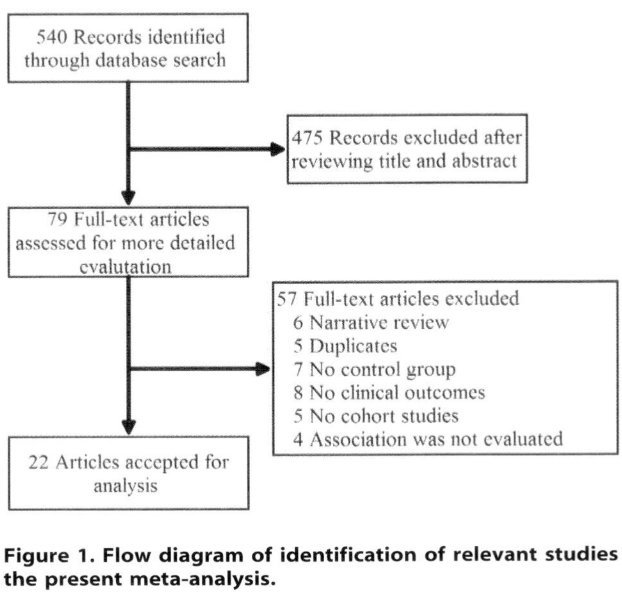

Figure 1. Flow diagram of identification of relevant studies in the present meta-analysis.

Table 1. Patient demographic and clinical characteristics.

First Author, Year(Ref.#)	Study type	Country	No.of patients			Mean age(year)			Outcomes meased
			RS	LS	OS	RS	LS	OS	
Veljovich et al., 2008	Prospective cohort	USA	25	4	131	59.5	54	63	BMI,OT,EBL,LOHS,complications, uterine weight
Boggess et al., 2008	Prospective cohort	USA	108	81	138	61.9	62.0	64.0	BMI,OT,LOHS,conversion,EBL,total nodes,stage,complication,transfusion
Bell et al.,2008	Retrospective cohort	USA	40	30	40	63.0	68.4	72.3	BMI,OT,EBL,TLNH,Uterine weight,average cost,LOHS
DeNardis et al., 2008	Retrospective cohort	USA	56	-	106	58.9	-	6.5	BMI,FIGO stage,Grade,OT,EBL,LOHS,Transfusion rate,TLNH
Magrina et al., 2008	Prospective cohort	USA	27	31	35	50	31	35	BMI,OT,EBL, LOHS,FIGO stage,transfusion,readmission, TLNH
Seamon[1] et al.,2009	Prospective cohort	USA	32	17	14	55.0	52.8	42.0	BMI,FIGO stage,OT,EBL,TLNH,Surgical margins,Depth of invasion,complications,transfusions,LOHS,Follow-up,Survival status
Seamon[2] et al.,2009	Prospective cohort	USA	92	-	162	58	-	62	BMI,TLNH,conversion,transfusion,complications,OT,LOHS
Hoekstra1 et al.,2009	Prospective cohort	USA	32	7	26	62	59	56	BMI,Grade,Stage,OT,EBL,TLNH,LOHS,Conversion,Complications
Cardenas-Goicoechea et al.,2010	Retrospective cohort	USA	102	173	-	62	59.6	-	BMI,Tumor type,TLNH,Uterine weight,FIGO stage,Surgical time,Conversion,Blood transfusion,Estimated blood loss,LOHS
Sarlos et al., 2010	Prospective cohort	Switzerland	40	40	-	47	43.6	-	BMI,OT,EBL,Uterus weight,LOHS,Wound infection,Personnel costs
Jung et al.,2010	Prospective cohort	Korea	28	25	56	52.89	49.88	50.20	BMI,OT,Uterine weight,TLNH,Conversion, Overall complications,Transfusion,FIGO stage,LOHS
Göçmen et al., 2010	Prospective cohort	Turkey	10	-	12	55.7	-	56.4	BMI,EBL,Histology,FIGO stage,OT,conversions,LOHS,transfusion, complication,TLNH
Lim et al.,2010	Prospective cohort	USA	56	56	-	62.5	61.4	-	BMI,OT,EBL,TLNH,LOHS
Subramaniam et al., 2011	Retrospective cohort	USA	73	-	104	57	-	61.3	BMI,Grade,Uterine weight,TLNH,OT,EBL,LOHS,Wound complications,30 Day mortality
Goel et al.,2011	Retrospective clinical data	USA	59	-	38	66.5	-	59.5	BMI,OT,TLNH,EBL,Weight of uterus,FIGO stage,LOHS,Grade
Martino et al., 2011	Retrospective cohort	USA	101	114	-	61.8	63.6	-	BMI,Stage,TLNH,Total drug interventions
Coronado et al.,2012	Retrospective cohort	Spain	71	84	192	67.3	65.9	64.7	BMI,Grade,Stage,TLNH,OT,EBL,transfusions,conversion, complications,LOHS,Intra-operative
ElSahwi et al., 2012	Retrospective cohort	USA	155	-	150	62.4	-	65	BMI,LOHS,Stage,Grade,Uterine weight,TLNH,EBL,OT, Conversion
Venkat et al., 2012	Retrospective cohort	USA	27	27	-	58.2	60.2	-	BMI,Height,Weight,Hypertension,Smoker,TLNH,Uterine weight,LOSH,EBL,Stage,Grade,histology
Wright et al., 2012	Perspective	USA	1437	1027	-	-	-	-	Complication,Transfusion,LOHS,hospital cost

Table 1. Cont.

First Author, Year(Ref.#)	Study type	Country	No.of patients			Mean age(year)			Outcomes meased
			RS	LS	OS	RS	LS	OS	
Seror et al.,2013	Retrospective cohort	France	40	106	-	66.27	66.91	-	BMI,Height,Weight,Hypertension,Hereditary history,OT,LOHS,Transfusion,FIGO stage,Complications
Fagotti et al., 2013	Retrospective case-controlled	Italy	19	38	-	62.0	61.9	-	BMI,OT,EBL,LOHS,complications

BMI(kg/m2):body mass index;OT(min):operating time; EBL(ml):estimated blood loss; FIGO: International Federation of Gynecology and Obstetrics;LOHS(h):length of hospital stay;TLNH(%): total lymph nodes harvested;RS:robotic surgery;LS: laparoscopy surgery;OS: open surgery;-:not available;

was attained by eight studies [11,13,18,19,25–27], a score of 8 was attained by seven studies [10,12,14–16,20,22], and a score of 9 was attained by seven studies [2,9,17,21,23,24,28].

Publication bias

Funnel plot analysis was performed for those studies that compared the numbers of overall complications, conversions, and transfusions between robotic surgery and laparoscopy. None of the studies lay outside the limits of the 95% CIs, and there was no evidence of publication bias among the studies (Fig. 2). The funnel plot for robotic surgery versus laparotomy showed no publication bias because there were no studies with a smaller mean difference (0–50) or higher variability (SE 16–20).

Operative outcomes of robotic surgery versus laparoscopy

OT. Thirteen studies showed no statistically significant differences in OT between robotic surgery and laparoscopy. Analysis of the pooled results also showed that the two types of surgery did not significantly differ in this regard (WMD, 10.19; 95% CI, −12.30–32.68; $p = 0.37$) (Fig. 3A).

Complications. Twelve studies showed a significantly higher number of complications in robotic surgery than in laparoscopy. Analysis of the pooled results also showed that the number of complications was significantly lower in robotic surgery than in laparoscopy (OR, 0.62; 95% CI, 0.50–0.77; $p<0.0001$) (Fig. 3B).

LOHS. Twelve studies showed no significant difference in LOHS between robotic surgery and laparoscopy. Analysis of the pooled results also showed that the two types of surgery did not significantly differ in this regard (WMD, −0.23; 95% CI, −0.47–0.02; $p = 0.07$) (Fig. 3C).

EBL. Ten studies showed significantly lower EBL in robotic surgery than in laparoscopy. Analysis of the pooled results also showed significantly lower EBL in robotic surgery than in laparoscopy (WMD, −59.67; 95% CI, −107.41–11.94; $p = 0.01$) (Fig. 3D).

Transfusion. Nine studies showed no significant difference in the number of transfusions between robotic surgery and laparoscopy. Analysis of the pooled results also showed that the two types of surgery did not significantly differ in this regard (OR, 0.60; 95% CI, 0.34–1.08; $p = 0.09$) (Fig. 3E).

TLNH. Seven studies showed no significant difference in the TLNH between robotic surgery and laparoscopy. Analysis of the pooled results also showed that the two types of surgery did not significantly differ in this regard (WMD, −1.71; 95% CI, −6.61–3.19; $p = 0.49$) (Fig. 3F).

Conversions. Seven studies showed significantly fewer conversions in robotic surgery than in laparoscopy. Analysis of the pooled results also showed that the number of conversions was significantly lower in robotic surgery than in laparoscopy (OR, 0.38; 95% CI, 0.21–0.67; $p = 0.0008$) (Fig. 3G).

Operative outcomes of robotic surgery versus laparotomy

OT. Thirteen studies showed that the OT was significantly longer in robotic surgery than in laparotomy. Analysis of the pooled results also showed that the OT was significantly longer in robotic surgery than in laparotomy (WMD, 53.69; 95% CI, 32.7–74.68; $p<0.00001$) (Fig. 4A).

Complications. Fourteen studies showed significantly fewer complications in robotic surgery than in laparotomy. Analysis of the pooled results also showed significantly fewer complications in robotic surgery than in laparotomy (WMD, 0.26; 95% CI, 0.17–0.41; $p<0.00001$) (Fig. 4B).

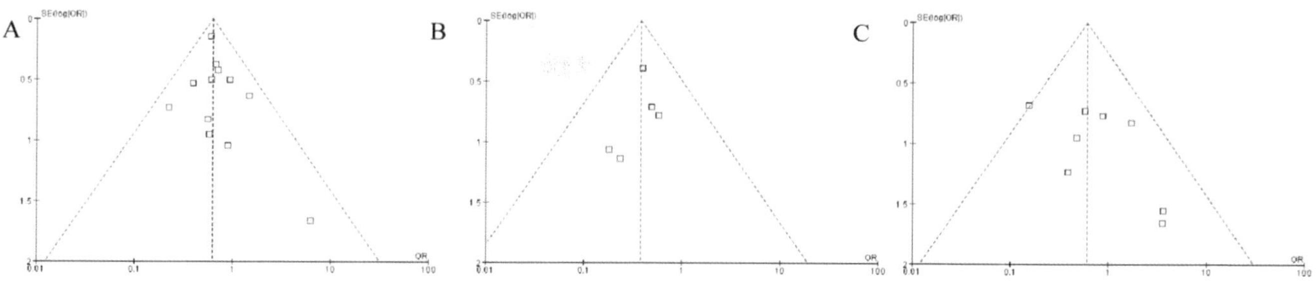

Figure 2. Funnel plot for main operative outcomes (complications, conversions, and transfusions) among all studies that compared robotic surgery and laparoscopy. (A) Publication bias regarding complications (Begg's test: $Z = 0.48$, $p = 0.63$; Egger's test: $t = 1.03$, $p = 0.032$). (B) Publication bias regarding conversions (Begg's test: $Z = 1.22$, $p = 0.022$; Egger's test: $t = -1.64$, $p = 0.20$). (C) Publication bias regarding transfusions (Begg's test: $Z = 0.62$, $p = 0.54$; Egger's test: $t = 1.55$, $p = 0.17$).

LOHS. Twelve studies showed that the LOHS was significantly shorter in robotic surgery than in laparotomy. Analysis of the pooled results also showed that the LOHS was significantly shorter in robotic surgery than in laparotomy (WMD, −2.78; 95% CI, −3.28 to −2.29; p<0.00001) (Fig. 4C).

EBL. Eleven studies showed significantly lower EBL in robotic surgery than in laparotomy. Analysis of the pooled results also showed significantly lower EBL in robotic surgery than in laparotomy (WMD, −130.41; 95% CI, −168.87 to −91.95; p< 0.00001) (Fig. 4D).

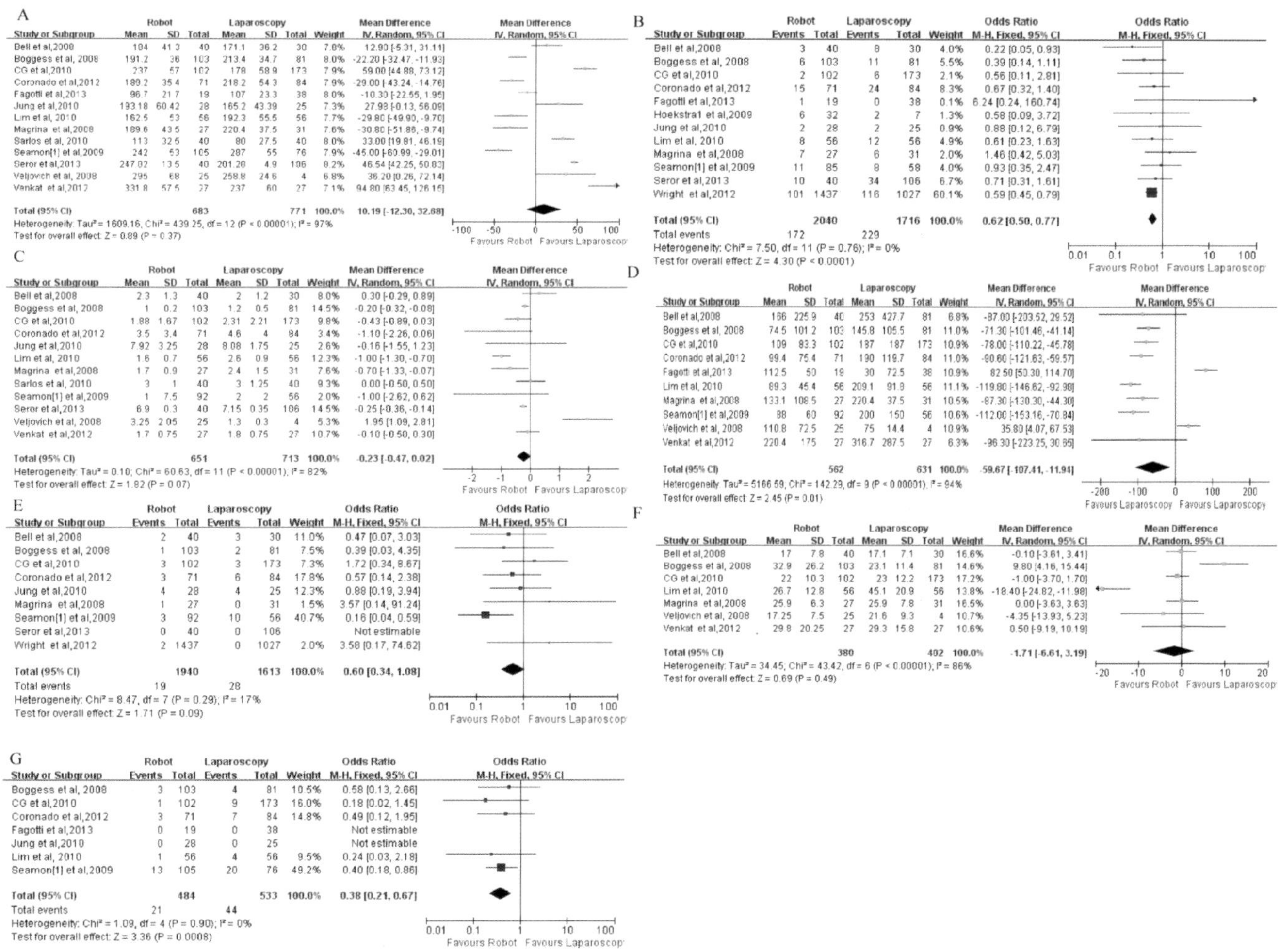

Figure 3. Comparison of robotic surgery and laparoscopy with respect to (A) operating time, (B) complications, (C) length of hospital stay, (D) estimated blood loss, (E) transfusions, (F) total number of lymph nodes harvested, and (G) conversions. OR: odds ratio; WMD: weighted mean difference.

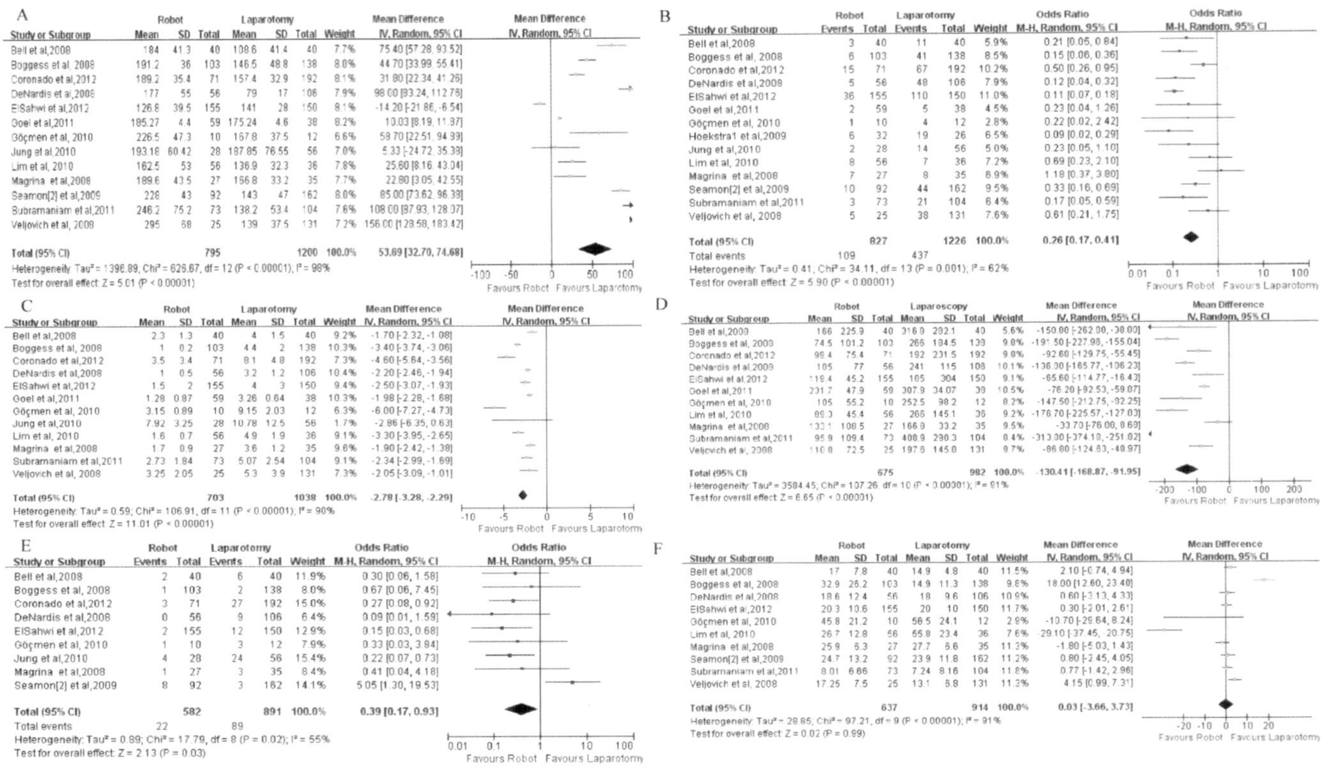

Figure 4. Comparison of robotic surgery and laparotomy with respect to (A) operating time, (B) complications, (C) length of hospital stay, (D) estimated blood loss, (E) transfusions, and (F) total number of lymph nodes harvested. OR: odds ratio; WMD: weighted mean difference.

Transfusion. Nine studies showed significantly fewer transfusions in robotic surgery than in laparotomy. Analysis of the pooled results also showed significantly fewer transfusions in robotic surgery than in laparotomy (WMD, 0.39; 95% CI, 0.17–0.93; p = 0.03) (Fig. 4E).

TLNH. Ten studies showed no significant difference in TLNH between robotic surgery and laparotomy. Analysis of the pooled results also showed that the two types of surgery did not differ in this regard (WMD, 0.03; 95% CI, −3.66–3.73; p = 0.99) (Fig. 4F).

Discussion

Surgical management has long been the primary therapy for endometrial cancer. Multiple surgical approaches to endometrial cancer have been available since newly developed methods of minimally invasive surgery were introduced. The choice of the most appropriate surgical method is becoming increasingly more important with growth in the obese and morbidly obese populations. To the best of our knowledge, this is the first comprehensive meta-analysis to compare robotic surgery with both laparoscopy and laparotomy for treatment of endometrial cancer. The results of this study show that robotic surgery is superior to laparotomy in terms of the number of complications, LOHS, EBL, and number of transfusions but is inferior to laparotomy in terms of the OT. Additionally, robotic surgery is superior to laparoscopy in terms of the EBL and number of conversions but is generally equivalent to laparoscopy in terms of the OT, number of complications, LOHS, and number of transfusions.

Robotic surgery may offer benefits over laparotomy in terms of reduced numbers of complications and transfusions, shorter LOHS, and lower EBL. The results of this study are consistent with those of previous studies [4]. In addition, the OT was longer in robotic surgery than in laparotomy. However, there was no significant difference in the TLNH between robotic surgery and laparoscopy. The numbers of conversions to laparotomy and complications are critical in minimally invasive surgical procedures for endometrial cancer. They are the most commonly reported outcomes because patients who have undergone conversion to laparotomy have higher complication rates [29]. The number of complications was significantly lower in robotic surgery than in laparoscopy. This result was due to both the inferior visualization of the laparoscopic videoscope and the superior ability of the three-dimensional robotic surgical platform, which enhances operative visualization [11]. Jung *et al.* [25] found that the high rate of operative complications among patients who underwent laparotomy was caused by the operative wound associated with the procedure.

In the present study, robotic surgery generally resulted in fewer conversions and lower EBL than did laparoscopy. These results can be explained by the robotic platform, which offers increased precision and dexterity, and are consistent with the results of previous studies [2,23,25,29]. There were no significant differences in the OT or LOHS between robotic surgery and laparoscopy. Boggess *et al.* [2] and Jung *et al.* [25], however, found that robotic surgery was associated with a shorter LOHS and OT than was laparoscopy. Seamon *et al.* [30] noted that the OT is not consistently defined, making it difficult to compare this parameter between robotic surgery and laparoscopy in the face of heterogeneous data involving either a lack of the definition of OT in a given publication or the presence of data collection bias (retrospectively versus prospectively collected data). In another study [15], the OT included the time required to place the laparoscopic ports and uterine manipulator with colpotomy ring as well as the robotic docking time. However, other studies did not include these factors in the definition of OT. One possible explanation for the discrepant conclusions among various studies is the learning curve for robotic surgery in the treatment of endometrial cancer. Differences in the LOHS may be explained by differences in the medical insurance systems and cultures of the various countries in which each study was performed. In the present meta-analysis, the number of complications was significantly higher in laparoscopy than in robotic surgery; this may be associated with the OT and LOHS, neither of which showed a significant difference between robotic surgery and laparoscopy.

Our meta-analysis indicates that robotic surgery is associated with fewer complications than is laparotomy. This is similar to the findings of other investigators. Frigerio *et al.* [31] compared laparoscopy and laparotomy and found fewer postoperative complications among patients who underwent laparoscopic-assisted vaginal hysterectomy. Gil-Moreno *et al.* [32] compared laparoscopy and laparotomy and found that the amount of blood loss, number of blood transfusions required, and LOHS were significantly lower in the laparoscopic group; however, the OT was significantly longer. On the other hand, we found significantly more complications in robotic surgery than in laparoscopy. This is not completely different from the results of other investigations [17,30]. Our data also showed a significantly lower EBL, shorter LOHS, and fewer transfusions in robotic surgery than in laparotomy. These findings are also not different from those of other investigations. Bell *et al.* [23] showed that the transfusion rate was not statistically different between robotic surgery and laparotomy. Finally, our study demonstrated that robotic surgery was associated with more complications than in laparoscopy but fewer complications than in laparotomy.

More prospective studies are needed to fully compare the effectiveness of robotic surgery with that of laparoscopy and laparotomy. The results of this study should be interpreted while taking its limitations into account. First, the data used for the WMD statistical analysis were median and range rather than mean and SD. The mean and SD must be estimated from the median and range, which may result in error or inaccuracy. Second, the learning curve is very important, especially for inexperienced surgeons, and affects the training curve for robotic surgery. As experience with robotic systems increases, the natural expectation is that the OT, LOHS, and transfusion rate will tend to decrease [24]. Finally, this meta-analysis was characterized by heterogeneity in the OT, LOHS, EBL, TLNH, and conversion rate because it was impossible to match the patient characteristics among all studies. Additionally, the random-effects model took between-study variation into consideration, which may have had a limited influence on the results.

In summary, this is the first meta-analysis to compare three conventional surgical approaches to endometrial cancer (robotic surgery, laparoscopy, and laparotomy) with respect to OT, complications, LOHS, EBL, transfusions, TLNH, and conversions. Overall, the present study has shown that robotic surgery is a feasible and promising method for the treatment of endometrial cancer compared with both laparoscopy and laparotomy. Some articles [13,18,19,26] have reported that the costs associated with robotic surgery are higher than those associated with laparoscopy; however, we believe that robotic surgery can be a feasible alternative technique when robotic costs are reduced. No randomized controlled trials were available for inclusion in this study, which may have biased the interpretation of the results. Randomized controlled trials must be included in future studies to more fully assess the long-term results of this new technology in the field of endometrial cancer.

Author Contributions

Conceived and designed the experiments: LKR JJ YX. Performed the experiments: LKR JJ YX. Analyzed the data: LKR JJ YQB. Contributed reagents/materials/analysis tools: JJ YX. Wrote the paper: LKR YQB FZS.

References

1. Ahmedin Jemal DVM, Siegel R, Xu J (2010) Cancer statistics, 2010. CA Cancer J Clin 5: 277–300.
2. Boggess JF, Gehrig PA, Cantrell L, Shafer A, Ridgway M, et al. (2008) A comparative study of 3 surgical methods for hysterectomy with staging for endometrial cancer: robotic assistance, laparoscopy, laparotomy. Am J Obstet Gynecol 199: 360 e361–369.
3. Herron DM, Marohn M, SAGES-MIRA Robotic Surgery Consensus Group (2008) A consensus document on robotic surgery. Surg Endosc 2: 313–325.
4. Reza M, Maeso S, Blasco JA, Andradas E (2010) Meta-analysis of observational studies on the safety and effectiveness of robotic gynaecological surgery. Br J Surg 97: 1772–1783.
5. O'Neill M, Moran PS, Teljeur C, O'Sullivan OE, O'Reilly BA, et al. (2013) Robot-assisted hysterectomy compared to open and laparoscopic approaches: systematic review and meta-analysis. Arch Gynecol Obstet 287: 907–918.
6. Peiretti M, Zanagnolo V, Bocciolone L, Landoni F, Colombo N, et al. (2009) Robotic surgery: changing the surgical approach for endometrial cancer in a referral cancer center. J Minim Invasive Gynecol 16: 427–431.
7. Hozo SP, Djulbegovic B, Hozo I (2005) Estimating the mean and variance from the median, range, and the size of a sample. BMC Med Res Methodol 5: 13.
8. Wells GA, Shea B, Connell DO, Peterson J, Welch V, et al. (2007) The Newcastle-Ottawa Scale (NOS) for assessing the quality of nonrandomised studies in meta-analyses. Proceedings of the Third Symposium on Systematic Reviews Beyond the Basics: Improving Quality and Impact 7: 3–5.
9. Cardenas-Goicoechea J, Adams S, Bhat SB, Randall TC (2010) Surgical outcomes of robotic-assisted surgical staging for endometrial cancer are equivalent to traditional laparoscopic staging at a minimally invasive surgical center. Gynecol Oncol 117: 224–228.
10. Fagotti A, Corrado G, Fanfani F, Mancini M, Paglia A, et al. (2013) Robotic single-site hysterectomy (RSS-H) vs. laparoendoscopic single-site hysterectomy (LESS-H) in early endometrial cancer: a double-institution case-control study. Gynecol Oncol 130: 219–223.
11. Lim PC, Kang E, Park do H (2010) Learning curve and surgical outcome for robotic-assisted hysterectomy with lymphadenectomy: case-matched controlled comparison with laparoscopy and laparotomy for treatment of endometrial cancer. J Minim Invasive Gynecol 17: 739–748.
12. Martino MA, Shubella J, Thomas MB, Morcrette RM, Schindler J, et al. (2011) A cost analysis of postoperative management in endometrial cancer patients treated by robotics versus laparoscopic approach. Gynecol Oncol 123: 528–531.
13. Sarlos D, Kots L, Stevanovic N, Schaer G (2010) Robotic hysterectomy versus conventional laparoscopic hysterectomy: outcome and cost analyses of a matched case-control study. Eur J Obstet Gynecol Reprod Biol 150: 92–96.
14. Seror J, Bats AS, Huchon C, Bensaid C, Douay-Hauser N, et al. (2013) Laparoscopy vs Robotics in Surgical Management of Endometrial Cancer: Comparison of Intraoperative and Postoperative Complications. J Minim Invasive Gynecol.
15. Venkat P, Chen LM, Young-Lin N, Kiet TK, Young G, et al. (2012) An economic analysis of robotic versus laparoscopic surgery for endometrial cancer: costs, charges and reimbursements to hospitals and professionals. Gynecol Oncol 125: 237–240.
16. Wright JD, Burke WM, Wilde ET, Lewin SN, Charles AS, et al. (2012) Comparative effectiveness of robotic versus laparoscopic hysterectomy for endometrial cancer. J Clin Oncol 30: 783–791.
17. DeNardis SA, Holloway RW, Bigsby GEt, Pikaart DP, Ahmad S, et al. (2008) Robotically assisted laparoscopic hysterectomy versus total abdominal hysterec-

tomy and lymphadenectomy for endometrial cancer. Gynecol Oncol 111: 412–417.
18. Gocmen A, Sanlikan F, Ucar MG (2010) Comparison of robotic-assisted surgery outcomes with laparotomy for endometrial cancer staging in Turkey. Arch Gynecol Obstet 282: 539–545.
19. Seamon LG, Cohn DE, Henretta MS, Kim KH, Carlson MJ, et al. (2009) Minimally invasive comprehensive surgical staging for endometrial cancer: Robotics or laparoscopy? Gynecol Oncol 113: 36–41.
20. Subramaniam A, Kim KH, Bryant SA, Zhang B, Sikes C, et al. (2011) A cohort study evaluating robotic versus laparotomy surgical outcomes of obese women with endometrial carcinoma. Gynecol Oncol 122: 604–607.
21. Coronado PJ, Herraiz MA, Magrina JF, Fasero M, Vidart JA (2012) Comparison of perioperative outcomes and cost of robotic-assisted laparoscopy, laparoscopy and laparotomy for endometrial cancer. Eur J Obstet Gynecol Reprod Biol 165: 289–294.
22. Goel M, Zollinger TW, Moore DH (2011) Surgical staging of endometrial cancer: robotic versus open technique outcomes in a contemporary single surgeon series. J Robotic Surg 5: 109–114.
23. Bell MC, Torgerson J, Seshadri-Kreaden U, Suttle AW, Hunt S (2008) Comparison of outcomes and cost for endometrial cancer staging via traditional laparotomy, standard laparoscopy and robotic techniques. Gynecol Oncol 111: 407–411.
24. Hoekstra AV, Jairam-Thodla A, Rademaker A, Singh DK, Buttin BM, et al. (2009) The impact of robotics on practice management of endometrial cancer: transitioning from traditional surgery. Int J Med Robot 5: 392–397.
25. Jung YW, Lee DW, Kim SW, Nam EJ, Kim JH, et al. (2010) Robot-assisted staging using three robotic arms for endometrial cancer: comparison to laparoscopy and laparotomy at a single institution. J Surg Oncol 101: 116–121.
26. Magrina JF, Kho RM, Weaver AL, Montero RP, Magtibay PM (2008) Robotic radical hysterectomy: comparison with laparoscopy and laparotomy. Gynecol Oncol 109: 86–91.
27. Veljovich DS, Paley PJ, Drescher CW, Everett EN, Shah C, et al. (2008) Robotic surgery in gynecologic oncology: program initiation and outcomes after the first year with comparison with laparotomy for endometrial cancer staging. Am J Obstet Gynecol 198: 679 e671–679; discussion 679 e679–610.
28. ElSahwi KS, Hooper C, De Leon MC, Gallo TN, Ratner E, et al. (2012) Comparison between 155 cases of robotic vs. 150 cases of open surgical staging for endometrial cancer. Gynecol Oncol 124: 260–264.
29. Guillou PJ, Quirke P, Thorpe H, Walker J, Jayne DG, et al. (2005) Short-term endpoints of conventional versus laparoscopic-assisted surgery in patients with colorectal cancer (MRC CLASICC trial): multicentre, randomised controlled trial. Lancet 365: 1718–1726.
30. Seamon LG, Bryant SA, Rheaume PS, Kimball KJ, Huh WK, et al. (2009) Comprehensive surgical staging for endometrial cancer in obese patients: comparing robotics and laparotomy. Obstet Gynecol 114: 16–21.
31. Frigerio L, Gallo A, Ghezzi F, Trezzi G, Lussana M, et al. (2006) Laparoscopic-assisted vaginal hysterectomy versus abdominal hysterectomy in endometrial cancer. Int J Gynaecol Obstet 93: 209–213.
32. Gil-Moreno A, Diaz-Feijoo B, Morchon S, Xercavins J (2006) Analysis of survival after laparoscopic-assisted vaginal hysterectomy compared with the conventional abdominal approach for early-stage endometrial carcinoma: a review of the literature. J Minim Invasive Gynecol 13: 26–35.

Does Minimally-Invasive Pancreaticoduodenectomy Have Advantages over Its Open Method?

Han Qin[1], Jianguo Qiu[2], Yiyang Zhao[3], Gang Pan[1], Yong Zeng[1]*

1 Department of Hepatic Surgery, West China Hospital, Sichuan University, Chengdu, Sichuan, P. R. China, **2** Department of Hepatobiliary Surgery, The First Affiliated Hospital, Chongqing Medical University, Chongqing, P. R. China, **3** Department of Pediatric Surgery, West China Hospital, Sichuan University, Chengdu, Sichuan, P. R. China

Abstract

Background: While more and more open procedures now routinely performed using laparoscopy, minimally invasive pancreaticoduodenectomy (MIPD) remains one of the most challenging abdominal procedures. Therefore, we carried out this meta-analysis to evaluate whether MIPD is safe, feasible and worthwhile.

Methods: PubMed, EMBASE, and Cochrane Library were searched to identify studies published between January 1994 and November 2013 comparing MIPD with open pancreaticoduodenectomy (OPD). Intraoperative outcomes, oncologic safety, postoperative complications, and postoperative recovery were evaluated.

Results: 11 retrospective studies representing 869 patients (327 MIPDs, 542 OPDs) were included. MIPD was associated with a reduction in estimated blood loss (MD −361.93 ml, 95% CI −519.22 to −204.63 ml, $p<0.001$, $I^2=94\%$), wound infection (OR 0.41, 95% CI 0.22 to 0.78, $p=0.007$, $I^2=0\%$), and hospital stay (MD −2.64 d, 95% CI −4.23 to −1.05 d, $p=0.001$, $I^2=78\%$). However, it brings longer operative time (MD 105 min, 95% CI 49.73 to 160.26 min, $p<0.001$, $I^2=93\%$). There were no significant differences between the two procedures in likelihood of overall complications ($p=0.05$), pancreatic fistula (PF) ($p=0.86$), delayed gastric empting (DGE) ($p=0.96$), positive surgical margins ($p=0.07$), retrieval of lymph nodes ($p=0.48$), reoperation ($p=0.16$) and mortality ($p=0.64$).

Conclusions: Our results suggest that MIPD is currently safe, feasible and worthwhile. But considering the selection bias, complexity of MIPD and lack of long-term oncologic outcomes, we suggest it be performed in a high-volume pancreatic surgery center in selected patients.

Editor: Hana Algül, Technische Universität München, Germany

Funding: The authors have no support or funding to report.

Competing Interests: The authors have declared that no competing interests exist.

* Email: zengyonghxyy@163.com

Introduction

Laparoscopy has become widely accepted in many intra-abdominal surgeries and has proved to be beneficial to patients in terms of postoperative recovery, reduction of complications and hospital stay [1–5] on various occasions. And laparoscopic cholecystectomy has even become the gold standard for surgical removal of the gallbladder. Even though, MIPD is still not universally practiced, because the complexity of the procedure has questioned the safety and advantages over its open counterpart. With the maturation of surgeons' laparoscopic skills and advances in technology, including surgical robotics, MIPD now received more interest.

In recent years, a large number of single-institution series of MIPD have been performed and a variety of studies have been reported [6–10]. However, there is currently no powerful evidence that informs the advantages of using laparoscopy over conventional OPD.

The purpose of our study is to critically evaluate whether MIPD, including laparoscopic and robot-assisted laparoscopic, is safe, feasible and worthwhile. Therefore, we carried out a systematic review of the literatures and a meta-analysis of MIPD vs OPD to evaluate the intraoperative outcomes, postoperative complications, postoperative recovery, and oncologic safety. To our knowledge, this meta-analysis is the first to expound this important issue in different subgroups.

Methods

A systematic review was conducted according to a prespecified protocol based on guidance from the Centre for Reviews and Dissemination [11] and the Cochrane Handbook [12]. The review is reported on the basis of the PRISMA (Preferred Reporting Items for Systematic Reviews and Meta-Analyses) guidelines [13]. We defined MIDP as: using laparoscopy or robot to complete resection of the head of pancreas and duodenum, as well as reconstruction of digestive duct's continuity.

Eligibility Criteria

Eligibility criteria for all included studies were: (1) meeting the definition of MIPD; (2) comparing MIPD with OPD [acceptable study designs were prospective controlled trials (CTs), cohort studies, and case control studies]; (3) reporting at least one of the outcomes of interest, such as: intraoperative outcomes, oncologic safety, postoperative complications, and postoperative recoveries.

No limits were placed on publication status or language. Translators were consulted as necessary. We excluded studies with any of the following: (1) nonhuman subjects; (2) it was impossible to extract appropriate data from the published articles; (3) there was considerable overlap between authors, institutes, or patients in the published literatures.

Search Strategy

In accordance with the prespecified study protocol, PubMed, EMBASE, and Cochrane Library were systematically searched with the assistance of 2 independent reviewers (Gang Pan and Yiyang Zhao) from January 1, 1994 (the year MIPD first reported) to November 17, 2013(the day we completed the literature search). The prespecified search terms were grouped in 3 areas: the "minimally invasive" terms (minimally invasive/laparoscopic/laparoscopy/robotic/Da Vinci/robotic-assisted/laparoscopic-assisted), the "open" terms (open/conventional), and the "pancreaticoduodenectomy" terms (pancreaticoduodenectomy/whipple/duodenopancreatectomy/pancreatectomy/pancreatic).

Study Selection

The study selection process took place in 2 consecutive steps. In Phase 1, a manual selection of the potentially relevant articles was performed by scanning their title and abstract. In Phase 2, the full-text versions of articles selected in Phase 1 were assessed. Two reviewers (Qiang Liu and Jinhai Gou) independently evaluated all retrieved articles using prespecified eligibility criteria. In case of disagreement, a consensual decision was made.

Data Extraction

Two reviewers (Gang Pan and Yiyang Zhao) extracted data from all selected studies in RevMan 5.0 software independently. The same consensus process mentioned above was used to resolve disagreements. The data extracted included year of study publication, study country, study type, patient demographics, definitions of PF&DGE, conversion rate, intraoperative outcomes, oncologic safety, postoperative complications, and postoperative recovery. If possible, the first or corresponding author was contacted to obtain supplementary information when there were missing data or inaccuracy in the information. If the author failed to respond, the study was excluded from the outcome analysis.

Quality Assessment

The quality of the studies was assessed by using the Modified Newcastle–Ottawa Score [14], which allocates a maximum of 9 points each to patient selection, the comparability of the two groups (MIPD and OPD), and outcome assessment. Two authors (Han Qin and Jianguo Qiu) examined the studies independently. The same consensus process mentioned above was used to resolve disagreements.

Statistical Methods

This meta-analysis was performed in line with recommendations from the Cochrane Collaboration [15] and the Quality of Reporting of Meta-analyses [16] guidelines. The statistical software Review Manager version 5.0 (The Cochrane Collaboration, Oxford, United Kingdom) was used to perform all statistical analyses. I^2 values were used for quantification of statistical inconsistency, defined as the percentage of variation between studies due to heterogeneity [17]. And a value exceeding 50% was considered to represent significant heterogeneity. A random-effects model was used to report the results of heterogeneous data, otherwise a fixed-effects model was used. Continuous variables was conducted with the Inverse-Variance statistical method by using weighted mean difference (MD), and dichotomous variables were analyzed with the Mantel-Haenszel statistical method using odds ratio (OR) as the summary statistic, and both were reported with 95% confidence intervals (CI). Funnel plots were constructed to detect and assess publication bias and any associations between treatment estimates and sample size. Forest plots were constructed, and the value of $P<0.05$ was considered to indicate statistical significance.

Results

The literature search yielded 649 studies initially. No other eligible studies were found from other sources. In phase 1 of the study selection process, 19 potential eligible articles were included for a full-text version after screening their titles and abstracts. Of these, we excluded 5 [18–22], because they were reviews of MIPD. Nakamura M et al [23] was excluded for it was a meta-analysis of laparoscopic pancreatic resection vs open pancreatic resection. Gumbs AA et al [24] was excluded because the data was not extractable and the authors could not be reached to provide additional information. Another study [25] in which no comparison was found was also excluded. Finally, this left a total of 11 studies [26–36] representing 869 patients for inclusion in the meta-analysis. The PRISMA flow chart of literature search strategies is illustrated in **Figure 1.**

Study Characteristics

Characteristics of included studies are presented in **Table 1**. All eleven were retrospective studies of variable quality that compared consecutive cases of MIPD with either consecutive or matched OPD performed during the same period. They were varied with respect to age, gender, body mass index (BMI), American Society of Anesthesiologists (ASA) score, and operation indication. For example, Buchs NC et al [36] reported that the ASA score was 2.5 ± 0.5 in the MIPD group, while it was 2.15 ± 0.7 in the OPD group ($p=0.01$). And the percentage of patients with pancreatitis was 3.36% in the MIPD group, while it was 6.83% in the OPD group. Most of the referred studies used the definitions from ISGPF&ISGPS [37,38] to define pancreatic fistula and delayed gastric emptying, but some might use the others like the definition from Suc B et al [39]. All the conversions were included in the MIPD group. The majority of cases were performed for malignancy, but no report of long-term oncologic result. In most cases, the selection criteria for patients to undergo MIPD were not reported.

Quality Assessment

Evaluation of methodological quality based on the Cochrane risk of bias tool was not performed, because there was no RCT. However, we used the Modified Newcastle–Ottawa Score instead. The quality of the studies was evaluated by examining three

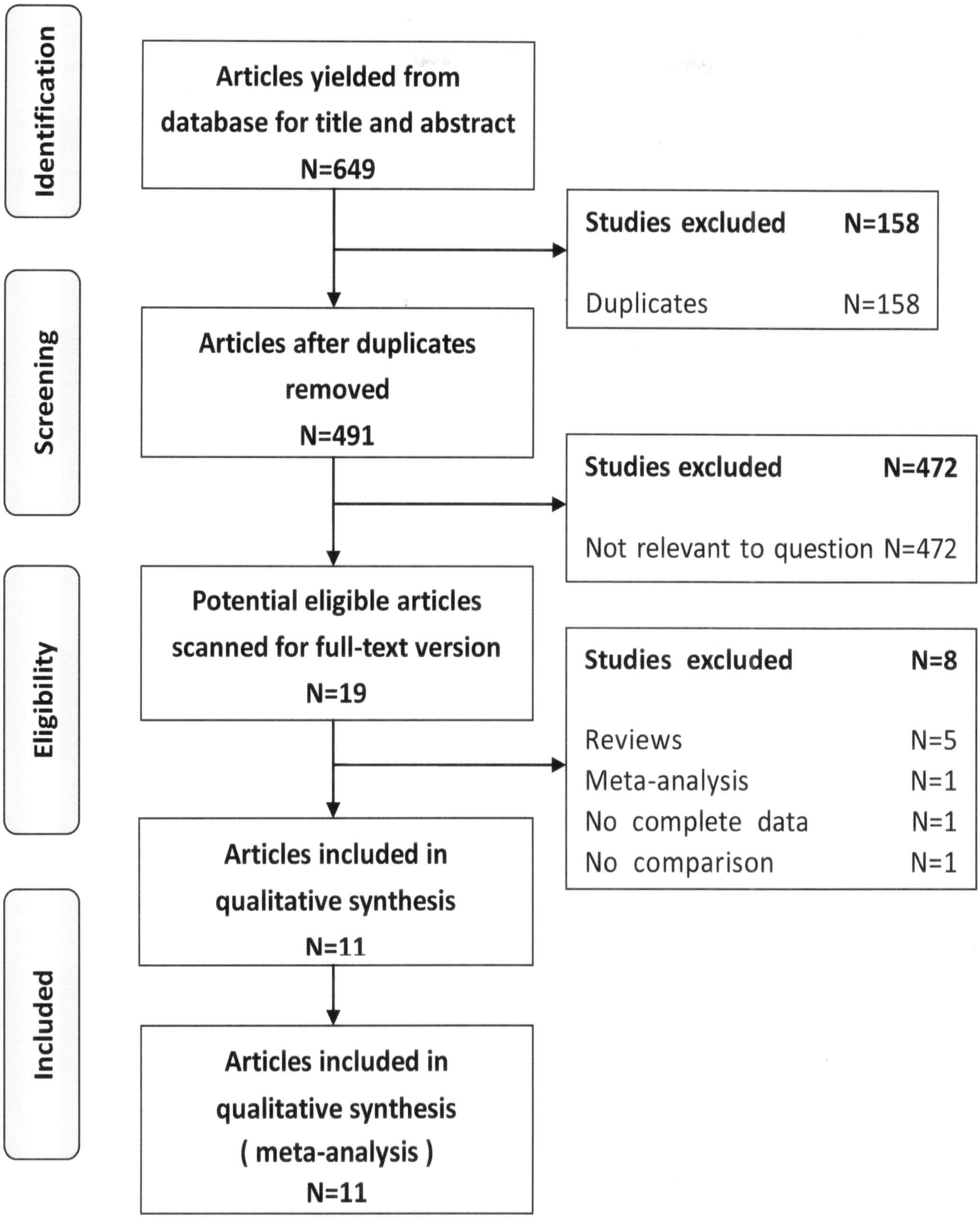

Figure 1. The PRISMA flowchart of literature review.

Table 1. Characteristics of included studies.

Study	Year	Country	No. Patients		Mean Age(Yrs)		Male(%)		Definition of PF	Definition of DGE	Conversion rate, (%)	Quality scores	Type of MIPD	Operation indications
			MIPD	OPD	MIPD	OPD	MIPD	OPD						
Kuroki T et al.[26]	2012	Japan	20	31	71.2±8.8	73.5±7.3	55	68	ISGPF	ISGPS	0	6	NRA	1,2,3,4,5,7
Zureikat AH et al.[27]	2011	USA	14	14	79.8±10.2	67.4±11	79	50	ISGPF	NR	14	4	NRA	1,2,3,4,6,7,8
Cho A et al.[28]	2009	Japan	15	15	64±10	68±9	40	47	ISGPF	ISGPS	0	6	NRA	1,2,3,4,5,8,9
Asbun HJ et al.[29]	2012	USA	53	215	62.9±14.14	67.3±11.53	55	44	ISGPF	ISGPS	15	8	NRA	1,2,3,4,5,7,8,9
Mesleh MG et al.[30]	2013	USA	75	48	NR	NR	57	48	ISGPF	ISGPS	13	4	NRA	3,4,9
Li Y et al.[31]	2013	China	20	47	57±11	58±10	60	68	NR	ISGPS	0	3	NRA	1,2,3,6,7
Chalikonda S et al.[32]	2012	USA	30	30	62±11.4	61±12.7	54	54	ISGPF	ISGPS	10	6	RA	1,2,3,4
Zhou NX et al.[33]	2011	China	8	8	64.38±9.08	59.38±9.38	63	50	Suc B et al.	NR	0	5	RA	1,2,3,8,9
Bao PQ et al.[34]	2013	USA	28	28	68.0±11.2	67.7±12.5	46	46	ISGPF	ISGPS	14	8	RA	1,2,3,4,5,6,7,8
Lai EC et al.[35]	2012	Hong Kong	20	67	66.4±11.9	62.1±11.2	60	57	NR	NR	5	6	RA	1,2,3,4,5,6,7,8,9
Buchs NC et al.[36]	2011	USA	44	39	63±14.5	56±15.8	50	36	ISGPF	NR	4.5	7	RA	1,2,3,4,5,7,8,9

NR, no record; NRA, no robot-assisted; RA, robot-assisted; Operation indications: 1.Cholangiocarcinoma 2.Pancreatic adenocarcinoma 3.Periampullar adenocarcinoma 4.Intraductal pancreatic mucinous neoplasm 5.pancreatic neuroendocrine tumor 6.gastrointestinal stromal tumor 7.Pancreatitis 8.Periampullar adenoma 9.Else.

Table 2. Comparison of MIPD Versus OPD (Pooled Analysis).

Outcome of interest	Studies, n	Patients, n	OR/MD	95% CI	P value	Heterogeneity Test	
						P value	I^2
Intraoperative outcomes							
Operative time,min	11	869	105	(49.73, 160.26)	**<0.001**	<0.001	93%
Estimated blood loss, mL	10	746	−361.93	(−519.22 −204.63)	**<0.001**	<0.001	94%
Postoperative outcomes							
Morbidity, (%)	9	762	0.73	(0.53, 1.00)	0.05	0.35	10%
Wound infection, n	6	584	0.41	(0.22, 0.78)	**0.007**	0.86	0%
Overall pancreatic fistula, n	10	802	0.96	(0.65, 1.44)	0.86	0.88	0%
Grade A	5	486	0.88	(0.47, 1.66)	0.7	0.86	0%
Grade B	6	548	1.01	(0.46, 2.20)	0.98	0.89	0%
Grade C	6	525	0.83	(0.37, 1.85)	0.64	0.87	0%
Overall delayed gastric emptying, n	11	869	0.99	(0.62, 1.56)	0.96	0.76	0%
Grade A	3	386	0.82	(0.31, 2.19)	0.69	0.49	0%
Grade B	4	446	0.77	(0.29, 2.02)	0.59	0.93	0%
Grade C	3	365	1.23	(0.41, 3.71)	0.71	0.8	0%
Reoperation, n	8	721	0.63	(0.34, 1.19)	0.16	0.73	0%
Mortality, (%)	7	582	0.82	(0.37, 1.85)	0.64	0.93	0%
Length of stay, d	10	818	−2.64	(−4.23, −1.05)	**0.001**	<0.001	78%
Oncologic outcomes							
Retrieved lymph nodes, n	7	612	1.15	(−2.02, 4.32)	0.48	<0.001	83%
Positive surgical margins,n	7	451	0.57	(0.31, 1.04)	0.07	0.12	40%

factors: patient selection, comparability of the study groups and assessment of outcomes. A score of 0–9 was allocated to each study. In general, 7 studies were considered to be of high quality by achieving a score of ≥6. The scores of those studies are also presented in **Table 1**. Results from the meta-analysis with regard to intraoperative outcomes, postoperative outcomes, and oncologic safety are summarized in **Table 2**.

Pooled Analysis

Intraoperative Outcomes

All the eleven studies reported data on operative time, and when a random-effects model was used, the meta-analysis showed that the use of minimally invasive procedures brings longer operative time (MD 105 min, 95% CI 49.73 to 160.26 min, $p<0.001$, $I^2=93\%$). Estimated blood loss was reported in ten studies[26~29, 31~36] which included 746 patients. The meta-analysis showed that MIPD gives a reduction in intraoperative estimated blood loss (MD −361.93 ml, 95% CI −519.22 to −204.63 ml, $p<0.001$, $I^2=94\%$)

Postoperative Outcomes

Nine studies[27~33, 34, 35] representing 746 patients reported overall complications, and the meta-analysis showed there was no statistical difference between MIPD and OPD (OR 0.73, 95% CI 0.53 to 1.00, $p=0.05$, $I^2=10\%$). Six studies[28, 29, 32, 34~36] showed that MIPD has fewer wound infections (OR 0.41, 95% CI 0.22 to 0.78, $p=0.007$, $I^2=0\%$). The meta-analysis of ten studies including 802 patients indicated that there was no significant statistical difference between MIPD and OPD in the incidence of neither overall pancreatic fistula (OR 0.96, 95% CI 0.65 to 1.44, $p=0.86$, $I^2=0\%$) (Fig. 2) nor overall delayed gastric emptying (OR 0.99, 95% CI 0.62 to 1.56, $p=0.96$, $I^2=0\%$). Besides, when dividing PF&DGE into 3 subgroups of Grade A, B, and C, according to the guidelines of ISGPF& ISGPS[37, 38] respectively, there was still no statistical difference between MIPD and OPD. Eight studies[27, 29, 30, 32~36] representing 721 patients reported the incidence of reoperation, the meta-analysis showed there was no statistical difference between the two procedures (OR 0.63, 95% CI 0.34 to 1.19, $p=0.16$, $I^2=0\%$). The meta-analysis of seven studies[27, 29, 31~35] including 582 patients showed there was no statistical difference in mortality (OR 0.82, 95% CI 0.37 to 1.85, $p=0.64$, $I^2=0\%$). Length of stay was shorter by 2.64 days for the MIPD group, and the difference was statistically significant (MD −2.64 d, 95% CI −4.23 to −1.05 d, $p=0.001$, $I^2=78\%$) (**Fig. 3**).

Oncologic Outcomes

The number of retrieved lymph nodes was mentioned in 7 studies[27~29, 32, 34~36], representing 612 patients. The meta-analysis showed there was no significant statistical difference between MIPD and OPD (MD 1.15, 95% CI −2.02 to 4.32, $p=0.48$, $I^2=83\%$). As to the rate of positive surgical margins, which mean they were not R0 resections, the meta-analysis showed there was no statistical difference (OR 0.57, 95% CI 0.31 to 1.04, $p=0.07$, $I^2=40\%$). (**Fig. 4**)

Sensitivity Analysis

The sensitivity analysis included the following: (1) NRA: 6 studies which did not use robot; (2) RA: 5 studies which used robot; (3) HQ: 7 studies of high quality (with quality score of 6 or more using the modified Newcastle-Ottawa scale); and (4) large sample size (LSS): 4 studies with at least 30 patients in each procedure. Results from sensitivity analysis were summarized in **Table 3**.

NRA subgroup

When only studies without robot were analyzed, it comes out that there was no statistical difference in length of stay (MD −1.85 d, 95% CI, −3.80 to 0.11 d, $P=0.06$, $I^2=84\%$) and wound infection (OR 0.47, 95% CI 0.19 to 1.13, $p=0.09$, $I^2=0\%$). The heterogeneity of length of stay increased a little. The rest of the outcomes were consistent with the overall analysis. Heterogeneity of estimated blood loss and overall complications increased, while it reduced in retrieved lymph nodes.

RA subgroup

When only studies with robot were analyzed, it comes out that there was no statistical difference in operative time (MD 100.71 min, 95% CI −35.12 to 236.54 min, $p=0.15$, $I^2=96\%$), and there was an increase in the degree of heterogeneity. There were not enough studies referred to the three grades of delayed gastric emptying, so no meta-analysis was carried out. The rest of the outcomes were consistent with the overall analysis. And except for oncologic outcomes, the heterogeneity reduced. Though the heterogeneity of positive surgical margins increased significantly ($I^2=51\%$), no difference was found when a random-effects model was used ($p=0.54$).

HQ subgroup

7 studies were considered to be of high quality by achieving a score of ≥6. Difference in operative time became nonsignificant (MD 77.03 min, 95% CI −5.14 to 159.21 min, $p=0.07$, $I^2=95\%$). Complications were fewer in the MIPD group (OR 0.62, 95% CI 0.42 to 0.92, $p=0.02$, $I^2=0\%$). The other variables remained similar to the original MIPD versus OPD analysis. Heterogeneity of operative time, Grade A of pancreatic fistula, length of stay, and retrieved lymph nodes increased a little, while heterogeneity of estimated blood loss reduced. Although the heterogeneity of positive surgical margins increased significantly ($I^2=58\%$), no difference was found when a random-effects model was used ($p=0.39$).

LSS subgroup

Four studies with more than 30 patients in each procedure were also compared. No statistical difference was found in operative time (MD 84.06 min, 95% CI −27.20 to 195.32 min, $p=0.14$, $I^2=97\%$) and the rate of wound infection (OR 0.44, 95% CI 0.19 to 1.00, $p=0.05$, $I^2=0\%$), while complications were fewer in the MIPD group (OR 0.62, 95% CI 0.42 to 0.92, $p=0.02$, $I^2=0\%$). For there was only one study which mentioned Grade A&C delayed gastric emptying, no meta-analysis was carried out. Besides, the meta-analyses showed MIPD has an advantage over OPD in oncologic outcomes, including both retrieved lymph nodes (MD 4.5, 95% CI 1.12 to 7.89, $p=0.009$, $I^2=73\%$) and positive surgical margins (OR 0.27, 95% CI 0.10 to 0.73, $p=0.01$, $I^2=0\%$). The remaining results were similar to the original analysis. Heterogeneity of operative time and length of stay increased a little, while heterogeneity of estimated blood loss, overall complications, and oncologic outcomes reduced.

Publication bias

The funnel plot of this study based on overall complications is shown in **Figure 5**. All studies lay inside the limits of the 95% CIs and distributed evenly about the vertical, showing no evidence of publication bias.

Study or Subgroup	MIPD Events	MIPD Total	OPD Events	OPD Total	Weight	Odds Ratio M-H, Fixed, 95% CI
4.1.1 No robot-assisted						
Asbun HJ et al.	7	53	29	215	20.5%	0.98 [0.40, 2.37]
Cho A et al.	2	15	2	15	3.6%	1.00 [0.12, 8.21]
Mesleh MG et al.	3	75	3	48	7.2%	0.63 [0.12, 3.23]
T. Kuroki et al.	9	20	12	31	10.6%	1.30 [0.41, 4.05]
Zureikat AH et al.	5	14	6	14	7.9%	0.74 [0.16, 3.39]
Subtotal (95% CI)		**177**		**323**	**49.8%**	**0.96 [0.54, 1.69]**
Total events	26		52			
Heterogeneity: Chi² = 0.64, df = 4 (P = 0.96); I² = 0%						
Test for overall effect: Z = 0.15 (P = 0.88)						
4.1.2 Robot-assisted						
Bao PQ et al.	8	28	10	28	14.7%	0.72 [0.23, 2.22]
Buchs NC et al.	8	44	8	39	14.3%	0.86 [0.29, 2.56]
Chalikonda S et al.	3	30	5	30	9.2%	0.56 [0.12, 2.57]
Lai EC et al.	7	20	12	67	7.4%	2.47 [0.81, 7.50]
Zhou NX et al.	2	8	3	8	4.6%	0.56 [0.06, 4.76]
Subtotal (95% CI)		**130**		**172**	**50.2%**	**0.97 [0.55, 1.71]**
Total events	28		38			
Heterogeneity: Chi² = 3.80, df = 4 (P = 0.43); I² = 0%						
Test for overall effect: Z = 0.10 (P = 0.92)						
Total (95% CI)		**307**		**495**	**100.0%**	**0.96 [0.65, 1.44]**
Total events	54		90			
Heterogeneity: Chi² = 4.44, df = 9 (P = 0.88); I² = 0%						
Test for overall effect: Z = 0.18 (P = 0.86)						

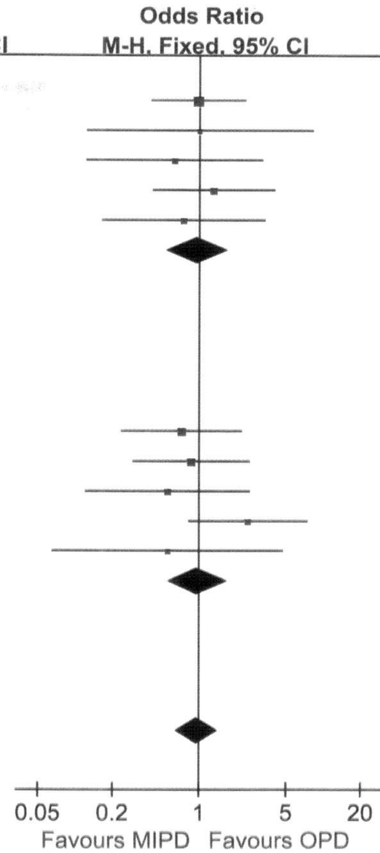

Figure 2. Pooled meta-analysis of pancreatic fistula, comparing MIPD with OPD.

Study or Subgroup	MIPD Mean	MIPD SD	MIPD Total	OPD Mean	OPD SD	OPD Total	Weight	Mean Difference IV, Random, 95% CI
17.1.1 No robot-assisted								
Asbun HJ et al.	8	3.2	53	12.4	8.5	215	13.7%	-4.40 [-5.83, -2.97]
Cho A et al.	16.4	3.7	15	15.6	1.3	15	12.4%	0.80 [-1.18, 2.78]
Li Y et al.	13	3.5	20	16.3	3.9	47	12.6%	-3.30 [-5.20, -1.40]
Mesleh MG et al.	7	2.6	75	8	2.8	48	14.5%	-1.00 [-1.99, -0.01]
Zureikat AH et al.	8	8.5	14	8.5	3	14	6.5%	-0.50 [-5.22, 4.22]
Subtotal (95% CI)			**177**			**339**	**59.7%**	**-1.85 [-3.80, 0.11]**
Heterogeneity: Tau² = 3.80; Chi² = 24.54, df = 4 (P < 0.0001); I² = 84%								
Test for overall effect: Z = 1.85 (P = 0.06)								
17.1.2 Robot-assisted								
Bao PQ et al.	7.4	4.6	28	8.1	3.7	28	11.9%	-0.70 [-2.89, 1.49]
Buchs NC et al.	13	7.5	44	14.6	9.5	39	8.4%	-1.60 [-5.31, 2.11]
Chalikonda S et al.	9.79	5.1	30	13.26	6.2	30	10.2%	-3.47 [-6.34, -0.60]
Lai EC et al.	13.7	6.1	20	25.8	23.1	67	4.7%	-12.10 [-18.24, -5.96]
Zhou NX et al.	16.38	4.14	8	24.25	7.09	8	5.2%	-7.87 [-13.56, -2.18]
Subtotal (95% CI)			**130**			**172**	**40.3%**	**-4.29 [-7.58, -1.00]**
Heterogeneity: Tau² = 9.81; Chi² = 15.99, df = 4 (P = 0.003); I² = 75%								
Test for overall effect: Z = 2.55 (P = 0.01)								
Total (95% CI)			**307**			**511**	**100.0%**	**-2.64 [-4.23, -1.05]**
Heterogeneity: Tau² = 4.31; Chi² = 41.54, df = 9 (P < 0.00001); I² = 78%								
Test for overall effect: Z = 3.25 (P = 0.001)								

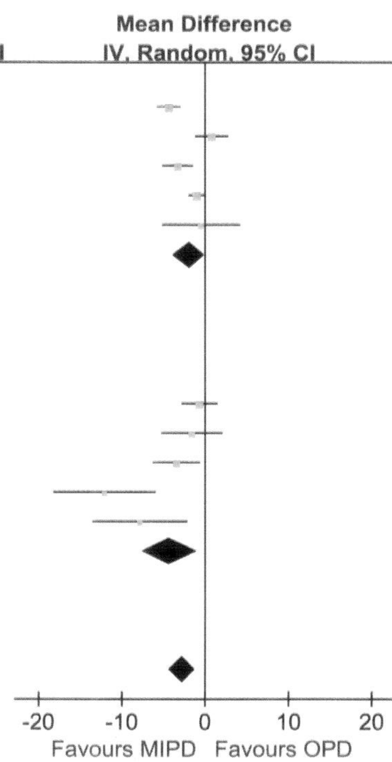

Figure 3. Pooled meta-analysis of length of stay, comparing MIPD with OPD.

Study or Subgroup	MIPD Events	MIPD Total	OPD Events	OPD Total	Weight	Odds Ratio M-H, Fixed, 95% CI
2.1.1 Not robot-assisted						
Asbun HJ et al.	2	39	24	141	32.8%	0.26 [0.06, 1.17]
Zureikat AH et al.	0	12	1	12	4.8%	0.31 [0.01, 8.31]
Subtotal (95% CI)		**51**		**153**	**37.6%**	**0.27 [0.07, 1.05]**
Total events	2		25			
Heterogeneity: Chi² = 0.01, df = 1 (P = 0.93); I² = 0%						
Test for overall effect: Z = 1.89 (P = 0.06)						
2.1.2 Robot-assisted						
Bao PQ et al.	7	19	3	26	5.3%	4.47 [0.98, 20.49]
Buchs NC et al.	3	33	5	27	16.6%	0.44 [0.09, 2.04]
Chalikonda S et al.	0	30	4	30	14.7%	0.10 [0.00, 1.88]
Lai EC et al.	4	15	19	53	20.4%	0.65 [0.18, 2.33]
Zhou NX et al.	0	8	1	6	5.3%	0.22 [0.01, 6.31]
Subtotal (95% CI)		**105**		**142**	**62.4%**	**0.75 [0.38, 1.51]**
Total events	14		32			
Heterogeneity: Chi² = 8.15, df = 4 (P = 0.09); I² = 51%						
Test for overall effect: Z = 0.80 (P = 0.42)						
Total (95% CI)		**156**		**295**	**100.0%**	**0.57 [0.31, 1.04]**
Total events	16		57			
Heterogeneity: Chi² = 10.05, df = 6 (P = 0.12); I² = 40%						
Test for overall effect: Z = 1.82 (P = 0.07)						

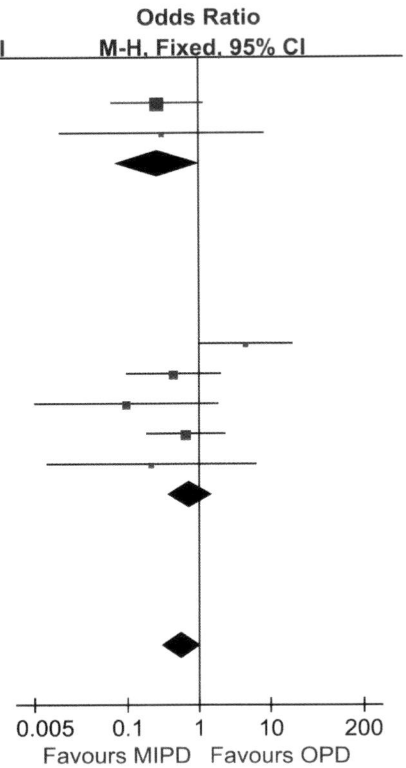

Figure 4. Pooled meta-analysis of positive surgical margins, comparing MIPD with OPD.

Discussion

Summary of Evidence

The evolution of minimally invasive approaches represents one of the most significant advances in the field of general surgery. Till now, it has proved to be beneficial to patients in terms of postoperative recovery, reduction of complications and hospital stay [1–5] on various occasions. With the maturation of surgeons' laparoscopic skills and advances in technology, including surgical robotics, it becomes possible in complex operations. As a new progression strategy, MIPD for pancreatic surgery is still in its early stages, and information regarding the comparison of using minimally invasive procedures over conventional OPD is rare. In the present study, a deliberate evaluation and meta-analysis using the largest available dataset of published studies were made. Gumbs AA [19] reported the rate of conversion to an open procedure was 9% after reviewing 285 published cases of MIPD. In line with it, the mean rate of the eleven studies was about 9.5%. The results demonstrated that MIPD was associated with a reduction in estimated blood loss, wound infection, and a shorter hospital stay. However, the use of minimally invasive procedures brings longer operative time. There were no significant differences between the two procedures in the likelihood of the overall complications, pancreatic fistula, delayed gastric emptying, reoperation, mortality, and oncologic outcomes. The findings of sensitivity and subgroup analysis are in most cases consistent with the pooled analysis, implying the credibility of our results.

Operative time was shown to be longer in MIPD in the pooled analysis. This is often attributed to the complexity of the procedure, including difficulties in access and exposure of the pancreas, hemorrhage control from major vasculature, particularly the reconstruction of a technically demanding reconstruction of the biliary and pancreatic remnants. But because of surgical robotics, it may make it possible to reduce the time. As expected, there was no statistical difference in the RA subgroup between MIPD&OPD, while it was statistically longer in the NRA subgroup. Considering the factor of experience, surgeons who performed more MIPD may be more skilled, the outcome from the large sample size subgroup is well explained. So we can see Buchs N C et al [36] reported that the time they spent on MIPD (444±93.5 min) was less than that on OPD (559±135 min). However, we can still find there's a trend that MIPD may cost longer operative time in all the four subgroups because the surgeons are not experienced enough.

Intraoperative blood loss was proved to be lower in the pooled analysis and all the four subgroups. This is often attributed to the magnified view afforded by laparoscopy which enhances the surgeon's view of the structures surrounding the specimen, allowing precise dissection along appropriate planes. But it also needs to be noticed that during preoperative assessment, those with expected bleeding or vascular involvement were directly decided to receive an open PD by the surgeons. It obviously led to selection bias, because these patients were expected with more blood loss. However, hemorrhage control during MIPD is extremely important or it may lead to massive bleeding. And blood loss during MIPD will obscure the view of laparoscopy, so the surgeon must perform a more careful dissection.

Overall complications should be investigated and reported out past the standard inpatient or 30-day hospitalization, which all the included studies didn't follow. Besides, it's hard for clinicians to observe and record all complications by the same criteria after such a complex operation. What's more, patients' characteristics, especially their ASA score, chronic pancreatitis and pancreatic trauma, have high influences on postoperative complications, but

Table 3. Comparison of MIPD Versus OPD (Sensitivity Analysis).

Outcome of interest	Studies, n	Patients, n	OR/MD	95% CI	P value	Heterogeneity Test	
						P value	I^2
Analysis of NRA subgroup							
Intraoperative outcomes							
Operative time,min	6	567	119.46	(77.61, 161.30)	**<0.001**	<0.001	82%
Estimated blood loss, mL	5	444	−451.62	(−867.47, −35.77)	**0.03**	<0.001	96%
Postoperative outcomes							
Morbidity, (%)	5	516	0.8	(0.53, 1.19)	0.27	0.27	22%
Wound infection, n	2	298	0.47	(0.19, 1.13)	0.09	0.8	0%
Overall pancreatic fistula, n	5	500	0.96	(0.54, 1.69)	0.88	0.96	0%
Grade A	3	347	1.09	(0.50, 2.35)	0.83	0.84	0%
Grade B	3	349	1.06	(0.35, 3.18)	0.92	0.82	0%
Grade C	3	326	0.83	(0.26, 2.61)	0.75	0.6	0%
Overall delayed gastric emptying, n	6	567	1.11	(0.65, 1.90)	0.7	0.51	0%
Grade A	3	386	0.82	(0.31, 2.19)	0.69	0.49	0%
Grade B	3	386	0.74	(0.26, 2.09)	0.57	0.81	0%
Grade C	3	365	1.23	(0.41, 3.71)	0.71	0.8	0%
Reoperation, n	3	419	0.79	(0.27, 2.32)	0.67	0.63	0%
Mortality, (%)	3	363	0.77	(0.27, 2.21)	0.63	0.66	0%
Length of stay, d	5	516	−1.85	(−3.80, 0.11)	0.06	<0.001	84%
Oncologic outcomes							
Retrieved lymph nodes, n	3	326	1.86	(−3.86, 7.59)	0.52	0.009	79%
Positive surgical margins,n	2	204	0.27	(0.07, 1.05)	0.06	0.93	0%
Analysis of RA subgroup							
Intraoperative outcomes							
Operative time,min	5	302	100.71	(−35.12, 236.54)	0.15	<0.001	96%
Estimated blood loss, mL	5	444	−287.51	(−454.84, −120.18)	**<0.001**	<0.001	91%
Postoperative outcomes							
Morbidity, (%)	4	246	0.62	(0.36, 1.06)	0.08	0.35	8%
Wound infection, n	4	286	0.35	(0.14, 0.90)	**0.03**	0.64	0%
Overall pancreatic fistula, n	5	302	0.97	(0.55, 1.71)	0.92	0.43	0%
Grade A	2	139	0.58	(0.20, 1.74)	0.34	0.74	0%
Grade B	3	199	0.96	(0.32, 2.89)	0.95	0.54	0%
Grade C	3	199	0.82	(0.27, 2.55)	0.73	0.67	0%
Overall delayed gastric emptying, n	5	302	0.71	(0.28, 1.76)	0.45	0.73	0%
Grade A	0	0	/	/	/	/	/
Grade B	1	60	/	/	/	/	/
Grade C	0	0	/	/	/	/	/
Reoperation, n	5	302	0.56	(0.26, 1.22)	0.15	0.51	0%
Mortality, (%)	4	219	0.92	(0.25, 3.30)	0.89	0.79	0%
Length of stay, d	5	302	−4.29	(−7.58, −1.00)	**0.01**	0.003	75%
Oncologic outcomes							
Retrieved lymph nodes, n	4	286	1.15	(−3.32, 4.59)	0.75	<0.001	85%
Positive surgical margins,n	5	247	0.75	(0.38, 1.51)	0.42	0.09	51%
Analysis of HQ subgroup							
Intraoperative outcomes							
Operative time,min	7	635	77.03	(−5.14, 159.21)	0.07	<0.001	95%
Estimated blood loss, mL	7	635	−493.46	(−735.81, −251.12)	**<0.001**	<0.001	92%
Postoperative outcomes							
Morbidity, (%)	5	528	0.62	(0.42, 0.92)	**0.02**	0.76	0%

Table 3. Cont.

Outcome of interest	Studies, n	Patients, n	OR/MD	95% CI	P value	Heterogeneity Test	
						P value	I^2
Wound infection, n	6	584	0.41	(0.22, 0.78)	**0.007**	0.86	0%
Overall pancreatic fistula, n	7	635	1.04	(0.67, 1.61)	0.86	0.72	0%
Grade A	3	402	0.97	(0.46, 2.05)	0.93	0.71	0%
Grade B	6	548	1.01	(0.46, 2.20)	0.98	0.89	0%
Grade C	5	497	0.89	(0.39, 2.05)	0.78	0.84	0%
Overall delayed gastric emptying, n	7	635	0.89	(0.49, 1.63)	0.71	0.89	0%
Grade A	2	319	0.62	(0.16, 2.39)	0.49	0.27	17%
Grade B	3	379	0.94	(0.28, 3.14)	0.92	0.92	0%
Grade C	2	298	1.32	(0.41, 4.29)	0.64	0.56	0%
Reoperation, n	5	554	0.57	(0.28, 1.16)	0.12	0.54	0%
Mortality, (%)	4	471	0.8	(0.32, 2.01)	0.63	0.83	0%
Length of stay, d	6	584	−2.86	(−5.39, −0.33)	**0.03**	<0.001	83%
Oncologic outcomes							
Retrieved lymph nodes, n	6	584	1.38	(−2.13, 4.89)	0.44	<0.001	85%
Positive surgical margins,n	5	413	0.61	(0.32, 1.13)	0.12	0.05	58%
Analysis of LSS subgroup							
Intraoperative outcomes							
Operative time,min	4	534	84.06	(−27.20, 195.32)	0.14	<0.001	97%
Estimated blood loss, mL	3	411	−546.47	(−874.87, −218.08)	**0.001**	<0.001	86%
Postoperative outcomes							
Morbidity, (%)	4	534	0.62	(0.42, 0.92)	**0.02**	0.61	0%
Wound infection, n	3	411	0.44	(0.19, 1.00)	0.05	0.57	0%
Overall pancreatic fistula, n	4	534	0.82	(0.45, 1.48)	0.51	0.92	0%
Grade A	2	351	0.77	(0.30, 2.00)	0.6	0.81	0%
Grade B	3	411	1.08	(0.32, 3.69)	0.9	0.57	0%
Grade C	3	411	0.85	(0.31, 2.30)	0.74	0.71	0%
Overall delayed gastric emptying, n	4	534	1.02	(0.53, 1.96)	0.96	0.69	0%
Grade A	1	268	/	/	/	/	/
Grade B	2	328	0.84	(0.22, 3.25)	0.81	0.89	0%
Grade C	1	268	/	/	/	/	/
Reoperation, n	54	534	0.51	(0.23, 1.12)	0.09	0.62	0%
Mortality, (%)	2	328	0.78	(0.26, 2.34)	0.65	0.36	0%
Length of stay, d	4	534	−2.64	(−4.79, −0.49)	**0.02**	0.001	81%
Oncologic outcomes							
Retrieved lymph nodes, n	3	411	4.5	(1.12, 7.89)	**0.009**	0.02	73%
Positive surgical margins,n	3	300	0.27	(0.10, 0.73)	**0.01**	0.65	0%

they were not well matched in these studies. Therefore, the real result of overall complications needs more data or studies to be evaluated.

Considering no RCT was available and information about definitions of wound infection, as well as antibiotics used in the perioperative period were not mentioned in most of the eleven studies, this question remains to be research.

The most severe complications of pancreaticoduodenectomy are pancreatic fistula and delayed gastric emptying, which have a close relationship with postoperative recovery and mortality. Our meta-analyses showed there were no statistical differences in neither overall pancreatic fistula and its three grades nor delayed gastric emptying and its three grades. And there was no difference in mortality and rate of reoperation. These indeed proved the safety of MIPD. However, considering definitions of PF&DGE were not mentioned in some included studies (**Table 1**) and most of the cases didn't mention the softness of the pancreas and the diameter of the main pancreatic duct, which are tightly related to PF [40,41], there might be flaws in our analyses.

Our meta-analysis showed MIPD has a shorter length of stay. But it varies a lot inside the MIPD group as well as inside the OPD group. We think it may have been related to local preferences and different health care systems. A short hospital stay theoretically can

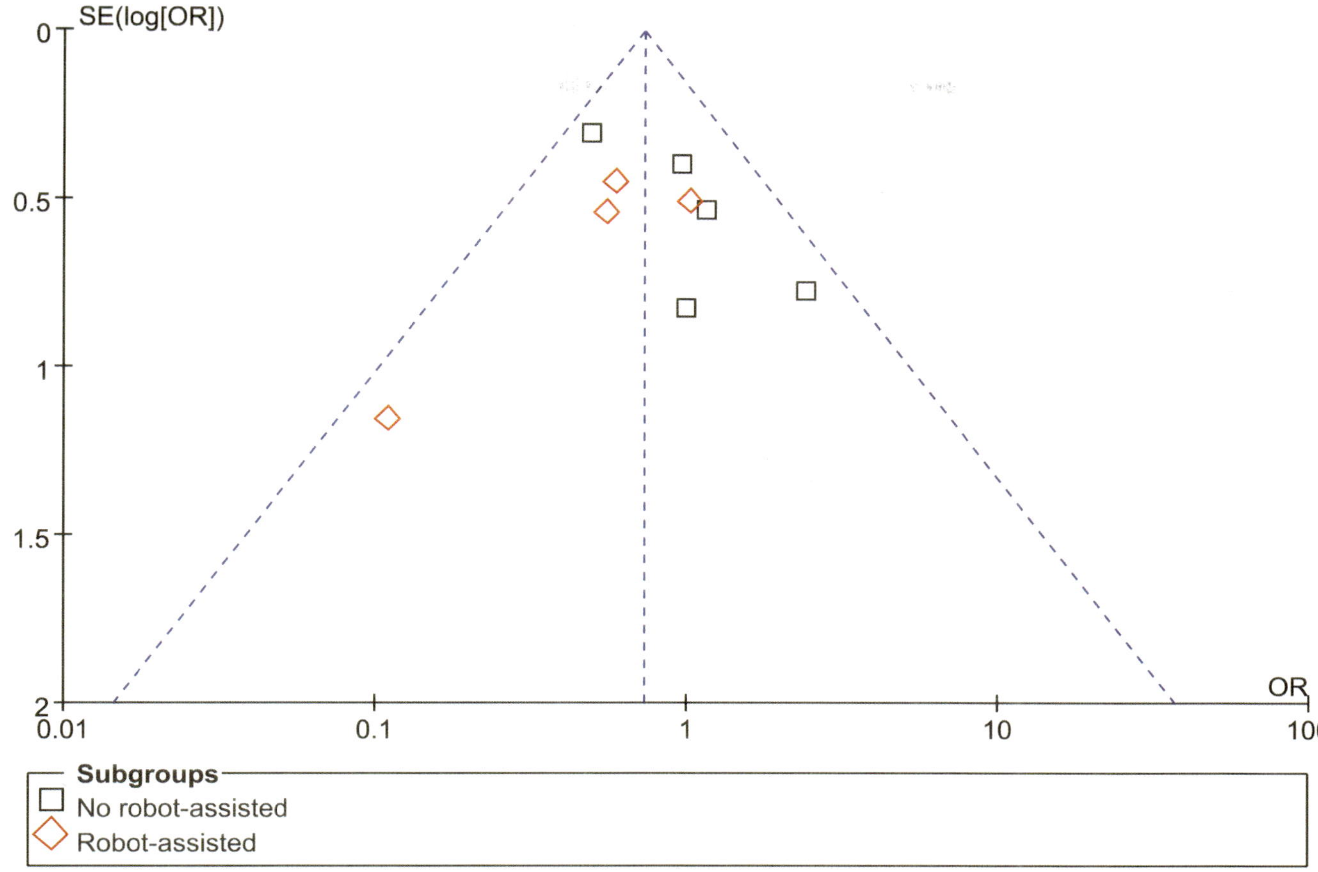

Figure 5. Funnel plot of overall complications in included studies, showing no publication bias.

decrease the pain of the patients and cost of the whole treatment, and therefore brings lots of benefits.

Considering that patients received pancreaticoduodenectomy were in most cases because of malignant tumors, comparison of oncologic safety between MIPD and OPD became important. In our pooled and sensitivity analyses, oncologic outcomes were not statistically different except in the large sample size subgroup, which showed either the number of retrieved lymph nodes or rate of R0 resection, was better in MIPD. But either the pooled or sensitive studies showed the trend that MIPD had better oncologic outcomes. However, the number of retrieved lymph nodes and rate of R0 resection can just speculate it indirectly; besides, long-term oncologic outcomes were not addressed in these referred studies. We need more long-term researches to answer this question.

Limitations

The strength of this review lies in that it provides a comprehensive comparison of MIPD with OPD. To our knowledge, this meta-analysis is the first to expound this important issue in different subgroups. This meta-analysis has some limitations that must be taken into account. The strengths and limitations of meta-analytical techniques have been a source of considerable debate. Besides, there were no RCT contained in the meta-analysis, and the calculated results from such trials may have many biases. For example, surgeons may avoid using laparoscopy on patients with larger and more advanced tumors, and most studies didn't mention how control groups were selected. So the included patients were not well matched in age, gender, BMI, ASA scores and so on. But as RCT similar to this meta-analysis is unattainable because of ethical problems, the outcomes from non-RCT would be valuable. Furthermore, we have no convincing evidence that the number of lymph nodes retrieved during a pancreaticoduodenectomy is associated with significant end-point outcome and in particular long term survival. So we need more researches in this field. Still, only one study [30] mentioned the cost and it showed LPD was associated with equivalent overall cost compared with OPD. Obviously there should be more studies to prove it. Ultimately, the analysis included only eleven studies. The sample size of this study was not large enough, and the results require confirmation in further high-quality trials.

Conclusions

Because of the advantages in intraoperative blood loss, wound complications, and length of stay, MIPD is worthwhile. However, considering the selection bias, the complexity of MIPD and lack of long-term oncologic outcomes, we suggest it be performed in a high-volume pancreatic surgery center in patients with light pancreatitis or small cancers distant from the major vessels. Further studies which control for biases and discuss the benefits and negatives of these procedures are needed.

Acknowledgments

We would like to thank the staff and our colleagues at the Chinese Cochrane Centre for their help and support. The work should be attributed to: West China Hospital, Chengdu, Sichuan, China.

Author Contributions

Conceived and designed the experiments: Y. Zeng HQ. Performed the experiments: HQ JQ. Analyzed the data: Y. Zhao GP. Contributed reagents/materials/analysis tools: Y. Zhao GP. Wrote the paper: HQ. Offered suggestions: Y. Zeng JQ.

References

1. Qiu J, Pankaj P, Jiang H, Zeng Y, Wu H (2013) Laparoscopy versus open distal gastrectomy for advanced gastric cancer: a systematic review and meta-analysis. Surg Laparosc Endosc Percutan Tech 23: 1–7.
2. Barlehner E, Anders S, Schwetling R (2002) Laparoscopic resection of the left pancreas: technique and indication. Dig Surg 19: 507–510.
3. Qiu JG, Wu H, Jiang H, Huang JW, Pankaj P, et al. (2011) Laparoscopic fenestration vs open fenestration in patients with congenital hepatic cysts: a meta-analysis. World J Gastroenterol 17: 3359–3365.
4. Huscher CG, Mingoli A, Sgarzini G, Sansonetti A, Di Paola M, et al. (2005) Laparoscopic versus open subtotal gastrectomy for distal gastric cancer: five-year results of a randomized prospective trial. Ann Surg 241: 232–237.
5. Qiu J, Chen S, Prasoon P, Wu H (2013) Meta-analysis of laparoscopic versus open distal pancreatectomy for pancreatic diseases. Surgical Practice 17: 49–57.
6. Palanivelu C, Rajan PS, Rangarajan M, Vaithiswaran V, Senthilnathan P, et al. (2009) Evolution in techniques of laparoscopic pancreaticoduodenectomy: a decade long experience from a tertiary center. J Hepatobiliary Pancreat Surg 16: 731–740.
7. Dulucq JL, Wintringer P, Mahajna A (2006) Laparoscopic pancreaticoduodenectomy for benign and malignant diseases. Surg Endosc 20: 1045–1050.
8. Zheng MH, Feng B, Lu AG, Li JW, Hu WG, et al. (2006) Laparoscopic pancreaticoduodenectomy for ductal adenocarcinoma of common bile duct: a case report and literature review. Med Sci Monit 12: CS57–60.
9. Palanivelu C, Jani K, Senthilnathan P, Parthasarathi R, Rajapandian S, et al. (2007) Laparoscopic pancreaticoduodenectomy: technique and outcomes. J Am Coll Surg 205: 222–230.
10. Pugliese R, Scandroglio I, Sansonna F, Maggioni D, Costanzi A, et al. (2008) Laparoscopic pancreaticoduodenectomy: a retrospective review of 19 cases. Surg Laparosc Endosc Percutan Tech 18: 13–18.
11. Tacconelli E (2010) Systematic reviews: CRD's guidance for undertaking reviews in health care. The Lancet Infectious Diseases 10: 226.
12. Higgins JP, Green S, Collaboration C (2008) Cochrane handbook for systematic reviews of interventions: Wiley Online Library.
13. Moher D, Liberati A, Tetzlaff J, Altman DG, Group P (2009) Preferred reporting items for systematic reviews and meta-analyses: the PRISMA statement. BMJ 339: b2535.
14. Athanasiou T, Al-Ruzzeh S, Kumar P, Crossman M-C, Amrani M, et al. (2004) Off-pump myocardial revascularization is associated with less incidence of stroke in elderly patients. The Annals of thoracic surgery 77: 745–753.
15. Clarke M, Horton R (2001) Bringing it all together: Lancet-Cochrane collaborate on systematic reviews. The Lancet 357: 1728.
16. Stroup DF, Berlin JA, Morton SC, Olkin I, Williamson GD, et al. (2000) Meta-analysis of observational studies in epidemiology: a proposal for reporting. Meta-analysis Of Observational Studies in Epidemiology (MOOSE) group. JAMA 283: 2008–2012.
17. Higgins JP, Thompson SG, Deeks JJ, Altman DG (2003) Measuring inconsistency in meta-analyses. BMJ 327: 557–560.
18. Farid S, Morris-Stiff G (2013) Laparoscopic vs open pancreaticoduodenectomy. J Am Coll Surg 216: 1220–1221.
19. Gumbs AA, Rodriguez Rivera AM, Milone L, Hoffman JP (2011) Laparoscopic pancreatoduodenectomy: a review of 285 published cases. Ann Surg Oncol 18: 1335–1341.
20. Lai EC, Tang CN (2013) Current status of robot-assisted laparoscopic pancreaticoduodenectomy and distal pancreatectomy: a comprehensive review. Asian J Endosc Surg 6: 158–164.
21. Kendrick ML, Cusati D (2010) Total laparoscopic pancreaticoduodenectomy: feasibility and outcome in an early experience. Arch Surg 145: 19–23.
22. Underwood RA, Soper NJ (1999) Current status of laparoscopic surgery of the pancreas. J Hepatobiliary Pancreat Surg 6: 154–164.
23. Nakamura M, Nakashima H (2013) Laparoscopic distal pancreatectomy and pancreatoduodenectomy: is it worthwhile? A meta-analysis of laparoscopic pancreatectomy. J Hepatobiliary Pancreat Sci 20: 421–428.
24. Gumbs AA, Gres P, Madureira FA, Gayet B (2008) Laparoscopic vs. open resection of noninvasive intraductal pancreatic mucinous neoplasms. J Gastrointest Surg 12: 707–712.
25. Dulucq JL, Wintringer P, Stabilini C, Feryn T, Perissat J, et al. (2005) Are major laparoscopic pancreatic resections worthwhile? A prospective study of 32 patients in a single institution. Surg Endosc 19: 1028–1034.
26. Kuroki T, Adachi T, Okamoto T, Kanematsu T (2012) A non-randomized comparative study of laparoscopy-assisted pancreaticoduodenectomy and open pancreaticoduodenectomy. Hepato-gastroenterology 59: 570–573.
27. Zureikat AH, Breaux JA, Steel JL, Hughes SJ (2011) Can laparoscopic pancreaticoduodenectomy be safely implemented? J Gastrointest Surg 15: 1151–1157.
28. Cho A, Yamamoto H, Nagata M, Takiguchi N, Shimada H, et al. (2009) Comparison of laparoscopy-assisted and open pylorus-preserving pancreaticoduodenectomy for periampullary disease. Am J Surg 198: 445–449.
29. Asbun HJ, Stauffer JA (2012) Laparoscopic vs open pancreaticoduodenectomy: overall outcomes and severity of complications using the Accordion Severity Grading System. J Am Coll Surg 215: 810–819.
30. Mesleh MG, Stauffer JA, Bowers SP, Asbun HJ (2013) Cost analysis of open and laparoscopic pancreaticoduodenectomy: a single institution comparison. Surg Endosc 27: 4518–4523.
31. Li Y, Wang X, Wang M, Yang Z, Peng B (2013) [Delayed gastric emptying after laparoscopic versus open pancreaticoduodenectomy: a comparative study]. Zhonghua wai ke za zhi [Chinese journal of surgery] 51: 304–307.
32. Chalikonda S, Aguilar-Saavedra JR, Walsh RM (2012) Laparoscopic robotic-assisted pancreaticoduodenectomy: a case-matched comparison with open resection. Surg Endosc 26: 2397–2402.
33. Zhou NX, Chen JZ, Liu Q, Zhang X, Wang Z, et al. (2011) Outcomes of pancreatoduodenectomy with robotic surgery versus open surgery. Int J Med Robot 7: 131–137.
34. Bao PQ, Mazirka PO, Watkins KT (2013) Retrospective Comparison of Robot-Assisted Minimally Invasive Versus Open Pancreaticoduodenectomy for Periampullary Neoplasms. J Gastrointest Surg.
35. Lai EC, Yang GP, Tang CN (2012) Robot-assisted laparoscopic pancreaticoduodenectomy versus open pancreaticoduodenectomy—a comparative study. Int J Surg 10: 475–479.
36. Buchs NC, Addeo P, Bianco FM, Ayloo S, Benedetti E, et al. (2011) Robotic versus open pancreaticoduodenectomy: a comparative study at a single institution. World J Surg 35: 2739–2746.
37. Bassi C, Dervenis C, Butturini G, Fingerhut A, Yeo C, et al. (2005) Postoperative pancreatic fistula: an international study group (ISGPF) definition. Surgery 138: 8–13.
38. Wente MN, Bassi C, Dervenis C, Fingerhut A, Gouma DJ, et al. (2007) Delayed gastric emptying (DGE) after pancreatic surgery: a suggested definition by the International Study Group of Pancreatic Surgery (ISGPS). Surgery 142: 761–768.
39. Suc B, Msika S, Fingerhut A, Fourtanier G, Hay JM, et al. (2003) Temporary fibrin glue occlusion of the main pancreatic duct in the prevention of intra-abdominal complications after pancreatic resection: prospective randomized trial. Ann Surg 237: 57–65.
40. Gouma DJ, Van Geenen RC, van Gulik TM, de Haan RJ, de Wit LT, et al. (2000) Rates of complications and death after pancreaticoduodenectomy: risk factors and the impact of hospital volume. Annals of surgery 232: 786.
41. Tranchart H, Gaujoux S, Rebours V, Vullierme MP, Dokmak S, et al. (2012) Preoperative CT scan helps to predict the occurrence of severe pancreatic fistula after pancreaticoduodenectomy. Ann Surg 256: 139–145.

A Meta-Analysis of Unilateral versus Bilateral Pedicle Screw Fixation in Minimally Invasive Lumbar Interbody Fusion

Zheng Liu[1], Qi Fei[2]*, Bingqiang Wang[2], Pengfei Lv[1], Cheng Chi[1], Yong Yang[2], Fan Zhao[2], Jisheng Lin[2], Zhao Ma[2]

1 Department of Orthopaedics, Peking University Shougang Hospital, Beijing, China, **2** Department of Orthopaedics, Beijing Friendship Hospital, Capital Medical University, Beijing, China

Abstract

Study Design: Meta-analysis.

Background: Bilateral pedicle screw fixation (PS) after lumbar interbody fusion is a widely accepted method of managing various spinal diseases. Recently, unilateral PS fixation has been reported as effective as bilateral PS fixation. This meta-analysis aimed to comparatively assess the efficacy and safety of unilateral PS fixation and bilateral PS fixation in the minimally invasive (MIS) lumbar interbody fusion for one-level degenerative lumbar spine disease.

Methods: MEDLINE/PubMed, EMBASE, BIOSIS Previews, and Cochrane Library were searched through March 30, 2014. Randomized controlled trials (RCTs) and controlled clinical trials (CCTs) on unilateral versus bilateral PS fixation in MIS lumbar interbody fusion that met the inclusion criteria and the methodological quality standard were retrieved and reviewed. Data on participant characteristics, interventions, follow-up period, and outcomes were extracted from the included studies and analyzed by Review Manager 5.2.

Results: Six studies (5 RCTs and 1 CCT) involving 298 patients were selected. There were no significant differences between unilateral and bilateral PS fixation procedures in fusion rate, complications, visual analogue score (VAS) for leg pain, VAS for back pain, Oswestry disability index (ODI). Both fixation procedures had similar length of hospital stay (MD = 0.38, 95% CI = −0.83 to 1.58; P = 0.54). In contrast, bilateral PS fixation was associated with significantly more intra-operative blood loss (P = 0.002) and significantly longer operation time (P = 0.02) as compared with unilateral PS fixation.

Conclusions: Unilateral PS fixation appears as effective and safe as bilateral PS fixation in MIS lumbar interbody fusion but requires less operative time and causes less blood loss, thus offering a simple alternative approach for one-level lumbar degenerative disease.

Editor: Mohammed Shamji, Toronto Western Hospital, Canada

Funding: The study was funded by Basic-Clinical Cooperation Project in Capital Medical University (NO. 13JL37) and Beijing Outstanding Talent Training Project (NO. 2013D003034000005). The funders had no role in study design, data collection and analysis, decision to publish, or preparation of the manuscript.

Competing Interests: The authors have declared that no competing interests exist.

* Email: spinefei@126.com

Introduction

Minimally invasive (MIS) lumbar interbody fusion is a popular technique used to treat various lumbar degenerative disorders. Over the traditional open surgery, MIS surgery offers multiple advantages; it not only reduces the approach-related muscle damage, blood loss, postoperative pain, length of hospital stay, and postoperative narcotic usage but also allows for early ambulation. Accordingly, MIS is popularized by most of the spine surgeons, especially when it is used with percutaneous pedicle screws [1].

Generally, bilateral pedicle screw (PS) fixation is accepted as a standard procedure in lumbar interbody fusion. Providing rigid fixation, bilateral PS have a great biomechanical stability and several clinical advantages [2]. Recently, unilateral PS fixation has been suggested as an effective approach as bilateral PS fixation in spinal fusion requiring significantly shorter operating time and hospital stay [3–5]. Ding et al. evaluated outcomes of patients with degenerative disc disease following unilateral and bilateral PS fixation procedures respectively and validated the efficacy and safety of unilateral PS fixation in traditional open lumbar interbody fusion. However, this meta-analysis included samples of patients with both one- and two-level degenerative lumbar spine diseases, which might increase the statistical heterogeneity [5]. No similar meta-analyses on unilateral versus bilateral PS fixation in MIS lumbar interbody fusion particularly for one-level degenerative lumbar spine disease are available in the current literature. The objective of this meta-analysis was to examine the effects of unilateral PS fixation and bilateral PS fixation in MIS lumber interbody fusion for one-level degenerative lumbar spine disease by contrasting and combining results from previously reported relevant randomized controlled trials (RCTs) and controlled clinical trials (CCTs).

Methods

Literature search

The MEDLINE (through PubMed), EMBASE, Ovid (BIOSIS Previews included), and Cochrane databases were searched through March 18, 2014 using combinations of such key terms as 'lumbar interbody fusion', 'pedicle screw fixation', 'minimally invasive', 'unilateral', and 'bilateral' with the Boolean operators 'AND', 'NOT', and 'OR'. Studies cited in the identified articles were also searched manually. The included studies were published in a peer-reviewed journal as a full article, excluding the gray literature and conference proceedings.

Inclusion and exclusion criteria

RCTs and CCTs were included if the following criteria were met: (1) they were published in full-text in English in peer-reviewed journals but not in the gray literature and conference proceedings; (2) subjects were diagnosed with one-level lumbar degenerative disease; (3) bilateral and unilateral pedicle screw fixation procedures were comparatively evaluated; and (4) RCTs and comparative observational studies (CCTs). The exclusion criteria were: (1) combined anterior and posterior surgery; (2) lumbar tumors; (3) conditions such as severe osteoporosis, active infection, metabolic disease or symptomatic vascular disease; (4) previous lumbar surgery; and (5) an average follow-up time of <6 months.

Data extraction

Two reviewers independently screened the titles and abstracts of the retrieved articles to ensure that both inclusion and exclusion criteria were met. Disagreements, if any, were resolved by a third reviewer. Data on the primary outcome measures including visual analogue leg pain score (VAS), Oswestry disability index (ODI), fusion rate and complications and the secondary outcome measures including intra-operative blood loss, operating time and hospital stay were extracted from the included studies and are presented in Table 1.

Study quality

The methodological quality of the included studies was assessed by two independent authors based on the physiotherapy evidence database (PEDro) scale [6]. This scale is based on a list of 11 criteria, each conferring 1 point to the total score. One criterion was excluded from our calculation of the total PEDro score, and, subsequently there was a potentially maximum total score of 10 points for each of the individual studies included in this meta-analysis. Two reviewers performed the assessment independently. The agreement between the 2 reviewers was evaluated with both the correlation coefficient (r) for interrater agreement and the intraclass correlation coefficient.

Statistical analysis

The summary statistic was calculated for each individual study using the meta-analysis program of the Cochrane Collaboration (Review Manager 5.2). Binary data (e.g., fusion rate, incidence rate of screw complications) were presented as odds ratio (OR) and 95% confidence intervals (CIs). Continuous outcomes (VAS, ODI, intra-operative blood loss, operative time, and hospital stay) were summarized using the mean difference (MD) and respective 95% CI. Data on the primary and secondary outcome measures were analyzed as continuous or dichotomized variables using random effect model or fixed effect model. When there was no difference between the findings derived with the 2 models, the results were reported using the fixed-effect model, indicating the absence of significant statistical heterogeneity. Random-effects model was used as a more conservative estimate, less likely to reveal a difference between 2 treatment approaches as compared with the fixed-effects model. When any difference between treatment approaches really existed, both models were used. The possibility of publication bias was assessed by funnel plots, showing the intervention effect from each study against the corresponding standard error. Symmetrical and any asymmetry plots would suggest absence and presence of publication bias respectively. The strength and robustness of the pooled results by sequential omission of individual studies were tested by the sensitivity analysis.

Results

Eligible studies

A total of 1070 relevant titles were identified through electronic and manual searches. After review of the abstracts and titles, 802 studies were excluded in that they were irrelevant, not on human

Table 1. Outcome measurements in the studies included in this meta-analysis.

Clinical outcome	Choi Y 2013	Dahdaleh N 2013	Dong J 2014	Lin B 2013	Shen X 2013	Sonmez E 2013
VAS	Yes	Yes	Yes	Yes	Yes	Yes
ODI	Yes	Yes	Yes	Yes	Yes	Yes
JOA	NR	NR	Yes	NR	NR	NR
SF-36	NR	Yes	NR	NR	NR	NR
mProlo scores	NR	NR	NR	NR	Yes	NR
Fusion rate	Yes	Yes	Yes	Yes	Yes	Yes
Complication rate	Yes	Yes	Yes	Yes	Yes	Yes
Operation time	Yes	NR	Yes	Yes	NR	Yes
Blood loss	Yes	Yes	Yes	Yes	NR	Yes
Hospital stay	NR	Yes	Yes	NR	NR	Yes

subjects, not comparative studies or other forms of investigation. Forty articles on bilateral and unilateral PS fixation procedures were retrieved from the databases, and six studies (5 RCTs and 1 CCT) met the inclusion criteria (Figure 1). The characteristics of these six studies [7–12] are summarized in Table 2, and no significant differences were found in the baseline characteristics between the two groups. The six studies included a total of 298 participants with 146 adults treated with unilateral PS fixation and 152 adults treated with bilateral unilateral PS fixation.

Methodological quality

The total scores for all included studies assessed by PEDro quality criteria ranged from 5 to 7 (Table 3). Five studies were considered as being high quality (PEDro score ≥6), and one study was of low quality (PEDro score <6). The two independent reviewers reached consensuses on the scoring of all items without any disagreement.

Postoperative functional performance (VAS and ODI)

VAS and ODI are the most frequently used variables to assess the postoperative function performance of patients. Five studies assessed VAS for back pain, which was not significantly different between bilateral and unilateral groups (MD = −0.02, 95% CI = −0.17 to 0.13; P = 0.77) (Figure 2a). Three studies assessed VAS for leg pain, which was not different between the two groups either (MD = −0.10, 95% CI = −0.20 to 0.01; P = 0.06) (Figure 2b). ODI scores were available in five trials [16,19–22] where no significant difference was detected between the two groups (MD = 0.31, 95% CI = −0.66 to 1.27; P = 0.54) (Figure 2c).

Fusion rate and complications

The overall fusion rate was 91.8% (134/146) in the unilateral group and 96.0% (146/152) in the bilateral group (OR = 0.47, 95% CI = 0.18–1.27, P = 0.14, Figure 3a). No nonunion case was reported in the study of Dong [9]. The overall incidence of complications in the unilateral and bilateral groups was 5.48% (8/146) and 4.61% (7/152), respectively, and the difference was not significant (OR = 1.25, 95% CI = 0.44–3.59, P = 0.67, Figure 3b). No complications were observed in two studies [8,9].

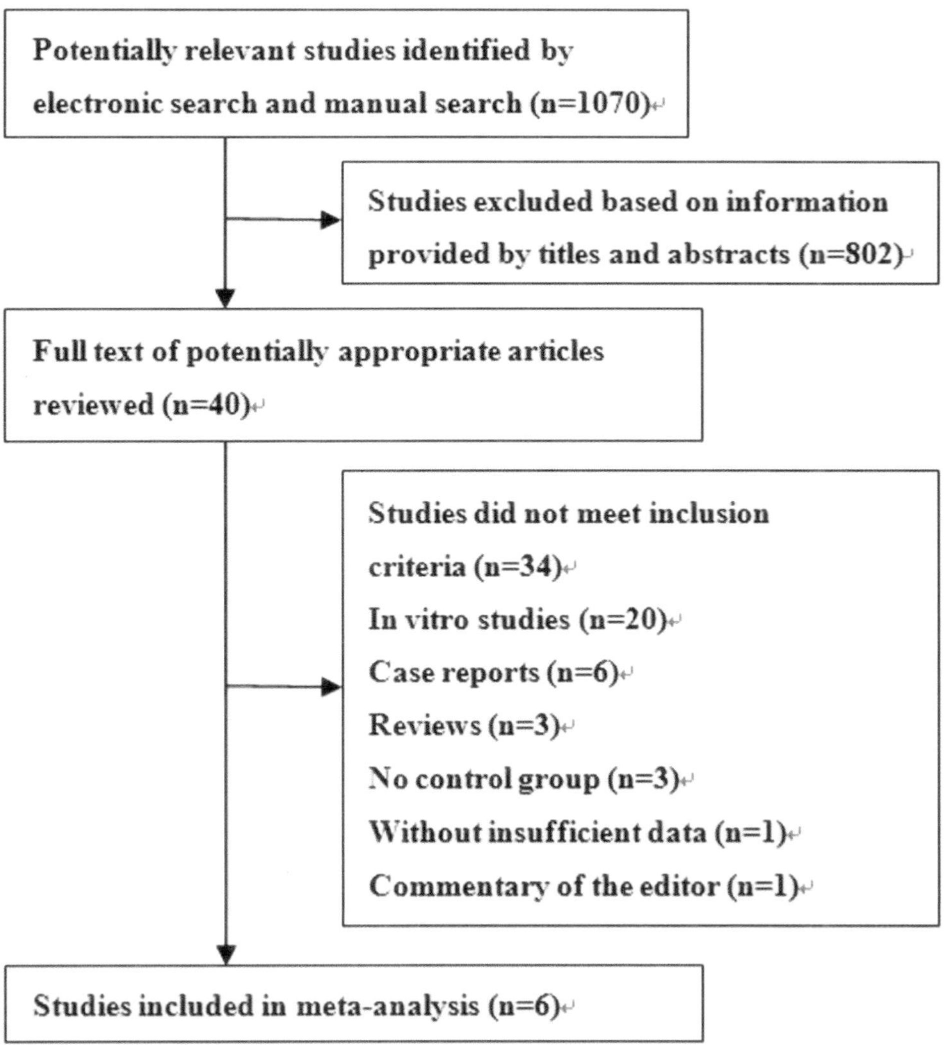

Figure 1. Flow diagram of study identification for this meta-analysis.

Table 2. Basic characteristics of the studies included in this meta-analysis.

Study	Time	Study design	Etiology	Case	Age	Follow-up	Fusion Technique
Choi Y	2013	RCT	disc herniation, spinal stenosis, degenerative spondylolisthesis, spondylolytic spondylolisthesis, and recurrent disc herniation	U:26	U: 53.39	U: 27.5 months	TLIF
				B:27	B: 56.22	B: 28.9 months	
Dahdaleh N	2013	RCT	single-level degenerative spondylosis or spondylolisthesis, Grade 1 or 2	U: 16	U: 62.2	U: 11.4 months	TLIF
				B: 20	B: 57.3	B: 12.4 months	
Dong J	2014	RCT	single-segment degenerative lumbar instability	U: 20	U: 54.0	U: 36 months	PLIF
				B: 19	B: 56.6	B: 36 months	
Lin B	2013	RCT	spinal canal stenosis,spondylolisthesis (grade I or II), and lumbar disk herniation	U: 43	U: 67	U: 26 months	TLIF
				B: 42	B: 65.5	B: 26 months	
Shen X	2013	RCT	Unilateral lumbar disc herniation, Foraminal stenosis	U: 31	U: 57.3	U: 26.6 months	TLIF
				B: 34	B: 58.9	B: 26.6 months	
Sonmez E	2013	CCT	single level recurrent disc herniation	U: 10	U: 47.3	U: 2 year	TLIF
				B: 10	B: 45.6	B: 2 year	

U unilateral fixation, B bilateral fixation.

Table 3. Methodological quality of the included studies assessed with the PEDro scale.

Study	Item PEDro score										Total score
	2	3	4	5	6	7	8	9	10	11	
Choi Y	+	–	+	–	–	+	+	+	+	+	7/10
Dahdaleh N	+	–	+	–	–	–	+	+	+	+	6/10
Dong J	+	–	+	–	–	–	+	+	+	+	6/10
Lin B	+	–	+	–	–	–	+	+	+	+	6/10
Shen X	+	–	+	–	–	–	+	+	+	+	6/10
Sonmez E	–	–	+	–	–	–	+	+	+	+	5/10

Operation time, blood loss and hospital stay

Operation time was assessed in four eligible studies and the results of the meta-analysis are presented in Figure 4a. Overall, unilateral PS fixation required a significantly less operative time as compared with bilateral PS fixation (MD = −30.17, 95% CI = −55.37 to −4.98; P = 0.02). Shown as a forest plot in Figure 4b are the results of meta-analysis of intra-operative blood loss; the amount of blood loss was significantly smaller in the unilateral group than in the bilateral group (MD = −99.06, 95% CI = −161.40 to −36.71; P = 0.002). Three studies reported the mean length of hospital stay where no significant difference was detected between the unilateral and bilateral groups (MD = 0.38, 95% CI = −0.83 to 1.58; P = 0.54).

Discussion

Bilateral PS fixation after lumbar interbody fusion is accepted as a standard procedure. Providing rigid fixation, bilateral PS fixation has a great biomechanical stability and clinical benefits. However, the rigidity of bilateral PS fixation can lead to device-related osteoporosis of the vertebrae [13] and makes the adjacent segment prone to load- and motion-induced degeneration [14]. To achieve optimal biomechanical conditions in the fused segment and minimize adverse effects in the adjacent levels caused by instrumentation, the use of less rigid systems of fixation has been advocated [15]. Some recent clinical and biomechanical studies on the suitability of unilateral PS fixation have demonstrated that a reliable fusion with fewer pedicle screws can be achieved [16,17]. Nevertheless, unilateral PS fixation may be detrimental to spine stability and the promotion for fusion as suggested by an *in vitro* study [18]. Therefore, the use of unilateral or bilateral PS fixation remains a matter of debate.

Numerous previous biomechanical and clinical studies attempted to comparatively evaluate unilateral and bilateral PS fixation approach and inconsistent results were obtained. Chen et al. [16] demonstrated that unilateral PS fixation was good enough to maintain the stability of the spine in a biomechanics study. Goel et al. [19] reported that the unilateral PS system was effective to reduce stress shielding of the vertebra and diminish peak stress arising in the adjacent levels above and below the fusion. Toyone and coauthors [20] recently reported that unilateral PS fixation was associated with a low incidence of adjacent-segment degeneration following posterior lumber interbody fusion. However, an increasing number of published studies have raised concerns over the clinical benefits of unilateral fixation. Yucesoy et al. [21] reported that unilateral PS fixation was inadequate to stabilize a 2-level unilateral lesion when compared with bilateral fixation. Aoki et al. [22] observed that unilateral fixation caused postoperative cage migration more frequently than bilateral fixation in patients who had scoliotic curvature with a Cobb angle >10°. In addition, Slucky et al. showed that unilateral PS fixation supplied only half of the improvement in stiffness compared bilateral PS fixation and caused significant off-axis rotational motions, which could hinder stability and the promotion for fusion after transforaminal lumbar interbody fusion (TLIF) [18].

However, unilateral PS fixation supplemented with translaminar facet screw fixation on the contralateral side offered stability comparable to that offered by bilateral PS fixation. Several other biomechanical and clinical studies also showed that supplementation of a contralateral facet screw might exert a similar effect as bilateral PS fixation on the stiffness or range of motion following TLIF [23–25]. Therefore supplementation of a contralateral facet

Study or Subgroup	unilateral pedicle screw fixation Mean	SD	Total	bilateral pedicle screw fixation Mean	SD	Total	Weight	Mean Difference IV, Fixed, 95% CI
Choi Y 2013	1.8	0.4	26	1.8	0.4	27	49.4%	0.00 [-0.22, 0.22]
Dahdaleh N 2013	2.6	2.4	16	2.1	2.1	20	1.0%	0.50 [-0.99, 1.99]
Lin B 2013	3.1	0.16	43	3.3	1.1	42	20.3%	-0.20 [-0.54, 0.14]
Shen X 2013	2	1.3	31	2.2	1.4	34	5.3%	-0.20 [-0.86, 0.46]
Sonmez E 2013	1.8	0.3	10	1.7	0.4	10	23.9%	0.10 [-0.21, 0.41]
Total (95% CI)			**126**			**133**	**100.0%**	**-0.02 [-0.17, 0.13]**

Heterogeneity: Chi² = 2.46, df = 4 (P = 0.65); I² = 0%
Test for overall effect: Z = 0.29 (P = 0.77)

(a)

Study or Subgroup	unilateral pedicle screw fixation Mean	SD	Total	bilateral pedicle screw fixation Mean	SD	Total	Weight	Mean Difference IV, Fixed, 95% CI
Choi Y 2013	1.7	0.2	26	1.8	0.2	27	92.9%	-0.10 [-0.21, 0.01]
Dahdaleh N 2013	2.6	3	16	2.1	2.8	20	0.3%	0.50 [-1.41, 2.41]
Sonmez E 2013	2.4	0.4	10	2.5	0.5	10	6.8%	-0.10 [-0.50, 0.30]
Total (95% CI)			**52**			**57**	**100.0%**	**-0.10 [-0.20, 0.01]**

Heterogeneity: Chi² = 0.38, df = 2 (P = 0.83); I² = 0%
Test for overall effect: Z = 1.86 (P = 0.06)

(b)

Study or Subgroup	unilateral pedicle screw fixation Mean	SD	Total	bilateral pedicle screw fixation Mean	SD	Total	Weight	Mean Difference IV, Fixed, 95% CI
Choi Y 2013	6.6	5.3	26	9.5	5.3	27	11.5%	-2.90 [-5.75, -0.05]
Dahdaleh N 2013	22.7	17.3	16	17.9	18.7	20	0.7%	4.80 [-6.99, 16.59]
Lin B 2013	15.67	2.3	43	14.93	2.6	42	86.0%	0.74 [-0.30, 1.78]
Shen X 2013	21.38	14.33	31	22.84	15.65	34	1.8%	-1.46 [-8.75, 5.83]
Sonmez E 2013	31	40	10	36	39	10	0.1%	-5.00 [-39.63, 29.63]
Total (95% CI)			**126**			**133**	**100.0%**	**0.31 [-0.66, 1.27]**

Heterogeneity: Chi² = 6.38, df = 4 (P = 0.17); I² = 37%
Test for overall effect: Z = 0.62 (P = 0.54)

(c)

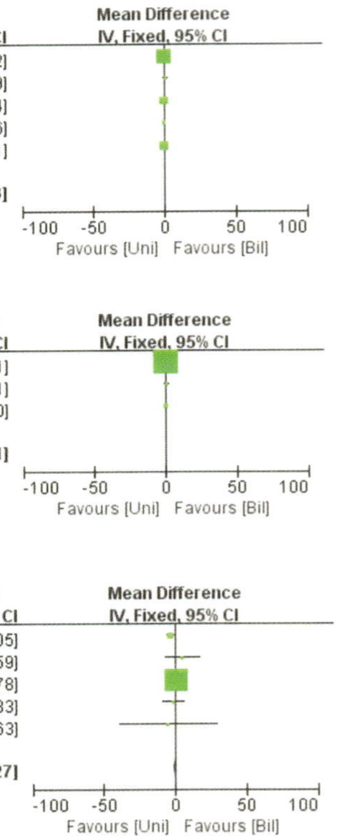

Figure 2. Forest plots for VAS for back pain (a), VAS for leg pain (b) and ODI (c) in patients undergoing unilateral and bilateral PS fixations respectively.

screw may possibly compensate the limitations of unilateral PS fixation in lumbar interbody fusion.

Spinal fusion can be achieved by both posterolateral and/or interbody fusion techniques [26]. However, conventional spinal fusion is related to significant muscle stripping and retraction that

Study or Subgroup	unilateral pedicle screw fixation Events	Total	bilateral pedicle screw fixation Events	Total	Weight	Odds Ratio M-H, Fixed, 95% CI
Choi Y 2013	22	26	26	27	32.7%	0.21 [0.02, 2.03]
Dahdaleh N 2013	15	16	19	20	8.8%	0.79 [0.05, 13.69]
Dong J 2014	20	20	19	19		Not estimable
Lin B 2013	39	43	39	42	30.6%	0.75 [0.16, 3.57]
Shen X 2013	30	31	34	34	12.9%	0.29 [0.01, 7.51]
Sonmez E 2013	8	10	9	10	15.0%	0.44 [0.03, 5.88]
Total (95% CI)		**146**		**152**	**100.0%**	**0.47 [0.18, 1.27]**
Total events	134		146			

Heterogeneity: Chi² = 1.03, df = 4 (P = 0.91); I² = 0%
Test for overall effect: Z = 1.49 (P = 0.14)

(a)

Study or Subgroup	unilateral pedicle screw fixation Events	Total	bilateral pedicle screw fixation Events	Total	Weight	Odds Ratio M-H, Fixed, 95% CI
Choi Y 2013	2	26	1	27	14.6%	2.17 [0.18, 25.46]
Dahdaleh N 2013	1	16	1	20	13.4%	1.27 [0.07, 21.97]
Dong J 2014	0	20	0	19		Not estimable
Lin B 2013	1	43	2	42	31.8%	0.48 [0.04, 5.46]
Shen X 2013	4	31	3	34	40.1%	1.53 [0.31, 7.46]
Sonmez E 2013	0	10	0	10		Not estimable
Total (95% CI)		**146**		**152**	**100.0%**	**1.25 [0.44, 3.59]**
Total events	8		7			

Heterogeneity: Chi² = 0.86, df = 3 (P = 0.84); I² = 0%
Test for overall effect: Z = 0.42 (P = 0.67)

(b)

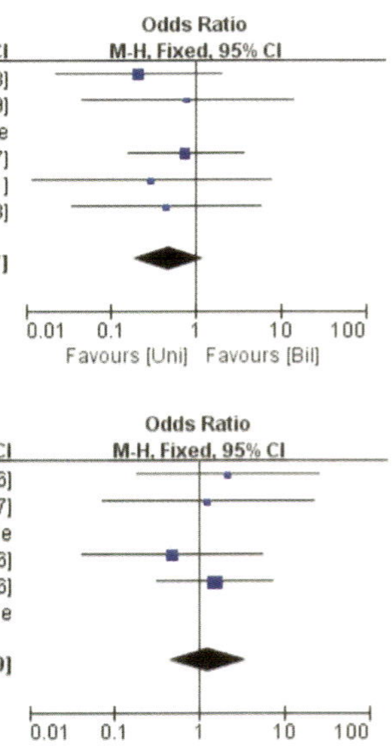

Figure 3. Forest plots for fusion rate (a) and incidence rate of complications (b) in patients undergoing unilateral and bilateral PS fixations respectively.

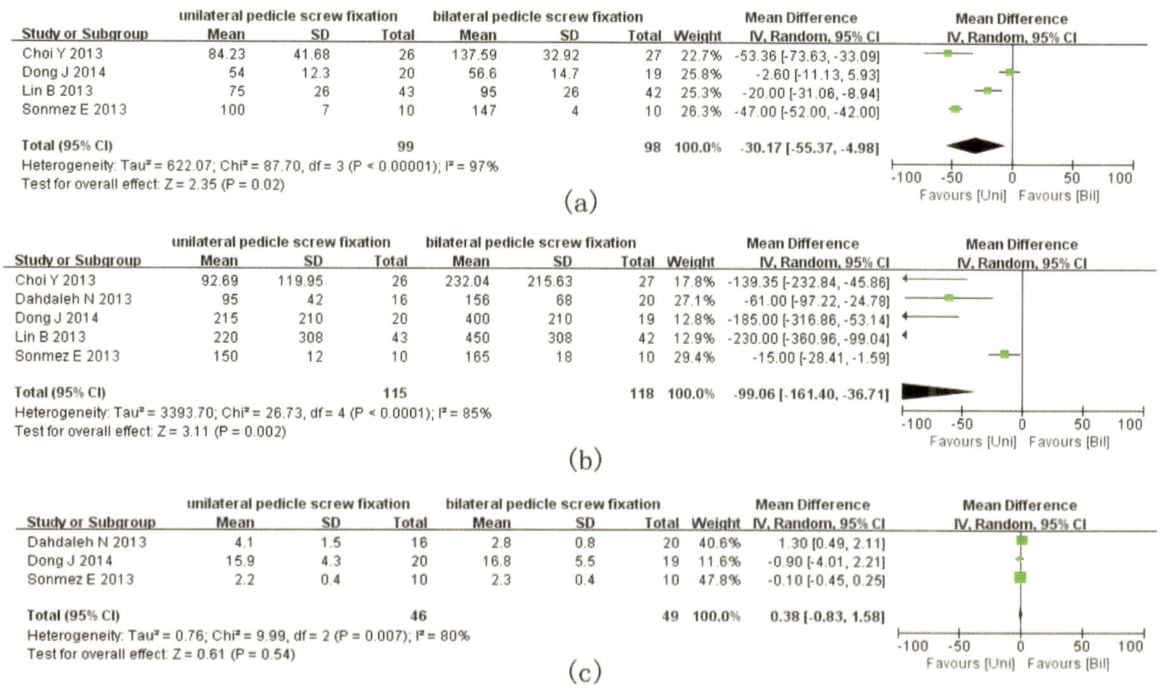

Figure 4. Forest plots for operation time (a), blood loss (b) and hospital stay (c) in patients undergoing unilateral and bilateral PS fixations respectively.

can adversely affect both short- and long-term patient outcomes [1]. In contrast, minimally invasive spinal fusion is performed by a muscle-dilating approach, which may significantly minimize or diminish the iatrogenic soft tissue injury, intra-operative blood loss, postoperative pain and the duration of hospital stays [27]. Accordingly, many surgeons prefer minimally invasive methods, such as TLIF with unilateral PS fixation [1,4,28], and believe that unilateral PS fixation is sufficient to accomplish spinal fusion. The objective of this meta-analysis was to systematically compare the efficiency and safety of unilateral and bilateral PS fixation procedures in MIS lumbar interbody fusion for one-level lumbar degenerative disease.

Our analysis suggested that there were no differences between unilateral PS fixation and bilateral PS fixation in VAS and ODI. This finding was in agreement with the results from some previous studies [9–11] where the patient outcomes were evaluated either using other assessment systems such as the Japanese Orthopaedic Association (JOA), 36-Item Short Form Healthy Survey version 2 (SF-36v2) and mProlo scores respectively or using radiographic parameters such as the whole lumbar lordosis, the segmental lordosis, fusion level disc space angle, lumbar scoliosis angle, and segmental scoliosis angle [11].

There were significantly less blood loss and significantly shorter operation time in the unilateral PS fixation group as compared with the bilateral PS fixation group in our meta-analysis. Unilateral PS fixation dissects soft tissue and insert pedicle screws only on one side and therefore it takes less time and decreases blood loss. Moreover, less soft tissue dissection may allow for early recovery [28]. However, the average length of hospital stay was similar in the two groups in our meta-analysis, which was inconsistent with the observation of a previous study where the hospital stay was shorter for unilateral fixation than for bilateral fixation due to early recovery and rehabilitation [7]. One of the reasons for the discrepancy might be the small number of studies included in our meta-analysis. Another reason might be the high heterogeneity among the included studies; in one study the hospital stay was longer in the unilateral group than in the bilateral group because of pulmonary edema in some patients.

Despite no statistical difference, the overall fusion rate was slightly lower in the unilateral group (91.8%) than in the bilateral group (96%). It was likely that less biomechanical stability in unilateral instrumentation might have negatively impacted the fusion. Because of this, supplementation of a contralateral facet screw has been proposed as a solution to compensate for the insufficient stability of unilateral PS fixation. The incidences of complications in unilateral and bilateral groups were 5.48% (8/146) and 4.61% (7/152), respectively. No single complication was identified in two studies. This finding was inconsistent with results from many previous studies where insufficient stability of unilateral PS fixation increased the incidence of cage migration [12,22].

Our study has a number of weaknesses. First of all, in some of the included studies, there were methodological limitations including failure to collect data prospectively, nonconsecutive enrollment of patients, inadequate baseline comparisons, and improper blinding or non-blinding. And these limitations somewhat reduced the level of evidence for this meta-analysis. Secondly, heterogeneity existed among the studies particularly when the continuous outcome measure variables were pooled. The heterogeneity might be attributable to differences among the included studies in the study design, study quality, patients' characteristics, and the diverse technical specifications. Thirdly, multiple assessment tools and fusion criteria were used in the included studies that might have confounded the combined results. Lastly, incomplete data recording was observed in some of the included studies. Pooling of such data might lead to bias.

In summary, through contrasting and combining results from 5 RCTs and 1 CCT on unilateral versus bilateral PS fixation in MIS lumbar fusion, this meta-analysis has shown that unilateral PS fixation may significantly reduce the intraoperative blood loss and shorten the operation time, somewhat improve the clinical outcome scores of ODI and VAS and fusion rate, and significantly decrease the incidence rate of complications while not affecting hospital stay as compared with bilateral PS fixation in patients with one-level lumbar degenerative disease. These findings suggest that unilateral PS fixation in MIS lumbar fusion is as effective and safe as but less time-consuming than bilateral PS fixation for one level lumbar degenerative disease. Nevertheless, this approach warrants further evaluations in high quality RCTs with large sample size and long-term follow-up before its wider clinical application.

Author Contributions

Analyzed the data: CC YY. Contributed to the writing of the manuscript: ZL. Conceived and designed the meta-analysis: QF. Performed the study: ZL. Screened data for analysis: BQW PFL. Conducted data extraction: FZ JSL ZM.

References

1. Foley KT, Holly LT, Schwender JD (2003) Minimally invasive lumbar fusion. Spine (Phila Pa 1976) 28: S26–S35.
2. Sim HB, Murovic JA, Cho BY, Lim TJ, Park J (2010) Biomechanical comparison of single-level posterior versus transforaminal lumbar interbody fusions with bilateral pedicle screw fixation: segmental stability and the effects on adjacent motion segments: laboratory investigation. Journal of Neurosurgery: Spine 12: 700–708.
3. Kasai Y, Inaba T, Kato T, Matsumura Y, Akeda K, et al. (2010) Biomechanical study of the lumbar spine using a unilateral pedicle screw fixation system. Journal of Clinical Neuroscience 17: 364–367.
4. Deutsch H, Musacchio Jr MJ (2006) Minimally invasive transforaminal lumbar interbody fusion with unilateral pedicle screw fixation. Neurosurgical Focus 20: 1–5.
5. Ding W, Chen Y, Liu H, Wang J, Zheng Z (2014) Comparison of unilateral versus bilateral pedicle screw fixation in lumbar interbody fusion: a meta-analysis. European Spine Journal 23: 395–403.
6. Verhagen AP, de Vet HC, de Bie RA, Kessels AG, Boers M, et al. (1998) The Delphi list: a criteria list for quality assessment of randomized clinical trials for conducting systematic reviews developed by Delphi consensus. Journal of clinical epidemiology 51: 1235–1241.
7. Lin B, Xu Y, He Y, Zhang B, Lin Q, et al. (2013) Minimally Invasive Unilateral Pedicle Screw Fixation and Lumbar Interbody Fusion for the Treatment of Lumbar Degenerative Disease. Orthopedics 36: e1071–e1076.
8. Hastaların İTY, Sonuçları YT (2013) Unilateral Percutaneous Pedicle Screw Instrumentation with minimally Invasive TLIF for the Treatment of Recurrent Lumbar Disk Disease: 2 Years Follow-Up. Turkish neurosurgery 23: 372–378.
9. Dong J, Rong L, Feng F, Liu B, Xu Y, et al. (2014) Unilateral pedicle screw fixation through a tubular retractor via the Wiltse approach compared with conventional bilateral pedicle screw fixation for single-segment degenerative lumbar instability: a prospective randomized study: Clinical article. Journal of Neurosurgery: Spine 20: 53–59.
10. Dahdaleh NS, Nixon AT, Lawton CD, Wong AP, Smith ZA, et al. (2013) Outcome following unilateral versus bilateral instrumentation in patients undergoing minimally invasive transforaminal lumbar interbody fusion: a single-center randomized prospective study. Neurosurgical Focus 35: E13.
11. Xiaolong S, Lei W, Hailong Z, Xin G, Guangfei G, et al. (2013) Radiographic Analysis of One-level Minimally Invasive Transforaminal Lumbar Interbody Fusion (MI-TLIF) With Unilateral Pedicle Screw Fixation for Lumbar Degenerative Diseases. Journal of spinal disorders & techniques.
12. Choi UY, Park JY, Kim KH, Kuh SU, Chin DK, et al. (2013) Unilateral versus bilateral percutaneous pedicle screw fixation in minimally invasive transforaminal lumbar interbody fusion. Neurosurgical Focus 35: E11.
13. McAfee PC, Farey ID, Sutterlin CE, Gurr KR, Warden KE, et al. (1991) The effect of spinal implant rigidity on vertebral bone density. A canine model. Spine (Phila Pa 1976) 16: S190–197.
14. Ha KY, Schendel MJ, Lewis JL, Ogilvie JW (1993) Effect of immobilization and configuration on lumbar adjacent-segment biomechanics. J Spinal Disord 6: 99–105.
15. Korovessis P, Papazisis Z, Koureas G, Lambiris E (2004) Rigid, semirigid versus dynamic instrumentation for degenerative lumbar spinal stenosis: a correlative radiological and clinical analysis of short-term results. Spine (Phila Pa 1976) 29: 735–742.
16. Chen HH, Cheung HH, Wang WK, Li A, Li KC (2005) Biomechanical analysis of unilateral fixation with interbody cages. Spine (Phila Pa 1976) 30: E92–96.
17. Xue H, Tu Y, Cai M (2012) Comparison of unilateral versus bilateral instrumented transforaminal lumbar interbody fusion in degenerative lumbar diseases. Spine J 12: 209–215.
18. Slucky AV, Brodke DS, Bachus KN, Droge JA, Braun JT (2006) Less invasive posterior fixation method following transforaminal lumbar interbody fusion: a biomechanical analysis. Spine J 6: 78–85.
19. Goel VK, Lim TH, Gwon J, Chen JY, Winterbottom JM, et al. (1991) Effects of rigidity of an internal fixation device. A comprehensive biomechanical investigation. Spine (Phila Pa 1976) 16: S155–161.
20. Toyone T, Ozawa T, Shiboi R, Kamikawa K, Watanabe A, et al. Adjacent Segment Degeneration Occured 3-Times More 5-Years After Bilateral Instrumented Plif Than Unilateral Instrumented Plif: 27; 2010. LWW. 27.
21. Yücesoy K, Yüksel KZ, Baek S, Sonntag VK, Crawford NR (2008) Biomechanics of unilateral compared with bilateral lumbar pedicle screw fixation for stabilization of unilateral vertebral disease.
22. Aoki Y, Yamagata M, Nakajima F, Ikeda Y, Shimizu K, et al. (2010) Examining risk factors for posterior migration of fusion cages following transforaminal lumbar interbody fusion: a possible limitation of unilateral pedicle screw fixation. J Neurosurg Spine 13: 381–387.
23. Chen S-H, Lin S-C, Tsai W-C, Wang C-W, Chao S-H (2012) Biomechanical comparison of unilateral and bilateral pedicle screws fixation for transforaminal lumbar interbody fusion after decompressive surgery–a finite element analysis. BMC musculoskeletal disorders 13: 72.
24. Awad BI, Lubelski D, Shin JH, Carmody MA, Hoh DJ, et al. (2013) Bilateral Pedicle Screw Fixation versus Unilateral Pedicle and Contralateral Facet Screws for Minimally Invasive Transforaminal Lumbar Interbody Fusion: Clinical Outcomes and Cost Analysis. Global spine journal 3: 225–230.
25. Hsiang J, Yu K, He Y (2013) Minimally invasive one-level lumbar decompression and fusion surgery with posterior instrumentation using a combination of pedicle screw fixation and transpedicular facet screw construct. Surgical neurology international 4.
26. Chen Z, Zhao J, Liu A, Yuan J, Li Z (2009) Surgical treatment of recurrent lumbar disc herniation by transforaminal lumbar interbody fusion. International orthopaedics 33: 197–201.
27. Holly LT, Schwender JD, Rouben DP, Foley KT (2006) Minimally invasive transforaminal lumbar interbody fusion: indications, technique, and complications. Neurosurg Focus 20: 1–5.
28. Beringer WF, Mobasser J-P (2006) Unilateral pedicle screw instrumentation for minimally invasive transforaminal lumbar interbody fusion. Neurosurgical Focus 20: 1–5.

21

Transperitoneal Mini-Laparoscopic Pyeloplasty and Concomitant Ureteroscopy-Assisted Pyelolithotomy for Ureteropelvic Junction Obstruction Complicated by Renal Caliceal Stones

Zhi Chen[1], Peng Zhou[2], Zhong-Qing Yang[1], Yang Li[1], Yan-Cheng Luo[1], Yao He[1], Nan-Nan Li[1], Chao-Qun Xie[1], Chen Lai[1], Xiao-Long Fang[1], Xiang Chen[1]*

1 Department of Urology, Xiangya Hospital, Central South University, Changsha, Hunan, China, **2** Department of General Surgery, Xiangya Hospital, Central South University, Changsha, Hunan, China

Abstract

Objective: To present our experience of combining transperitoneal mini-laparoscopic pyeloplasty (mini-LP) and concomitant ureteroscopy-assisted pyelolithotomy (U-P) for ureteropelvic junction obstruction (UPJO) complicated by renal caliceal stones in the same session.

Methods: Between May 2007 and December 2011, mini-LP and concomitant U-P was performed in nine patients with UPJO and ipsilateral renal caliceal stones. Stone location and burden were preoperatively assessed. After pyelotomy with appropriate length (about 4 mm), a 16-Fr catheter sheath replaced the uppermost or lowermost laparoscopic trocar and was introduced directly into the renal pelvis under the guidance of a guide wire and laparoscopic vision. A 7.5F rigid ureteroscopy passed through the catheter sheath into the plevis. Intracorporeal lithotripsy and/or pressure irrigation via a pump was used for caliceal stone removal. Subsequently, laparoscopic pyeloplasty was performed in a standard fashion. Postoperative imaging was assessed.

Results: The calculi sizes ranged from 2 to 11 mm (mean, 7.1 mm) and an average of 3 stones per patient was removed (range, 1 to 6 stones). Complete stone clearance confirmed by postoperative imaging was achieved in all patients. Mean operative time was 210 minutes, and estimated blood loss was 20 mL. Mean hospital stay was 5 days (4–7). Stent was removed after 4–8 weeks. No intraoperative or postoperative complications were noted during a mean follow-up of 18.5 months (range, 6 to 24 months).

Conclusions: Mini-LP and concomitant U-P are simple and effective alternatives for the simultaneous management of UPJO complicated by coexisting ipsilateral renal caliceal stones.

Editor: Nick Ashton, The University of Manchester, United Kingdom

Funding: The authors have no support or funding to report.

Competing Interests: The authors have declared that no competing interests exist.

* E-mail: cxiang1007@126.com

Introduction

Ureteropelvic junction obstruction (UPJO) complicated by the presence of ipsilateral calculus disease, especially renal caliceal calculus, poses a technically challenging situation for the urologist. Although the surgical treatment of UPJ obstruction associated with renal calculi has evolved significantly over the past 2 decades [1,2,3,4,5,6,7,8,9,10,11,12,13,14,15], there is still therapeutic controversy regarding the ideal minimally invasive management. In the present study, we report a minimally invasive and reproducible technique that greatly facilitates the surgical treatment of this morbidity, using a 7.5F rigid ureteroscopy during mini-laparoscopic pyeloplasty for caliceal stone removal.

Patients and Methods

Patients

Between May 2007 and December 2011, nine patients with UPJO and ipsilateral renal caliceal stones underwent transperitoneal mini-laparoscopic pyeloplasty (mini-LP) and concomitant ureteroscopy-assisted pyelolithotomy (U-P) at our institution. This study obtained ethics approval from the ethics committee at Xiangya Hospital, Central South University, Changsha, Hunan Province, China. Also, we obtained informed consent from the adult participants or from the parents of the children participants in our study. The informed consent was written and specified in the operative consent. The patients included 5 men and 4 women, with an average age of 26.1 years (range, 16–42 years). Of the 9 patients, 7 had UPJO on the left side and 2 on the right side. All patients presented with mild to moderate flank pain. No patients had undergone previous abdominal surgery in our series. Stone location and burden were preoperatively assessed. **(Figure 1)** A combination of diuretic renal scans, intravenous urography (IVU), kidney–ureter–bladder X-ray and/or CT was postoperatively performed to assess the drainage pattern and to evaluate any residual stones.

Operative Technique

Under general endotracheal anesthesia, patients were placed in a 45° lateral decubitus position. We used the three-port tranperitoneal approach. The pneumoperitoneum was obtained by carbon dioxide insufflation through a Veress needle at 12–14 mm Hg of intraabdominal pressure. A 5-mm port was placed infraumbilically for the camera and one 5-mm port and one 3-mm port in the midclavicular line ipsilaterally under direct vision using the laparoscope. **(Figure 2)**.

After the laparoscopic instruments were introduced, the line of Toldt was incised to reflect the colon medially and the kidney was exposed using standard laparoscopic techniques. The dilated renal pelvis was easily identified and carefully dissected down to the proximal ureter. Any crossing vessel at the UPJ was carefully dissected free from the UPJ if present. Whether a crossing vessel was required for transposition was determined based on individual anatomy. Then a pyelotomy was preformed with appropriate length (about 4 mm) to achieve the pyeloplasty. **(Figure 3)** A guide wire was passed through the uppermost (for middle or lower caliceal calculus) or lowermost (for middle or upper caliceal calculus) laparoscopic trocar and pyelotomy, directly into the renal pelvis under laparoscopic vision. The trocar was removed and a 16-Fr catheter sheath with a core was introduced under the guidance of the guide wire. After the guide wire and core was removed, a 7.5F rigid ureteroscopy was introduced through the catheter sheath into the plevis and the abdominal pressure was routinely decreased to 6–8 mmHg. **(Figure 4)** If the calculus was big, intracorporeal lithotripsy was routinely performed. **(Figure 5)** Otherwise, pressure irrigation via a pump was used to flush out the small calculus. The irrigant was aspirated by the suction probe placed just below the pyelotomy through the other laparoscopic port. **(Figure 6)**.

Subsequently, laparoscopic pyeloplasty was performed in a standard fashion. In brief, the pelvis was partly divided using a "cold" scissors through the lowermost trocar, from the most dependent part, cephalad toward the pelvis. The most lateral extent of the pelvis was left attached to the ureter for traction, which serves as a handle that can stabilize the ureter during subsequently spatulating, suturing and excising. The scissors was introduced through the uppermost trocar and the ureter was easily spatulated laterally. This change greatly facilitates this step because the axis of the scissors was almost in line with the ureteral axis.

A 4-0 Vicryl (Ethicon) suture was used for anastomosis. The most dependent part of the pyelotomy was sutured to the apex of the spatulated ureter. The UPJ and the redundant pelvis were excised. After completion of the posterior anastomosis with an interrupted suture and the remaining pyelotomy anastomosis with a running suture, a Double-J stent was placed in an antegrade manner. Subsequently, the anterior wall is closed with an interrupted suture. **(Figure 7)** A drain was placed through the lowermost port.

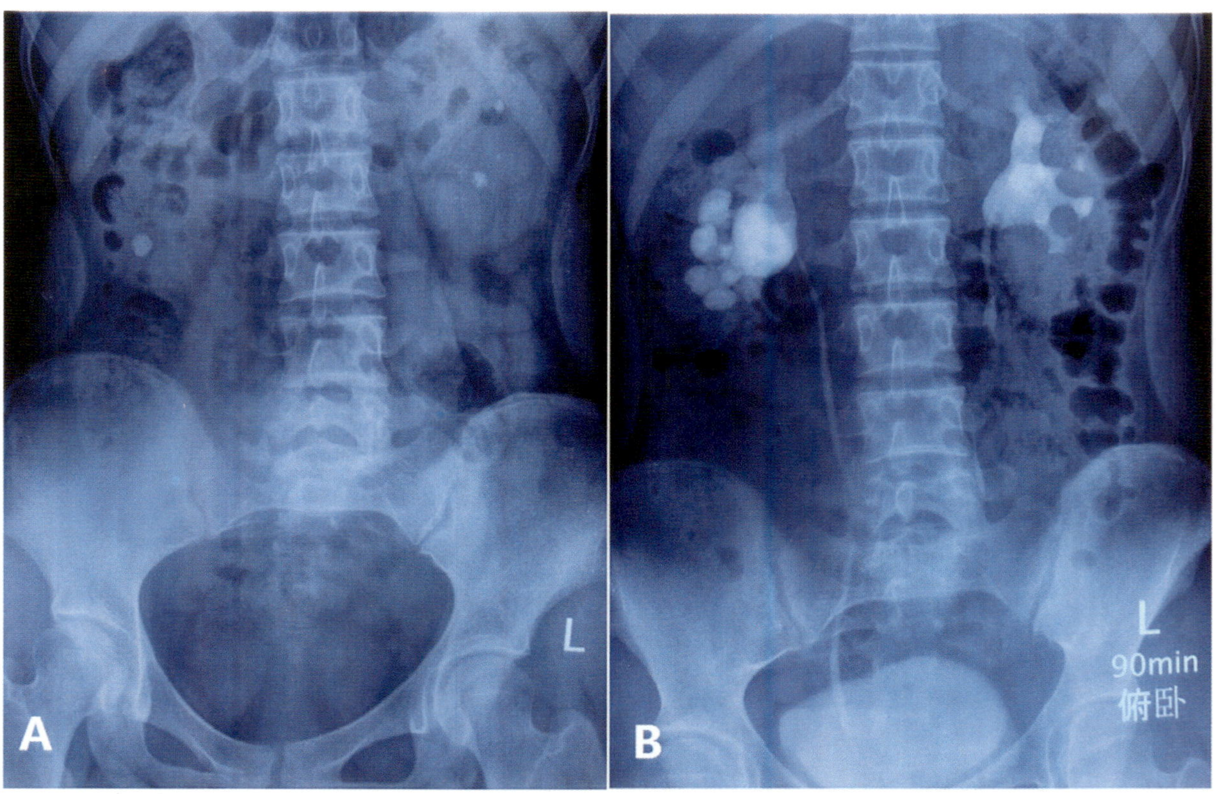

Figure 1. Preoperative assessment for stone location and burden. (A) Preoperative kidney–ureter–bladder X-ray. (B) Preoperative intravenous urography.

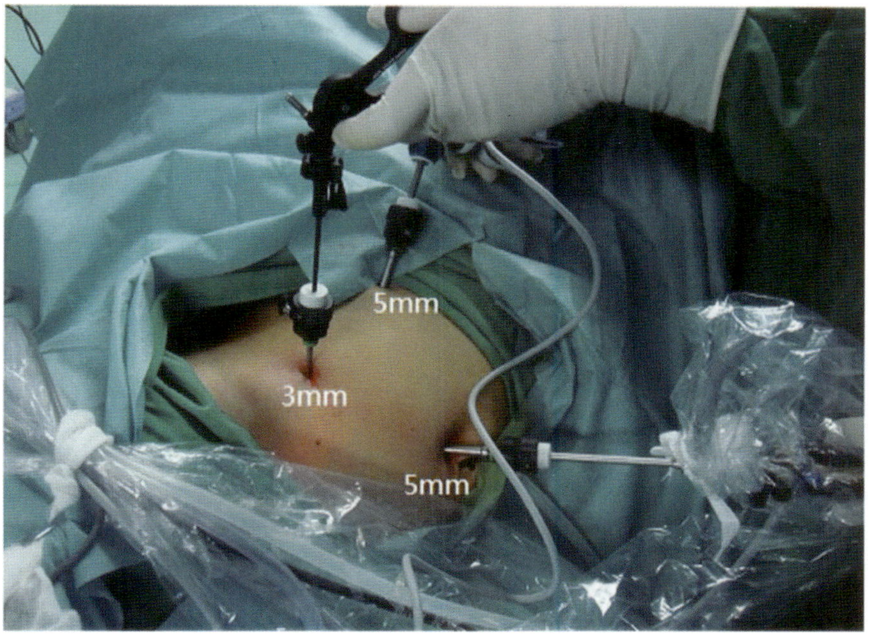

Figure 2. Port-placement for transperitoneal mini-laparoscopic pyeloplasty. A 5-mm port was placed infraumbilically for the camera (A) and one 5-mm port and one 3-mm port in the midclavicular line ipsilaterally (B and C). (right side).

Results

The calculi sizes ranged from 2 to 11 mm (mean, 7.1 mm) and an average of 3 stones per patient was removed (range, 1 to 6 stones). Mean operative time was 210 minutes, and estimated blood loss was 20 mL. In our initial 2 cases, a 16-Fr catheter sheath with a core was directly passed through the previous abdominal incision and pyelotomy into the renal pelvis without the guidance of a guide wire. Pelvis wall tear occurred during the procedure in the case 2. Thereafter, to decrease the risk of pelvis wall tear, we started the practice of routinely using a guide wire for the guidance of a 16-Fr catheter sheath with a core in the remaining 7 patients and experienced no that complication. In the case 5, the pyelotomy was unexpectedly preformed with a relatively longer length (about 8 mm). The opened up renal pelvis were partly closed by suturing with a 4-0 Vicryl suture (case 2) or

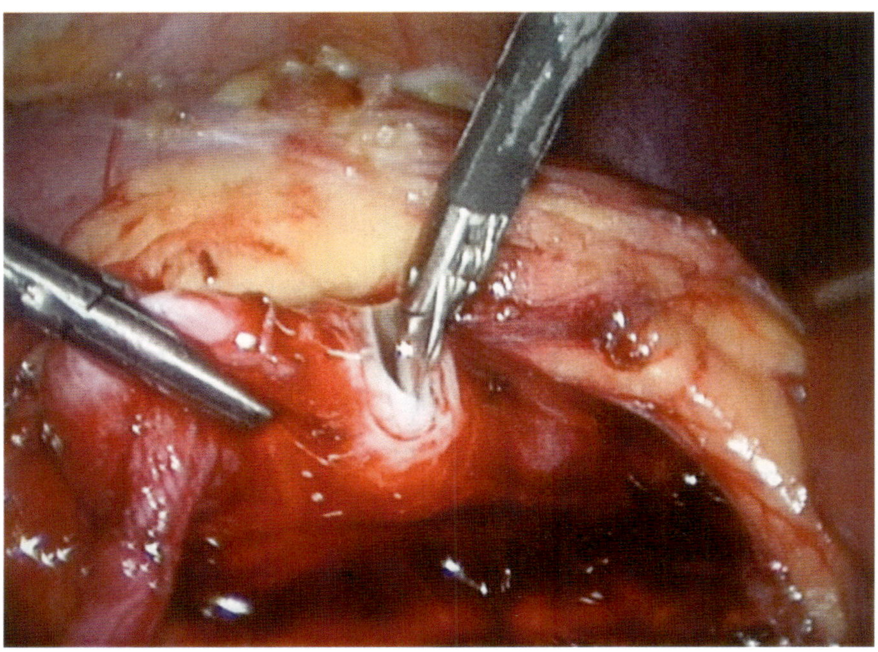

Figure 3. Performance of pyelotomy. A pyelotomy was preformed with appropriate length (about 4 mm) to achieve the pyeloplasty.

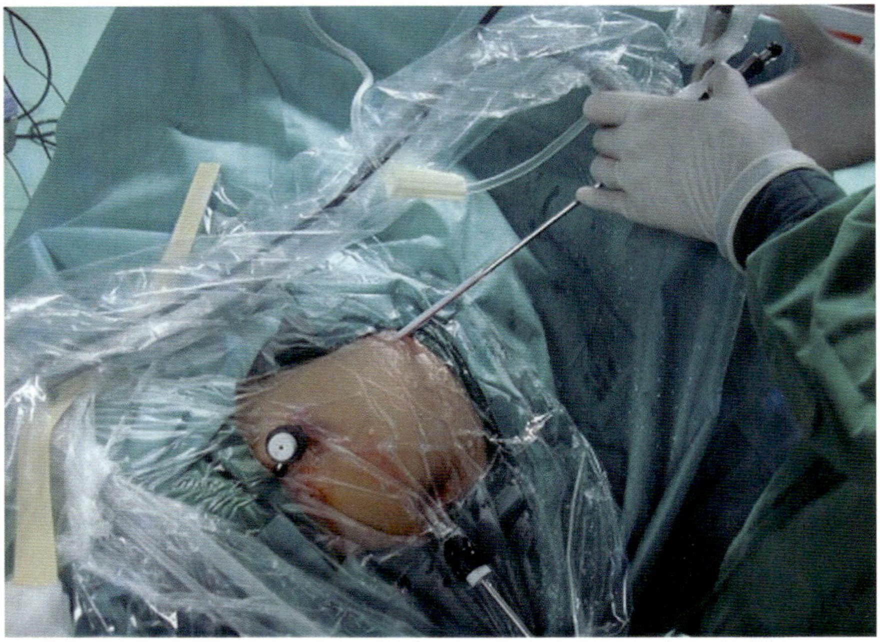

Figure 4. Introduction of rigid ureteroscopy. A 7.5F rigid ureteroscopy was introduced through the catheter sheath into the plevis.

holding the cut ends with the help of laparoscopic graspers (case 5) to keep the system distended for better visualization during ureteroscopy and minimize the chances of stone loss. In the case 6, we encountered problem in localizing the stones during the procedure, which was confirmed to located in the anterior middle calyces by preoperative CT. We struggled for a while before we realized that further mobilizing the kidney could significantly improve visualization angle of the ureteroscopy. These stones was successfully found and flushed out.

Complete stone clearance confirmed by postoperative imaging was achieved in all patients. Mean hospital stay was 5 days (4–7). Stent was removed after 4–8 weeks. No major intraoperative or postoperative complications were noted during a mean follow-up of 18.5 months (range, 6 to 24 months).

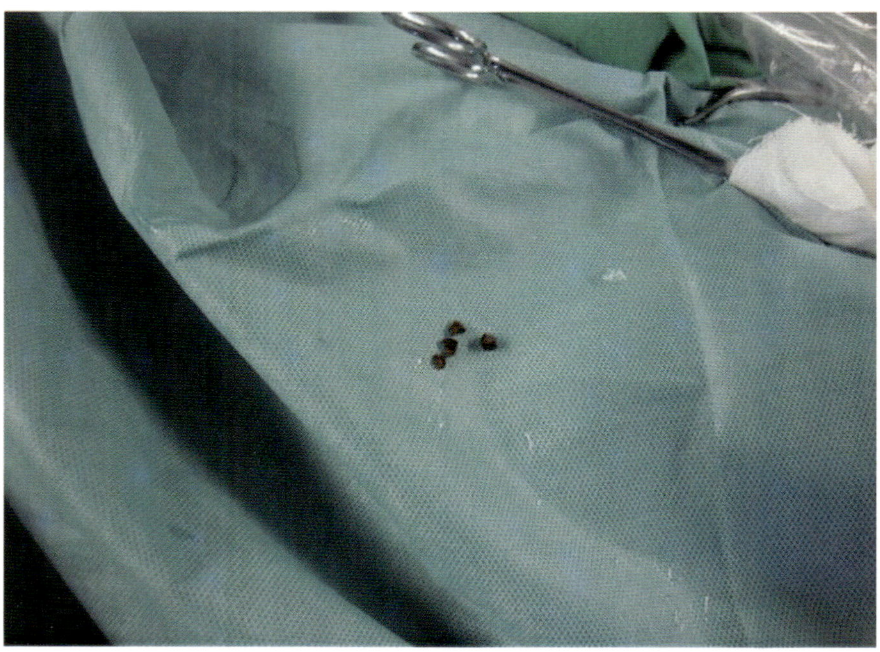

Figure 5. Renal caliceal calculus. Intracorporeal lithotripsy was performed and the calculus was flushed out.

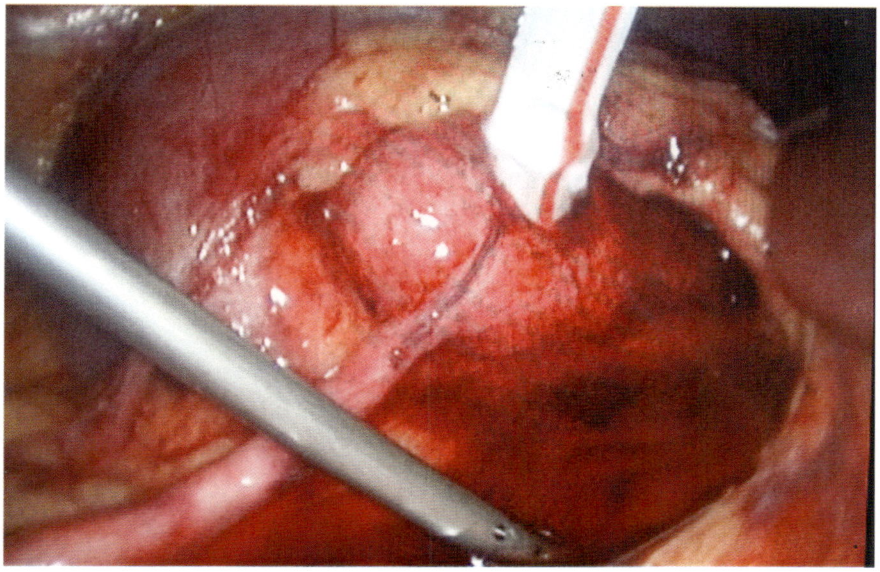

Figure 6. Aspiration of irrigant. The irrigant was aspirated by the suction probe placed just below the pyelotomy through the other laparoscopic port.

Discussion

Over the past 25 years, minimally invasive procedures (endopyelotomy and laparoscopic pyeloplasty) have replaced open pyeloplasty as the standard of care for UPJO. [5] However, presence of coexisting upper urinary tract stones in the patients with UPJO presents a therapeutic dilemma to the urologist. The surgical treatment for this morbidity has traditionally been open pyelolithotomy with pyeloplasty, but it is associated with considerable morbidity and protracted convalescence. Generally, the current concept in dealing with UPJO concomitant with renal stones could be that while taking into consideration the underlying anatomy, comorbidities, and patient preference, the surgeon can choose the most suitable operation to correct anatomical abnormality of UPJO that led to stasis and stone formation and concomitantly completely clear stones through minimally invasive surgery if surgery is indicated.

Laparoscopic pyeloplasty (LP) with concomitant pyelolithotomy [1,6,7,8,9,10,11], percutaneous nephrolithotomy (PNL) with endopyelotomy [3,12,13,14,15] or robotic assisted laparoscopic pyeloplasty (RALP) with concomitant pyelolithotomy [4] and PNL with LP [2] have been reported for treating UPJO concomitant with renal stones. Each of these methods has its own limitations.

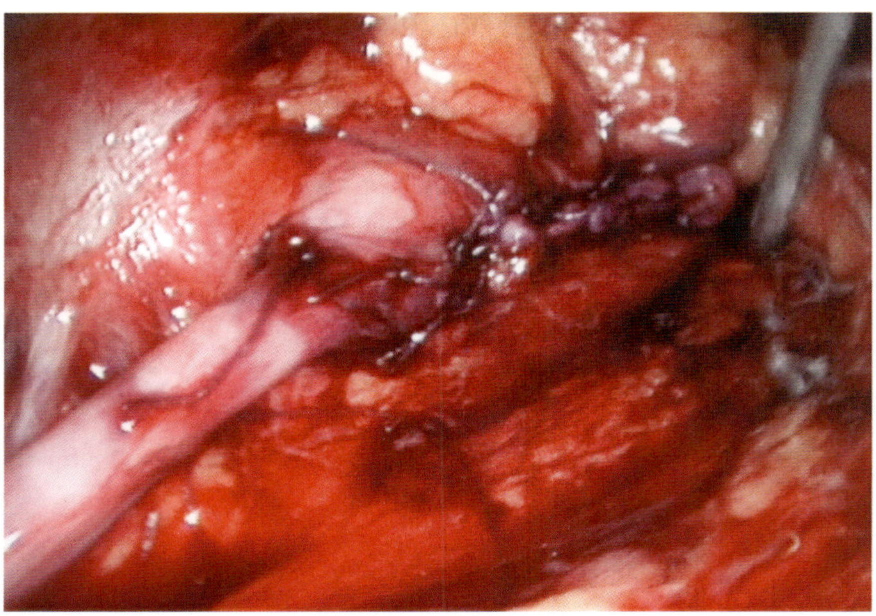

Figure 7. Ureteropelvic anastomosis. Anastomosis was completed using 4-0 Vicryl (Ethicon) sutures.

The overall success rates for patients treated with endopyelotomy are lower than those treated with open or laparoscopic pyeloplasty. [16] Several factors, including the presence of a crossing vessel, length of narrowing, preoperative split renal function, degree of hydronephrosis and the presence of contrast extravasation at the time of surgery, influence success rates for endopyelotomy, [17] Nonetheless, in a highly selective patient population, endopyelotomy can achieve equivalent success rates compared with laparoscopic pyeloplasty. [18,19] Therefore, PNL with endopyelotomy remains an effective alternative treatment for certain patients with UPJO complicated by renal stones, and can be easily performed by most urologists Although laparoscopic or assisted laparoscopic pyeloplasty produces success rates (87.5% to 100%) equivalent to open pyeloplasty with a 10% to 15% higher success rate when compared to endopyelotomy [20,21,22,23], it needs a steep learning curve or advanced laparoscopic training. In addition, in order to remove the stones, use of flexible nephroscopy during LP or RALP could also be very technically demanding. Furthermore, PNL with LP could be very cumbersome and time-consuming for requiring repositioning. Moreover, bleeding could occur and the nephrostomy catheter could exodus during laparoscopic manipulation. Guidelines on urolithiasis of European Association of Urology (EAU) recommends that simultaneous stone removal be performed with percutaneous or transureteral endopyelotomy and open or laparoscopic reconstructive surgery for patients with UPJO.

In our centre, LP has been the first choice for patients with UPJO. Because flexible nephroscopy are not covered by medical insurance in China for its expensive price and high deterioration, the patients have to bear these charges themselves. Therefore, we developed our own surgical technique to suit this technically challenging procedure. The key point of our technique is the use of the 7.5F rigid ureteroscopy. The option of the laparoscopic trocar, through which the ureteroscopy was introduced, was determined by the location of the caliceal stones. Generally, the uppermost trocar was for lower caliceal calculus and lowermost for upper caliceal calculus. For middle caliceal calculus, the both trocars seem reasonable. We believed that these modifications can achieve the advantages of flexible nephroscopy, but lower technically challenge was needed. In addition, proper preoperative identification of the stone-bearing calix was very important for successful stone extraction. [1] Furthermore, in our procedure, the introduction of 5-mm laparoscopy and 7.5F rigid ureteroscopy only need two 5-mm incisions and one 3-mm incision. Compared to the previous report [4], in which two 12-mm ports and two 8-mm ports were used, the surgical morbidity could be further reduced.

The length of pyelotomy before introducing the ureteroscopy should be appropriate (about 4 mm), which could decrease the spillage of the irrigant and maintain a certain pressure of the colleting system. This could be helpful to flush out the small calculus. In addition, the spillage of the irrigant can be aspirated by the suction probe placed just below the pyelotomy through the other laparoscopic port.

Mini-Laparoscopic pyeloplasty was successful in relieving obstruction in all patients (100%) in our series with a mean follow-up of 18.5 months and the stone-free rate was 100%. Although the present series included only 9 patients, we showed clearly that transperitoneal LP and concomitant U-P is technically feasible, safe and can be accomplished reasonably quickly and patients with UPJO and ipsilateral renal calculi can undergo simultaneous treatment of both conditions and expect good results in regard to resolution of obstruction and complete stone clearance. Our results were similar to the data reported in previous series. [1,2,4,13].

Stein et al. [1] reported a 5-mm atraumatic laparoscopic bowel grasper or lexible nephroscopy were used for extraction of renal caliceal stones during LP with concomitant pyelolithotomy. With a mean follow-up of 5.4 months, the obstruction relieving rate and stone-free rate was 93.3% (14/15) and 80% (12/15), respectively. Mean operative time was 174 minutes. Atug et al. [4] reported the use of robotic graspers in one patient and flexible nephroscopy in seven patients for pyelolithotomy during RALP. With a mean follow-up of 12.3 months, both the obstruction relieving rate and stone-free rate were 100%. Mean operative time was 275.8 minutes. Agarwal and coworkers [2] reported their experience of combining PNL with LP for UPJO with renal stones in the same session (8 cases) or staged manner (2 cases). Mean operative time was 234 minutes. At 6 months patients are stone free on ultrasound and show good drainage on renal scan. Berkman and colleagues [13] retrospectively reviewed patient data for all endoscopic pyeloplasties performed at a single institution over 10 years. Forty-one patients underwent simultaneous nephrolithotomy for ipsilateral renal calculi. Complete lithotomy was confirmed visually and with live fluoroscopy in all cases except those with radiolucent stones. [13] For 30 patients with>12 months of follow-up, the overall obstruction relieving rate was 90% in the nephrolithotomy and endopyelotomy group. Their operative time was not reported.

In the present study, the mean operative time was lower than that reported by Agarwal et al [2]and Atug et al [4] (210 vs 234 and 275.8 minutes, respectively). The reduction of the mean operative time may be explained by several reasons. First, our series only included the patients with UPJO and ipsilateral renal caliceal stones and the calculi sizes were small (2 to 11 mm). Therefore, our present series could be relatively easily managed. Second, with the use of the 7.5F rigid ureteroscopy, our technique could be less technical demanding. In addition, our mean operative time was higher than reported by Stein et al. [1], who used a laparoscopic grasper or pressure irrigation via a pump for removing stones in the majority of cases and intraoperative flexible nephroscopy was only used if the afore-mentioned techniques fail. That could explain the reduction of the mean operative time in their series. However, stone-free rate could be also reduced (93% vs 100%) for that. When compared to the results by PNL with endopyelotomy, the stone-free rate was equivalent (100%) and our obstruction relieving rate was higher (100% vs 90%) than that reported by Berkman and colleagues [13]. However, their cases included both primary and secondary UPJO while our series were all primary UPJO. Thus this difference could influence the success rate. Furthermore, their follow-up time was longer than ours. Therefore, long-term results of our series are awaited.

Our study also has some limitation. The use of the 2-camera system, allowing visualization and laparoscopic guidance of the rigid ureteroscopy, was required. However, this demand can be easily achieved in most medical centers.

Author Contributions

Conceived and designed the experiments: XC. Performed the experiments: ZC PZ ZQY YL YCL YH NNL CQX CL XLF XC. Analyzed the data: YCL YH NNL CQX CL XLF. Contributed reagents/materials/analysis tools: YCL YH NNL CQX CL XLF. Wrote the paper: ZC XC.

References

1. Stein RJ, Turna B, Nguyen MM, Aron M, Hafron JM, et al. (2008) Laparoscopic Pyeloplasty with Concomitant Pyelolithotomy: Technique and Outcomes. Journal of Endourology 22: 1251–1256.
2. Agarwal A, Varshney A, Bansal BS (2008) Concomitant Percutaneous Nephrolithotomy and Transperitoneal Laparoscopic Pyeloplasty for Ureteropelvic Junction Obstruction Complicated by Stones. Journal of Endourology 22: 2251–2256.
3. Bernardo NO (2008) Endopyelotomy: The Best Solution for Patients with Stones Associated with Ureteropelvic Junction Obstruction. Journal of Endourology 22: 1893–1896.
4. Atug F, Castle EP, Burgess SV, Thomas R (2005) Concomitant management of renal calculi and pelvi-ureteric junction obstruction with robotic laparoscopic surgery. BJU International 96: 1365–1368.
5. Jacobs BL, Kaufman SR, Morgenstern H, Hollenbeck BK, Wolf JS, et al. (2012) Trends in the Treatment of Adults with Ureteropelvic Junction Obstruction. J Endourol.
6. Nambirajan T, Jeschke S, Albqami N, Abukora F, Leeb K, et al. (2005) Role of laparoscopy in management of renal stones: single-center experience and review of literature. J Endourol 19: 353–359.
7. Micali S, Moore RG, Averch TD, Adams JB, Kavoussi LR (1997) The role of laparoscopy in the treatment of renal and ureteral calculi. J Urol 157: 463–466.
8. Ramakumar S, Lancini V, Chan DY, Parsons JK, Kavoussi LR, et al. (2002) Laparoscopic pyeloplasty with concomitant pyelolithotomy. J Urol 167: 1378–1380.
9. Srivastava A, Singh P, Gupta M, Ansari MS, Mandhani A, et al. (2008) Laparoscopic pyeloplasty with concomitant pyelolithotomy is it an effective mode of treatment? Urol Int 80: 306–309.
10. Ball AJ, Leveillee RJ, Patel VR, Wong C (2004) Laparoscopic pyeloplasty and flexible nephroscopy: simultaneous treatment of ureteropelvic junction obstruction and nephrolithiasis. JSLS 8: 223–228.
11. Inagaki T, Rha KH, Ong AM, Kavoussi LR, Jarrett TW (2005) Laparoscopic pyeloplasty: current status. BJU Int 95 Suppl 2: 102–105.
12. Minervini A, Davenport K, Keeley FX Jr, Timoney AG (2006) Antegrade versus retrograde endopyelotomy for pelvi-ureteric junction (PUJ) obstruction. Eur Urol 49: 536–542; discussion 542–533.
13. Berkman DS, Landman J, Gupta M (2009) Treatment outcomes after endopyelotomy performed with or without simultaneous nephrolithotomy: 10-year experience. J Endourol 23: 1409–1413.
14. Shalhav AL, Giusti G, Elbahnasy AM, Hoenig DM, McDougall EM, et al. (1998) Adult endopyelotomy: impact of etiology and antegrade versus retrograde approach on outcome. J Urol 160: 685–689.
15. Gupta M, Tuncay ÓL, Smith AD (1997) Open surgical exploration after failed endopyelotomy: a 12-year perspective. J Urol 157: 1613–1618; discussion 1618–1619.
16. Dimarco DS, Gettman MT, McGee SM, Chow GK, Leroy AJ, et al. (2006) Long-term success of antegrade endopyelotomy compared with pyeloplasty at a single institution. J Endourol 20: 707–712.
17. Samarasekera D, Chew BH (2011) Endopyelotomy still has an important role in the management of ureteropelvic junction obstruction. Can Urol Assoc J 5: 134–136.
18. el-Nahas AR, Shoma AM, Eraky I, el-Kenawy MR, el-Kappany HA (2006) Prospective, randomized comparison of ureteroscopic endopyelotomy using holmium:YAG laser and balloon catheter. J Urol 175: 614–618; discussion 618.
19. Stilling NM, Jung H, Norby B, Osther SS, Osther PJ (2009) Retrograde ureteroscopic holmium laser endopyelotomy in a selected population of patients with ureteropelvic junction obstruction. Scand J Urol Nephrol 43: 68–72.
20. Boylu U, Basatac C, Turan T, Onol FF, Gumus E (2012) Comparison of Surgical and Functional Outcomes of Minimally Invasive and Open Pyeloplasty. J Laparoendosc Adv Surg Tech A.
21. Ost MC, Kaye JD, Guttman MJ, Lee BR, Smith AD (2005) Laparoscopic pyeloplasty versus antegrade endopyelotomy: comparison in 100 patients and a new algorithm for the minimally invasive treatment of ureteropelvic junction obstruction. Urology 66: 47–51.
22. Riachy E, Cost NG, Defoor WR, Reddy PP, Minevich EA, et al. (2012) Pediatric Standard and Robot-Assisted Laparoscopic Pyeloplasty: A Comparative Single Institution Study. J Urol.
23. Doo CK, Hong B, Park T, Park HK (2007) Long-term outcome of endopyelotomy for the treatment of ureteropelvic junction obstruction: how long should patients be followed up? J Endourol 21: 158–161.

22

Comparison of Endoscopic Submuscosal Implantation vs. Surgical Intramuscular Implantation of VX2 Fragments for Establishing a Rabbit Esophageal Tumor Model for Mimicking Human Esophageal Squamous Carcinoma

Jin Huang[1,2], Yin Zhang[1], Hengao Zhong[1], Zhining Fan[1]*, Guobin Jiang[1], Yingzhou Shen[2], Hanming Song[2], Zhijian Tao[2], Kuangjing Wang[2]

1 Digestive Medical Center, The Second Affiliated Hospital of Nanjing Medical University, Nanjing, Jiangsu Province, China, **2** Division of Digestive Diseases, Renming Hospital of Ma Anshan, Ma Anshan City, Anhui Province, China

Abstract

Purpose: This study was undertaken to establish a rabbit esophageal tumor model for mimicking human esophageal squamous carcinoma (ESC) by endoscopic and surgical implantation of VX2 tumors.

Methods: Fragments of a VX2 tumour were endoscopically implanted in the submucosal layer of the thoracic esophagus of 32 New Zealand white rabbits, while 34 animals received surgical implantation into the muscular layer. Then, the animals were studied endoscopically and pathologically. The safety and efficiency of the two methods and the pathological features of the animal models were analyzed.

Results: Both the endoscopic and the surgical method had a relatively high success rate of tumor implantation [93.7% (30/32) vs. 97.1% (33/34)] and tumor growth [86.7% (26/30) vs. 81.8% (27/33)], and the variation in the results was not statistically significant ($P>0.05$). Compared with those produced by the surgical method, the models produced by the endoscopic method had a higher rate of severe esophageal stricture [61.5% (16/26) vs. 29.6% (8/27)] and of intra-luminal tumor growth [73.1% (19/26) vs. 37.0% (10/27)], and had a lower rate of tumor invasion of adjacent organs [53.8% (14/26) vs. 81.5% (22/27)]; all of these results were statistically significant ($P<0.05$). However, the difference in the survival time and the rates of tumor regional/distant metastasis [38.5% (10/26) vs. 51.8% (14/27)] between the two methods were not statistically significant ($P>0.05$).

Conclusion: The endoscopic and surgical methods are both safe and effective for establishment of VX2 tumors in the rabbit esophagus. The models produced by the two methods have different pathologic features mimicking that of human ESC. We recommend the models for studies on surgical procedures and minimally invasive treatments.

Editor: Wayne A. Phillips, Peter MacCallum Cancer Centre, Australia

Funding: This work was supported by the National Science Foundation of China under Grant No. 81172266/H1617 (www.nsfc.gov.cn/nsfc/cen/bsdt/jggb.html). The funders had no role in study design, data collection and analysis, decision to publish, or preparation of the manuscript.

Competing Interests: The authors have declared that no competing interests exist.

* E-mail: fanzhining5834@hotmail.com

Introduction

The annual incidence of esophageal cancer is as high as 30 to 800 per 100,000 people. Although the most common esophageal cancer in developed countries is adenocarcinoma, esophageal squamous carcinoma (ESC) remains an important clinical problem in China, Iran and parts of Africa [1,2]. For patients with advanced ESC, new therapeutic strategies are needed to prolong the survival time and improve the quality of life. However, the progress in relevant research is limited by the lack of a suitable moderate-to-large-sized animal model [3].

Although small animal model for esophageal cancer, such as rodent models, are available and wildly used in research [4–6], moderate-to-large-sized animal models are still desperately needed for preclinical studies. Theoretically, all therapeutic strategies that are systematically attempted in humans should be based on prior knowledge that has been conceived by sound science and tested in a model that has a reasonable chance of predicting at least the safety of the maneuver. Compared with the rodent tumor model, moderate-to-large-sized animal models can better simulate the human body environment and allow for research on surgical operations and minimally invasive treatments [7–9] such as endoscopic therapy, stent placement and intravascular interventional treatments.

The VX2 tumor model, in which the carcinoma is developed from papillomas in domestic rabbits and is proven histologically to be the squamous cell type, was originally proposed by Shope and

Hurst in 1933 [10,11], and is now used for studies involving many important organs in the human body, such as the liver, the lung, the kidney, the head and neck [12–14]. Rabbits are a moderate-to-large-sized animal, but they have rarely been used as an esophageal VX2 tumor model. Therefore, an effective modeling method and the pathological characteristics of the relevant model have not been introduced.

In this study, we endoscopically implanted VX2 fragments to the submuscosal layer and surgically into the muscular layer of thoracic esophagus of rabbits, and successfully established esophageal tumor models with the two methods. We investigated the safety and efficiency of the two methods, as well as the pathological characteristics of the models to provide detailed information on models and modeling methods for future research.

Materials and Methods

Animals and Tumors

A total of 66 male and female New Zealand White rabbits weighing between 2.5 and 3.0 kg were used in this study. Animals were obtained from the Jiangsu Agricultural Academy of Science in China and were allowed free access to food and water. The VX2 tumor was obtained from the Surgery Department in the First Affiliated Hospital of Nanjing Medical University.

This study was carried out in strict accordance with the recommendations in the Guide for the Care and Use of Laboratory Animals of the National Institutes of Health. The protocol was approved by the Animal Care and Use Subcommittee at Nanjing Medical University. All surgeries were performed under sodium pentobarbital anesthesia, and all efforts were made to minimize suffering.

Tumor propagation and maintenance

Rabbits with hind limb tumors (donors) were used to propagate and maintain VX2 tumors. Approximately two to three of thawed VX2 tumor tissue fragments (approximately 0.5 mm^3), previously stored in liquid nitrogen, were resuscitated and injected deep into the hind limb gluteal muscles of rabbits anesthetized by intramuscular injection of a 35-mg/kg pentobarbital sodium (Sigma Chemical Co., St. Louis, MO, USA). Three weeks after implantation, animals were sacrificed and hind limb tumors were harvested and processed immediately. The VX2 tumors were cleaned from the surrounding tissue and the gross necrotic portions of tumors were removed.

The collected tumors were cut into small pieces (approximately 0.5 mm^3) and preserved in saline for implantation: approximately 0.3 ml of saline solution with four pieces of tumor fragments were placed in a 2-ml syringe on ice until they were injected into the recipient rabbit's esophagus.

Endoscopic implantation of VX2 fragments

After 24 h of fasting with free access to water, the rabbits were anesthetized (as noted above) and then were placed in the left lateral decubitus position. The implantation site was approximately 5 cm away from the cardia, where was the equivalent of 15 cm away from the incisors of the rabbit. A slim endoscope (Olympus GIFXP260, Japan) was inserted into the thoracic esophagus. Using a fine needle (the inner core of an endoscopic needle, Olympus, MAJ-68, 23-gauge, Fig. 1A), 0.5 ml of saline was injected into the esophageal submucosal layer to elevate the mucosa layer. After that, a puncture was made across the mucosa into the submucosal layer using a large needle (a revised endoscopic needle, Olympus, MAJ-68, with an oblique cut in the front, Fig. 1B) and the success of the puncture was confirmed by further elevation of the mucosa when saline was injected. Approximately 0.3 ml of saline containing four VX2 pieces was then injected into the submucosal layer of the rabbits (Video S1).

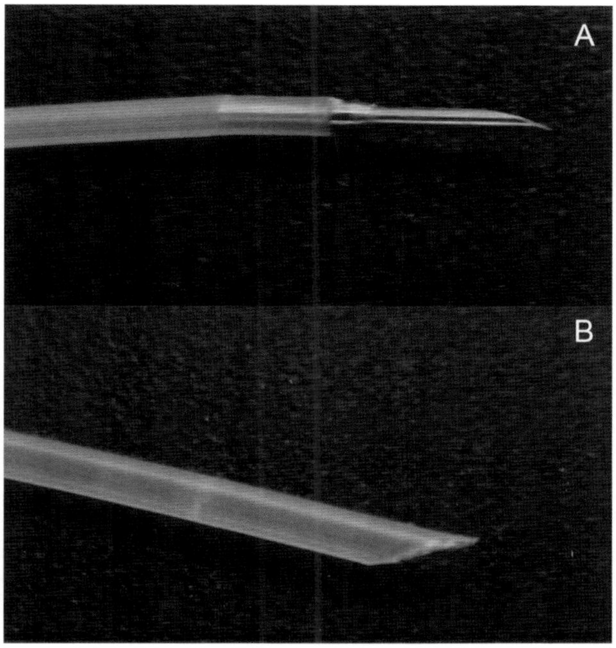

Figure 1. Needles for endoscopic implantation. (A) Tip of the endoscopic needle (fine needle). (B) Tip of the revised needle (large needle).

Surgical implantation of VX2 tumors

The rabbits were anesthetized (as mentioned previously) in the supine position and the hair over the abdominal region was molted with 8% sodium sulfide. Then, the abdominal region was cleaned with saline, which was followed by the disinfection of the operating site. The abdominal cavity was opened by the subxiphoid process, and the lower thoracic esophagus was pulled into the abdominal cavity and exposed. The implantation site was approximately 4–5 cm away from the cardia of the rabbit. A needle (20 G) was inserted into the muscular layer of the esophagus and VX2 fragments were injected (Fig. 2). As soon as the needle withdrew, manual pressure was applied to the surface of the esophageal wound for approximately 3 minutes to avoid the fragments falling out of the incision. Next the abdominal wall was closed in two layers. After the operation, the wound was kept sterile, and the antibiotic gentamicin (2.5mg/kg) was injected into the muscles to prevent infection of the wound and ensure wound healing.

Endoscopic follow up

All animals in this study received the implantation procedure only once, regardless of the implantation method. After implantation, an endoscopic examination was performed once a week to observe the tumor growth and the degree of esophageal stenosis. The anesthesia procedure was the same as that described before.

A diagnostic criteria for tumor growth was used in this study: tumor growth was determined by an endoscopic biopsy or by histologic sections. We conducted a biopsy when the diameter of the tumor at the widest part was larger than or equal to 0.3 cm under endoscopy. If the tumor diameter was less than 0.3 cm under endoscopy, we would depend on autopsy at the endpoint to

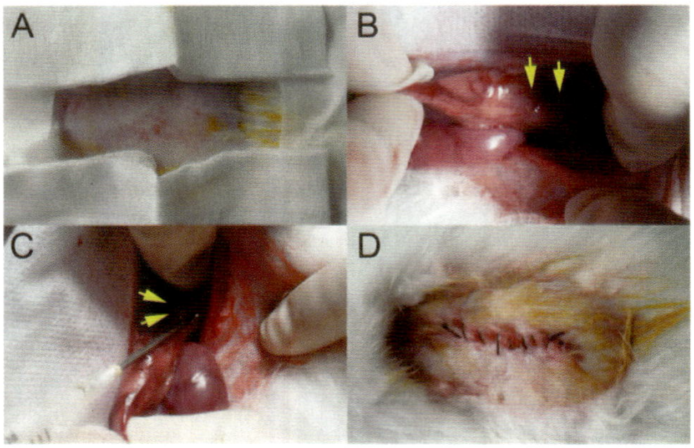

Figure 2. Procedure for surgical implantation. (A) Hair removal for the operation. (B)The lower thoracic esophagus (yellow arrows) was pulled into the abdominal cavity. (C) Using a 20 G needle, VX2 fragments were inoculated (yellow arrows) into the muscular layer of the esophagus. (D) The abdominal wall was closed.

prove tumor growth. If no sign of tumor intra-luminal growth or extrinsic compression occurred over four weeks, the rabbit was regarded as a failure animal and was dropped out of the study.

Three grades were used to evaluate the esophageal stenosis under endoscope: mild stenosis for tumors less than or equal to 1/3 of the luminal diameter; moderate stenosis for tumors more than 1/3 but less than or equal to 2/3 of the luminal diameter and severe stenosis for tumors more than 2/3 of the luminal diameter.

Survival time and Necropsy

Survival time was recorded for all of the rabbits with tumor growth, and the diagnostic criteria for tumor growth was as already described.

A humane endpoint was used in this study, at which the animal models would be humanely sacrificed when they would not eat any food or water for several days and their health was so weak that they could not stand.

Rabbits were fed separately in cages to observe daily the quantity of ingested food and water. Paste food or liquid food (vegetable juice) was provided for animals with dysphagia or a 50% reduction in food intake. The euthanasia procedure was as follows: the animal was first anesthetized by an intramuscular injection of a 35-mg/kg pentobarbital sodium through the ear venous and then was injected with 20 ml of air.

The tumor growth patterns including intra-luminal and extra-luminal growth were detected by endoscopy and necropsy. Tumor intra-luminal growth was defined as the condition when the size of the tumor body in the esophageal lumen was larger than its size outside of the esophageal lumen. Tumor extra-luminal growth was defined as the conditions when the size of the tumor body in the esophageal lumen was less than its size outside of the esophageal lumen.

Gross evidence for tumors was detected in organs such as the lung, pleura, pericardium, heart, trachea/bronchus, diaphragm, peritoneum, liver and kidney, and sections of the tissues associated with tumor invasion or metastasis were examined using hematoxylin and eosin (H&E) staining.

Data analysis

We calculated success rate of the implantation and the tumor growth, and the percentage of the varying degrees of esophageal stenosis and the patterns of tumor growth. The rates of tumor invasion into adjacent organs and regional/distant metastasis were also analyzed. The chi square test was used to determine the statistical significance of the differences between groups. The Kaplan-Meier method with log rank test was used to compare the survival. The statistical significance was set at the $P<0.05$ level. All statistical tests were performed with the software SPSS 16.0.

Results

Success rate of tumor implantation and tumor growth

Among the 66 animals that received VX2 fragments implantation, 32 rabbits received endoscopic implantation and 34 received surgical implantation. Two rabbits (6.3%) died of esophageal perforations from the endoscopic procedure, and one rabbit (2.9%) died from severe injury during surgical implantation. The success rates of tumor implantation for the two groups were 93.7% (30/32) and 97.1% (33/34), respectively. Four weeks after implantation, tumor growth was observed in 26/30 (86.7%) rabbits that received endoscopic implantation and in 27/33 (81.8%) rabbits that received surgical implantation. The difference in the success rates of implantation and tumor growth between the two methods was not statistically significant ($P>0.05$).

Degree of esophageal stricture

During the lifetimes of the animals, severe stricture was observed in 16/26 (61.5%) rabbits that received endoscopic implantation and in 8/27 (29.6%) rabbits that received surgical inoculation; mild-to-moderate stricture was observed in 10/26 (38.5%) and 19/27 (70.4%) rabbits in the two groups, respectively (Fig. 3). The difference in the rates of severe esophageal stricture between the two groups was 31.9% (95% CI, 6.5% to 57.3%). The results were statistically significant ($P=0.019$).

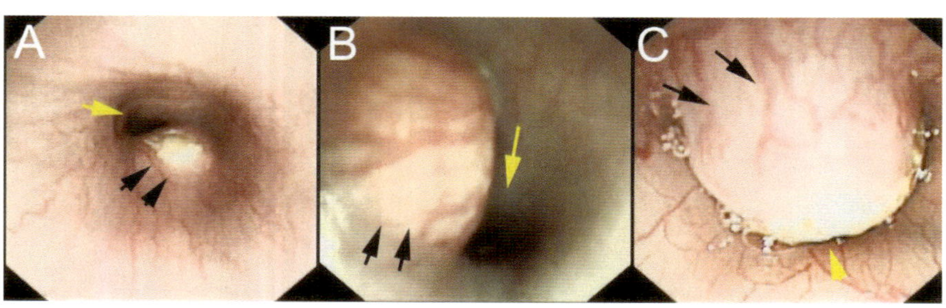

Figure 3. The degree of esophageal stenosis. Endoscopic view of (A) mild stricture, (B) moderate stricture and (C) severe stricture in a rabbit model produced by the endoscopic method. The black arrows point to the tumor and the yellow arrow points to the esophageal lumen.

Tumor growth patterns

Tumor intra-luminal growth (Fig. 4A, B) was detected in 19/26 (73.1%) rabbits that received endoscopic implantation and in 10/27 (37.0%) rabbits that received surgical implantation, whereas 7/26 (26.9%) and 17/27 (63.0%) rabbits had extra-luminal tumors (Fig. 4C, D) in the two groups, respectively. The difference in the rates of intra-luminal growth between the two groups was 36.1% (95% CI, 11.2% to 59.8%) and the results were statistically significant ($P = 0.008$).

Tumor invasion of adjacent tissue and metastasis

The rate of tumor invasion of adjacent tissues (Fig. 5) in the endoscopic group (Table S1) was 53.8% (14/26) and in surgical group (Table S2) was 81.5% (22/27). The difference in the rates between the two groups was 27.7% (95% CI, 3.5% to 51.9%), and the results were statistically significant ($P = 0.017$). The rate of tumor regional/distant metastasis (Fig. 6) in models produced by the endoscopic implantation (Table S1) was 38.5% (10/26) and 51.8% (14/27) by the surgical method (Table S2), and the difference was not significant ($P = 0.327$).

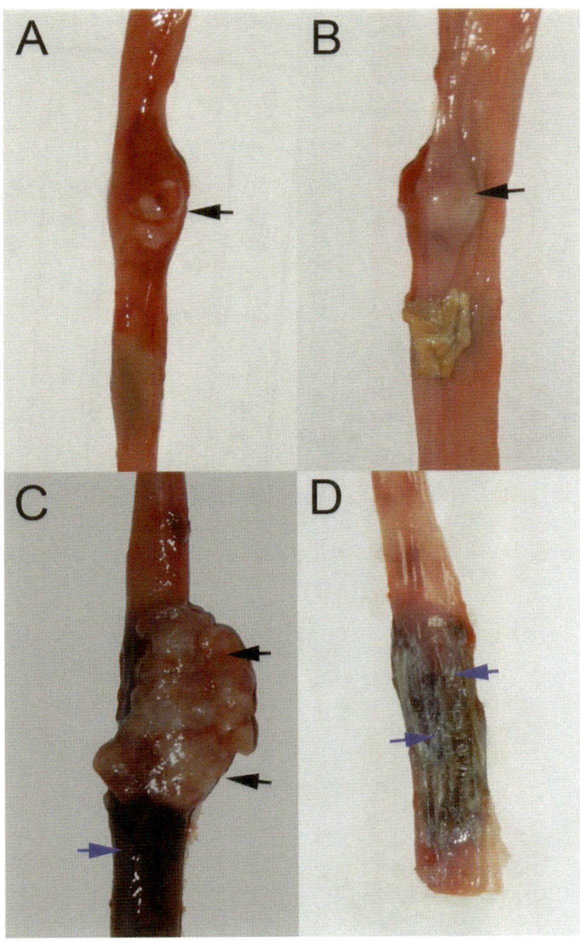

Figure 4. The tumor growth patterns. Tumor intra-luminal growth: (A) macroscopic external view of the esophageal tumor (black arrow) and (B) internal view of the esophageal tumor (black arrow) in a sacrificed animal model produced by the endoscopic method. Tumor extra-luminal growth: (C) macroscopic view of the tumor (black arrows) with esophageal congestion (blue arrow) from the external esophagus in a sacrificed animal model produced by the surgical method, and (D) macroscopic view of no tumor but esophageal congestion (blue arrows) from the internal esophagus.

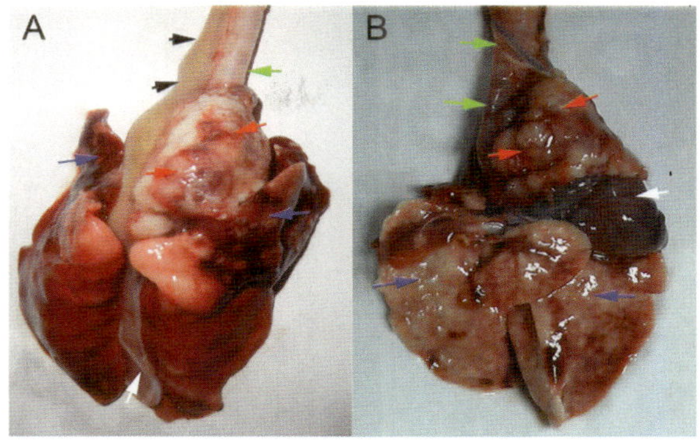

Figure 5. Tumor invasion of adjacent tissues. (A) Invasion was observed into the trachea/bronchus (green arrow) and the pleura and the lung in the upper lobes (blue arrows), but invasion of the heart and the pericardium (white arrow) was not observed. The black arrows point to the esophagus. (B) Tumor invasion was observed into the trachea/bronchus (green arrows) and the heart and the pericardium (white arrow), but invasion of the pleura and the lung (blue arrows) was not observed.

Survival time of the models

The longest survival time for rabbits that received endoscopic implantation was 81 days and the shortest was 26 days, with a median survival time of 50.0 (95% CI, 46.0 to 54.0) days. For the rabbits that received surgical implantation, the longest survival

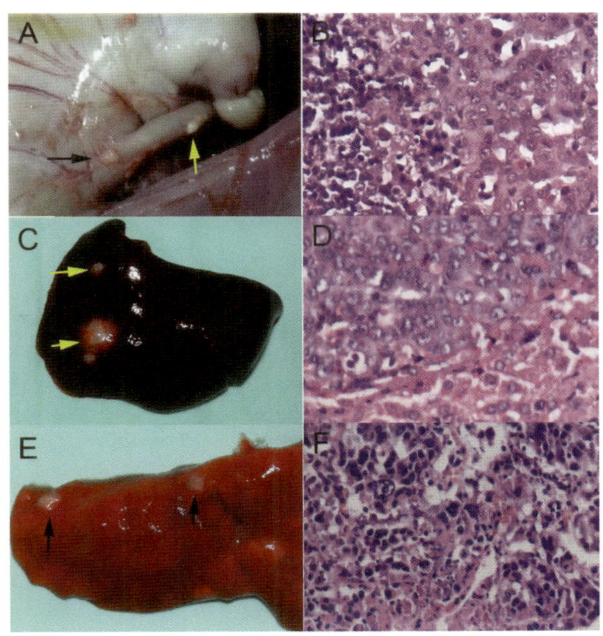

Figure 6. Tumor regional/distant metastases. (A) Macroscopic view of the lymph node metastases (black arrow) and the yellow arrow points to the esophageal tumor. (B) Microscopy observation of lymph node metastases (200x). (C) Macroscopic view of the liver metastases (yellow arrows). (D) Microscopy observation of liver metastases (200x). (E) Macroscopic view of the lung metastases (black arrows). (F) Microscopy view of lung metastases (200x).

time was 79 days and the shortest was 21 days, with a median survival time of 46.0 (95% CI, 42.0 to 50.0) days. The difference in the survival times between the two groups was not statistically significant ($P = 0.34$).

Discussion

The middle third of the esophagus is the most common site for human esophageal squamous carcinoma, so we implanted VX2 tumors in the rabbit thoracic esophagus in this study. Our models are moderate-to-large-sized and were histologically proven to be the squamous cell type. The pathologic features that the models showed such as different degree of esophageal stricture, different tumor growth patterns, with/without invasion of adjacent tissues and regional/distant metastasis, are extremely similar to the clinicopathologic characteristics of human ESC [15–17]. The findings indicate that our animal models are reliable for mimicking the disease of human ESC.

There are two types of tumor seeds to select for implantation: VX2 cells or fragments. VX2 cells were generally used for implantation in previous studies [18,19]. However, it has been reported that the success rate of tumor growth by the implantation of VX2 fragments was higher than by inoculation with intact VX2 cells [20–22] in organs such as the liver and the lung. Therefore, we selected VX2 fragments as the tumor seeds for the two implantation methods in this study.

There has not yet been a report on the establishment of an esophageal carcinoma model with VX2 fragments because it is more difficult to implant fragments than whole cells into the wall of the esophagus. The necessary open surgery for the implantation of VX2 fragments is more traumatic than whole cell implantation, and it risks post-surgical complications [23,24]. As an alternative, the endoscopic method is a minimally invasive procedure but increases the incidence of esophageal perforation when using large needles to implant the VX2 fragments. To avoid severe complications, we introduced a submucosal injection technique for endoscopic implantation [25,26] to enlarge the space between the mucosal and the muscular layer. When performing implantation with the surgical method, we selected an abdominal operation instead of thoracic surgery, which was accomplished by pulling down the lower thoracic esophagus into the abdominal cavity to decrease the mortality of animal. Although there is no data from other studies that can be used for comparison, the data from the current study indicates that both endoscopic and surgical implantation of VX2 fragments are safe and effective methods for establishment of rabbit esopgageal carcinoma models in the thoracic esophagus.

In current study, the models produced by two methods showed different pathologic features. We believe that the difference was not related to the two implantation procedures, but to the different sites of implantation: the submucosal layer for the endoscopic procedure and the muscular layer implantation for the surgical operation. There are technique limitations to selecting the same site for the two methods: the complication rates of esophageal perforation and mortality increase whether due to puncturing of the muscle layer under endoscopy or the submucosal layer during surgically, in our experience, because the wall of the esophagus is very thin. Our results indicate that implantation site may influence the tumor growth patterns and contribute to the formation of different pathologic characteristics. Thus the preferred model for future studies may depend upon the particular research question being addressed.

The models produced by the endoscopic method showed tumor intra-luminal growth and were generally complicated by severe stenosis, which may allow for research on surgical techniques, endoscopic procedures, stent placement, etc. The models produced by the surgical method showed tumor extra-luminal growth, which was frequently followed by tumor invasion of the adjacent organs and, therefore, can be used for studies on intravascular interventional treatment or palliative surgical procedures. In addition, the rabbits for modeling are animals with normal immunocompetence and their immune responses to therapeutic agents is more predictive of human responsiveness than those of immunodeficient rodent models. Therefore, our models could potentially be used for research on immunotherapy.

In conclusion, endoscopic submuscosal implantation and surgical intramuscular implantation are both safe and effective for establishment of VX2 tumours in the rabbit thoracic esophagus. The models produced by the two methods have different pathologic features, which are similar to that of human ESC, may be attributed to the different tumor implantation sites. We recommend the models for preclinical studies on surgical techniques and minimally invasive treatments.

Supporting Information

Video S1 Endoscopic Procedure for VX2 Fragments Implantation. Using a fine endoscopic needle, 0.5 ml of saline was first injected into the submucosal layer to elevate the mucosa layer. Then, a puncture was made using a large endoscopic needle (a revised needle) across the mucosa into the submucosal layer, and the success of the puncture was confirmed by further elevation of the mucosa when the saline was injected. Next, approximately 0.3 ml of saline containing four tumor pieces was injected into the submucosal layer. Finally, a second 0.3 ml portion of saline was injected to rinse the needles and collect the stuck pieces.

Table S1 The pathologic characteristics of the models produced by endoscopic method. For each rabbit, the degree of esophageal stricture, the tumor growth pattern, the status of tumor invasion of adjacent tissues and regional/distant metastasis are given.

Table S2 The pathologic characteristics of the models produced by surgical method. For each rabbit, the degree of esophageal stricture, the tumor growth pattern, the status of tumor invasion of adjacent tissues and regional/distant metastasis are given.

Acknowledgments

We thank Prof. Yi Miao at the First Affiliated Hospital of Nanjing Medical University for providing the VX2 tumor.

Author Contributions

Conceived and designed the experiments: ZF. Performed the experiments: JH YZ HZ. Analyzed the data: YS GJ ZT. Wrote the paper: HS KW.

References

1. Talukdar FR, Ghosh SK, Laskar RS, Mondal R (2013) Epigenetic, genetic and environmental interactions in esophageal squamous cell carcinoma from northeast India. PLoS One 8: e60996. doi: 10.1371/journal.pone.0060996.
2. Pennathur A, Gibson MK, Jobe BA, Luketich JD (2013) Oesophageal carcinoma. Lancet 381: 400–412.
3. Thomas GR, Smith LP (2006) Animal models for the study of squamous cell carcinoma of the upper aerodigestive tract: a historical perspective with review of their utility and limitations part B. Transgenic mouse models. Int J Cancer 118: 2379–2380.
4. Moriyama M, Shimada Y, Nagata T, Omura T, Sekine S, et al. (2013) Establishment and characterization of a novel xenograft model of human gastrointestinal stromal tumor in mice. Anticancer Res 33: 175–181.
5. Nishikawa T, Takaoka M, Ohara T, Tomono Y, Hao H, et al. (2013) Antiproliferative effect of a novel mTOR inhibitor temsirolimus contributes to the prolonged survival of orthotopic esophageal cancer-bearing mice. Cancer Biol Ther 14: 230–236.
6. Tian F, Fan T, Jiang Y, Zhang X, Wang X (2012) A small interfering RNA targeting NF-κB p65 alone or combined with 5-FU inhibits growth of esophageal squamous cell carcinoma in nude mice. Pathol Res Pract 208: 32–38.
7. Kim EY, Song HY, Kim JH, Fan Y, Park S, et al. (2013) IN-1233-eluting covered metallic stent to prevent hyperplasia: experimental study in a rabbit esophageal model.Radiology 267: 396–404.
8. Pauli EM, Schomisch SJ, Furlan JP, Marks AS, Chak A, et al. (2012) Biodegradable esophageal stent placement does not prevent high-grade stricture formation after circumferential mucosal resection in a porcine model. Surg Endosc 26: 3500–3508.
9. Ji JS, Lee BI, Kim HK, Cho YS, Choi H, et al. (2011) Antimigration property of a newly designed covered metal stent for esophageal stricture: an in vivo animal study. Gastrointest Endosc 74: 148–153.
10. Shope RE, Hurst EW (1933) Infectious papillomatosis of rabbits: with a note on the histopathology. J Exp Med 58: 607–624.
11. Selbie FR, Robinson RH (1948) Incidence of carcinoma in transmissible papillomatosis of the domestic rabbit. Br J Cancer 2: 48–59.
12. Stewart EE, Sun H, Chen X, Schafer PH, Chen Y, et al. (2012) Effect of an angiogenesis inhibitor on hepatic tumor perfusion and the implications for adjuvant cytotoxic therapy. Radiology 264: 68–77.
13. Valdivia Y Alvarado M, Wong K, He TC, Xue Z, Wong ST (2011) Image-guided fiberoptic molecular imaging in a VX2 rabbit lung tumor model. J Vasc Interv Radiol 22: 1758–1764.
14. Bruners P, Braunschweig T, Hodenius M, Pietsch H, Penzkofer T, et al. (2010) Thermoablation of malignant kidney tumors using magnetic nanoparticles: an in vivo feasibility study in a rabbit model. Cardiovasc Intervent Radiol 33: 127–134.
15. Ooki A, Yamashita K, Kobayashi N, Katada N, Sakuramoto S, et al. (2007) Lymph node metastasis density and growth pattern as independent prognostic factors in advanced esophageal squamous cell carcinoma. World J Surg 31: 2184–2191.
16. Seddik H, Rouibaa F, Massit H, El Hamdi FZ, Benkirane A (2011) Esophageal squamous cell carcinoma with extraluminal growth pattern. Presse Med 40: 889–890.
17. von Rahden BH, Brücher BL, Sarbia M (2006) Esophageal squamous cell carcinoma with entirely intramural growth pattern. Virchows Arch 448: 862–666.
18. Jumei Zhou, Ning Li, Qisheng Xia, Lehui Dua, Xiaowen Wang, et al. (2009) Hyperthermia by a nitinol stent in an alternating magnetic field: Safety and feasibility in rabbit esophageal cancer. Progress in Natural Science 19: 1713–1719.
19. Sheyhedin I, Okunaka T, Kato H, Yamamoto Y, Sakaniwa N, et al. (2000) Localization of experimental submucosal esophageal tumor in rabbits by using mono-L-aspartyl chlorin e6 and long-wavelength photodynamic excitation. Lasers Surg Med 26: 83–89.
20. Sun JH, Zhang YL, Nie CH, Yu XB, Xie HY, et al. (2012) Considerations for two inoculation methods of rabbit hepatic tumors: Pathology and image features. Exp Ther Med 3: 386–390.
21. Virmani S, Harris KR, Szolc-Kowalska B, Paunesku T, Woloschak GE, et al. (2008) Comparison of two different methods for inoculating VX2 tumors in rabbit livers and hind limbs. J Vasc Interv Radiol 19: 931–936.
22. Tu M, Xu L, Wei X, Miao Y (2009) How to establish a solitary and localized VX2 lung cancer rabbit model? A simple and effective intrapulmonary tumor implantation technique. J Surg Res 154: 284–292.
23. Bharat A, Crabtree T (2012) Management of advanced-stage operable esophageal cancer.Surg Clin North Am 92: 1179–1197.
24. Schubert D, Dalicho S, Flohr L, Benedix F, Lippert H (2012) Management of postoperative complications following esophagectomy. Chirurg 83: 712–718.
25. Soetikno R, Kaltenbach T. (2010) Dynamic submucosal injection technique. Gastrointest Endosc Clin N Am 20: 497–502.
26. Chávez Rossell M (2005) Endoscopic treatment of early gastric cancer: from Endoscopic Mucosal Resection (EMR) to Endoscopic Submucosal Dissection (ESD). Rev Gastroenterol Peru 25: 76–92.

Permissions

All chapters in this book were first published in PLOS ONE, by The Public Library of Science; hereby published with permission under the Creative Commons Attribution License or equivalent. Every chapter published in this book has been scrutinized by our experts. Their significance has been extensively debated. The topics covered herein carry significant findings which will fuel the growth of the discipline. They may even be implemented as practical applications or may be referred to as a beginning point for another development.

The contributors of this book come from diverse backgrounds, making this book a truly international effort. This book will bring forth new frontiers with its revolutionizing research information and detailed analysis of the nascent developments around the world.

We would like to thank all the contributing authors for lending their expertise to make the book truly unique. They have played a crucial role in the development of this book. Without their invaluable contributions this book wouldn't have been possible. They have made vital efforts to compile up to date information on the varied aspects of this subject to make this book a valuable addition to the collection of many professionals and students.

This book was conceptualized with the vision of imparting up-to-date information and advanced data in this field. To ensure the same, a matchless editorial board was set up. Every individual on the board went through rigorous rounds of assessment to prove their worth. After which they invested a large part of their time researching and compiling the most relevant data for our readers.

The editorial board has been involved in producing this book since its inception. They have spent rigorous hours researching and exploring the diverse topics which have resulted in the successful publishing of this book. They have passed on their knowledge of decades through this book. To expedite this challenging task, the publisher supported the team at every step. A small team of assistant editors was also appointed to further simplify the editing procedure and attain best results for the readers.

Apart from the editorial board, the designing team has also invested a significant amount of their time in understanding the subject and creating the most relevant covers. They scrutinized every image to scout for the most suitable representation of the subject and create an appropriate cover for the book.

The publishing team has been an ardent support to the editorial, designing and production team. Their endless efforts to recruit the best for this project, has resulted in the accomplishment of this book. They are a veteran in the field of academics and their pool of knowledge is as vast as their experience in printing. Their expertise and guidance has proved useful at every step. Their uncompromising quality standards have made this book an exceptional effort. Their encouragement from time to time has been an inspiration for everyone.

The publisher and the editorial board hope that this book will prove to be a valuable piece of knowledge for researchers, students, practitioners and scholars across the globe.

List of Contributors

San-Zhong Xu, Xiang-Jin Lin, Xiang Tong and Xuan-Wei Wang
Department of Orthopaedics, First Affiliated Hospital, College of Medicine, Zhejiang University, Hangzhou City, Zhejiang Province, China

Zachary A. Smith, Nader Dahdaleh and Richard G. Fessler
Northwestern Feinberg School of Medicine, Department of Neurological Surgery, Northwestern University, Chicago, Illinois, United States of America

Georgios A. Vastardis, Gerard Carandang, Robert M. Havey, Sean Hannon, Leonard I. Voronov and Avinash G. Patwardhan
Loyola University Stritch School of Medicine, Department of Orthopaedic Surgery, Maywood, Illinois, United States of America
Edward Hines Jr. VA Hospital, Hines, Illinois, United States of America

Baohui Yang, Haopeng Li, Xijing He, Guoyu Wang and Siyue Xu
Department of Orthopaedic Surgery, The 2nd Affiliated Hospital of Medical College, Xi'an Jiaotong University, Xi'an, Shaanxi Province, People's Republic of China

Zhi Chen, Zhong-Qing Yang, Yang Li, Yan-Cheng Luo, Yao He, Nan-Nan Li, Chao- Qun Xie, Chen Lai, Xiao-Long Fang and Xiang Chen
Department of Urology, Xiangya Hospital, Central South University, Changsha, Hunan, China

Peng Zhou
Department of General Surgery, Xiangya Hospital, Central South University, Changsha, Hunan, China

Yin Zhang, Hengao Zhong, Zhining Fan and Guobin Jiang
Digestive Medical Center, The Second Affiliated Hospital of Nanjing Medical University, Nanjing, Jiangsu Province, China

Jin Huang
Digestive Medical Center, The Second Affiliated Hospital of Nanjing Medical University, Nanjing, Jiangsu Province, China
Division of Digestive Diseases, Renming Hospital of Ma Anshan, Ma Anshan City, Anhui Province, China

Yan Xu
Department of Obstetrics and Gynecology, Southwest Hospital, Third Military Medical University, Chongqing, China

Charlotte S. Daniels
Department of Mechanical Engineering, University of California, Berkeley, California, United States of America

Boris Rubinsky
Department of Mechanical Engineering, University of California, Berkeley, California, United States of America
Graduate Program in Biophysics, University of California, Berkeley, California, United States of America

Haruki Funao
Department of Orthopaedic Surgery, Nerima General Hospital, Tokyo, Japan
Society for Minimally invasive spine Stabilization (Clinical research group)

Masaya Nakamura, Yoshiaki Toyama and Morio Matsumoto
Department of Orthopaedic Surgery, School of Medicine, Keio University, Tokyo, Japan

Ken Ishii, Akio Iwanami and Naobumi Hosogane
Department of Orthopaedic Surgery, School of Medicine, Keio University, Tokyo, Japan
Society for Minimally invasive spine Stabilization (Clinical research group)

Suketaka Momoshima
Department of Radiology, School of Medicine, Keio University, Tokyo, Japan

Kota Watanabe
Advanced Therapy for Spine and Spinal Cord Disorders, Keio University, Tokyo, Japan
Society for Minimally invasive spine Stabilization (Clinical research group)

Rens Wientjes, Herke J. Noordmans, Jerine A. J. van der Eijk and Henk van den Brink
University Medical Centre Utrecht, Utrecht, The Netherlands

Ai-Min Wu, Qing-Long Li, Yong-Long Jin, Peng Luo, Yong-Long Chi and Xiang-Yang Wang
The Department of Spinal Surgery, Second Affiliated Hospital of Wenzhou Medical University, Zhejiang Spinal Research Center, Wenzhou, Zhejiang, People's Republic of China

Yong Zhou
The First Medical College, Wenzhou Medical University, Wenzhou, Zhejiang, People's Republic of China

Xin-Lei Wu
Institute of Digitized Medicine, Wenzhou Medical University, Wenzhou, Zhejiang, People's Republic of China

Dehui Lai and Yuping Dai
Department of Urology, The First Affiliated Hospital of Sun Yat-sen University, Guangzhou, Guangdong, China

Yongzhong He and Xun Li
Department of Urology, The Fifth Affiliated Hospital of Guangzhou Medical University, Guangzhou, Guangdong, China

Weijun Fu, Xu Zhang, Peng Zhang, Jiangping Gao, Jun Dong, Guangfu Chen, Axiang Xu, Xin Ma, Hongzhao Li and Lixin Shi
Department of Urology, PLA General Hospital/ Medical school, Beijing, China

Xiaoyi Zhang
Department of Urology, The Second Artillery General Hospital of PLA, Beijing, China

Tuan-Jen Fang and Hsueh-Yu Li
Department of Otorhinolaryngology-Head and Neck Surgery, Chang Gung Memorial Hospital at Linkou, School of Medicine, College of Medicine, Chang Gung University, Taoyuan, Taiwan, R.O.C.
Sleep Center, Chang Gung Memorial Hospital at Linkou, Taoyuan, Taiwan, R.O.C.

Li-Ang Lee
Department of Otorhinolaryngology-Head and Neck Surgery, Chang Gung Memorial Hospital at Linkou, School of Medicine, College of Medicine, Chang Gung University, Taoyuan, Taiwan, R.O.C.
Sleep Center, Chang Gung Memorial Hospital at Linkou, Taoyuan, Taiwan, R.O.C.
Department of Otolaryngology, Xiamen Chang Gung Hospital, Xiamen, Fujian Province, China

Yu-Lun Lo and Ning-Hung Chen
Sleep Center, Chang Gung Memorial Hospital at Linkou, Taoyuan, Taiwan, R.O.C.
Department of Pulmonary and Critical Care Medicine, Chang Gung Memorial Hospital at Linkou, School of Medicine, College of Medicine, Chang Gung University, Taoyuan, Taiwan, R.O.C.

Jen-Fang Yu
Graduate Institute of Medical Mechatronics, Taiouan Interdisciplinary Otolaryngology Laboratory, Chang Gung University, Taoyuan, Taiwan, R.O.C.

Chung-Guei Huang
Department of Laboratory Medicine, Chang Gung Memorial Hospital at Linkou, College of Medicine, Chang Gung University, Taoyuan, Taiwan, R.O.C.

Wen-Nuan Cheng
Graduate School of Recreation and Sports Management, Taipei Physical Education College, Taipei, Taiwan, R.O.C.

Michiel van Elk
Center for Neuroprosthetics, School of Life Sciences, Ecole Polytechnique Fédé rale de Lausanne (EPFL), Lausanne, Switzerland
Laboratory of Cognitive Neuroscience, Brain Mind Institute, Ecole Polytechnique Fédé rale de Lausanne (EPFL), Lausanne, Switzerland

Ali Sengü and Giulio Rognini
Center for Neuroprosthetics, School of Life Sciences, Ecole Polytechnique Fédé rale de Lausanne (EPFL), Lausanne, Switzerland
Laboratory of Cognitive Neuroscience, Brain Mind Institute, Ecole Polytechnique Fédé rale de Lausanne (EPFL), Lausanne, Switzerland
Systems Robotic Laboratory, Ecole Polytechnique Fédé rale de Lausanne (EPFL), Lausanne, Switzerland

Olaf Blanke
Center for Neuroprosthetics, School of Life Sciences, Ecole Polytechnique Fédé rale de Lausanne (EPFL), Lausanne, Switzerland
Laboratory of Cognitive Neuroscience, Brain Mind Institute, Ecole Polytechnique Fédé rale de Lausanne (EPFL), Lausanne, Switzerland
Department of Neurology, University Hospital of Geneva (HUG), Geneva, Switzerland

Jane Elizabeth Aspell
Laboratory of Cognitive Neuroscience, Brain Mind Institute, Ecole Polytechnique Fédé rale de Lausanne (EPFL), Lausanne, Switzerland

Hannes Bleuler
Systems Robotic Laboratory, Ecole Polytechnique Fédé rale de Lausanne (EPFL), Lausanne, Switzerland

Jiangang Wang, Yan Li, Jie Han, Chunlei Xu, Changsheng Ma and Xu Meng
Department of Atrial Fibrillation Center, Beijing Anzhen Hospital, Capital Medical University, Beijing, China

Jiahai Shi
Department of Cardiothoracic Surgery, Affiliated Hospital of Nantong University, Nantong, China

Yon Cui, Wenzhou Cao, Hua Shen, Jianjun Xie and Qiang Shao
Department of Urology, Suzhou Municipal Hospital, Suzhou, China

Tamara S. Adams
Center for Cancer Genomics, Wake Forest University School of Medicine, Winston-Salem, North Carolina, United States of America

Yuanyuan Zhang
Wake Forest Institute for Regenerative Medicine, Wake Forest University Health Sciences, Winston-Salem, North Carolina, United States of America

Charlotte S. Daniels and Boris Rubinsky
Department of Mechanical Engineering, University of California, Berkeley, Berkeley, California, United States of America

Liang Zong, Yasuyuki Seto and Susumu Aikou
Department of Gastrointestinal Surgery, Graduate School of Medicine, University of Tokyo, Tokyo, Japan

Takamasa Takahashi
Division of Surgical Oncology, Department of Surgery, Nagoya University Graduate School of Medicine, Nagoya, Japan

Shaohui Zong, Li Du, Ye Fang and Taihang Gao
Department of Spine Osteopathia, the First Affiliated Hospital of Guangxi Medical University, Nanning, Guangxi, P.R. China

Gaofeng Zeng
College of Public Hygiene of Guangxi Medical University, Nanning, Guangxi, P.R. China

Jingmin Zhao
Department of Orthopaedics Trauma and Hand Surgery, the First Affiliated Hospital of Guangxi Medical University, Nanning, Guangxi, P.R. China

Mingjie Yang, Cheng Zeng, Song Guo, Jie Pan, Yingchao Han, Zeqing Li, Lijun Li and Jun Tan
Department of Spine Surgery, Shanghai East Hospital, Tongji University School of Medicine, Shanghai, People's Republic of China

Jia-Wei Wang, Jin-Ping Li, Ying-Lun Song, Ke Tan, Yu Wang, Tao Li, Peng Guo, Xiong Li, Yan Wang and Qi-Huang Zhao
Department of neurosurgery, Beijing Chao-Yang Hospital, Capital Medical University, Beijing, P. R. China

Jing Jin
Department of Bioinformatics, Chongqing Medical University, Chongqing, China

Longke Ran
Department of Bioinformatics, Chongqing Medical University, Chongqing, China
Molecular Medicine and Cancer Research Center, Chongqing Medical University, Chongqing, China

Youquan Bu and Fangzhou Song
Molecular Medicine and Cancer Research Center, Chongqing Medical University, Chongqing, China

Han Qin, Gang Pan and Yong Zeng
Department of Hepatic Surgery, West China Hospital, Sichuan University, Chengdu, Sichuan, P. R. China

Jianguo Qiu
Department of Hepatobiliary Surgery, The First Affiliated Hospital, Chongqing Medical University, Chongqing, P. R. China

Yiyang Zhao
Department of Pediatric Surgery, West China Hospital, Sichuan University, Chengdu, Sichuan, P. R. China

Zheng Liu, Pengfei Lv and Cheng Chi
Department of Orthopaedics, Peking University Shougang Hospital, Beijing, China

Qi Fei, Bingqiang Wang, Yong Yang, Fan Zhao, Jisheng Lin and Zhao Ma
Department of Orthopaedics, Beijing Friendship Hospital, Capital Medical University, Beijing, China

Yingzhou Shen, Hanming Song, Zhijian Tao and Kuangjing Wang
Division of Digestive Diseases, Renming Hospital of Ma Anshan, Ma Anshan City, Anhui Province, China